NURSING CARE
for Individuals with
Intellectual and Developmental Disabilities

NURSING CARE
for Individuals with
Intellectual and Developmental Disabilities

An Integrated Approach

edited by

Cecily L. Betz, Ph.D., RN, FAAN

University of Southern California
University Center for Excellence in Developmental Disabilities
Childrens Hospital Los Angeles

and

Wendy M. Nehring, Ph.D., RN, FAAN, FAAIDD

East Tennessee State University
College of Nursing

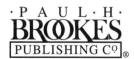

·P·A·U·L·H·
BROOKES
PUBLISHING CO®

Baltimore • London • Sydney

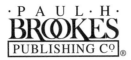

Paul H. Brookes Publishing Co.
Post Office Box 10624
Baltimore, Maryland 21285-0624
USA

www.brookespublishing.com

Typeset by Integrated Publishing Solutions, Grand Rapids, Michigan.
Manufactured in the United States of America by
Sheridan Books, Inc., Chelsea, Michigan.

Library of Congress Cataloging-in-Publication Data

Nursing care for individuals with intellectual and developmental disabilities : an integrated approach
/ edited by Cecily L. Betz and Wendy M. Nehring.
    p.   ; cm.
  Includes bibliographical references and index.
  ISBN-13: 978-1-55766-982-7
  ISBN-10: 1-55766-982-1
  1. Mental retardation—Nursing.   2. Developmental disabilities—Nursing.   I. Betz, Cecily Lynn.
II. Nehring, Wendy M., 1957–   III. Title. [DNLM: 1. Developmental Disabilities—nursing.
2. Learning Disorders—nursing.   3. Nursing Care—methods.
WY 160 N97421 2010]
RC570.2.N87 2010
616.85'880231—dc22   2009046531

British Library Cataloguing in Publication data are available from the British Library.

Contents

About the Editors vii

Contributors. ix

Preface xi

1   Historical Perspective and Emerging Trends
    Wendy M. Nehring. 1

2   Theoretical Models Guiding Care
    Pamela P. DiNapoli 19

3   Systems of Care for Individuals with Intellectual
    and Developmental Disabilities
    Cecily L. Betz 31

4   Developmental Transitions for Children with Intellectual
    and Developmental Disabilities: Prenatal to School-Age Period
    Marilyn J. Krajicek and Dalice L. Hertzberg 45

5   Developmental Transitions for Individuals with Intellectual
    and Developmental Disabilities: Adolescence and Beyond
    Mary Theresa Urbano 69

6   Continuum of Nursing Care
    Dalice L. Hertzberg. 91

7   Psychosocial Issues
    J. Carolyn Graff. 109

8   Physical Care of Individuals with Intellectual
    and Developmental Disabilities
    Lee Barks 131

9   Nursing Care Approaches: Clinical and Practical Considerations
    Cecily L. Betz and Martha Wilson Jones 147

10 Genetics
    Felissa R. Lashley 173

11 Intellectual and Developmental Disabilities
    Sandra A. Faux and Wendy M. Nehring. 193

12 Down Syndrome
Wendy M. Nehring and Cecily L. Betz 211

13 Cerebral Palsy
Martha Wilson Jones and Elaine Morgan 235

14 Mental and Behavioral Health Disorders in Individuals
with Intellectual and Developmental Disabilities
Sarah H. Ailey and Tanya Melich-Munyan 257

15 Autism
Jean E. Beatson 277

16 Fragile X Syndrome
Rebecca Kronk and Janice S. Dorman 311

17 Sensory Impairment
Joni Bosch and Sandie M. Bass-Ringdahl 333

18 Policies, Legislation, and Ethical/Legal Issues
Kathryn Smith and Teresa A. Savage 355

Index 371

About the Editors

Cecily L. Betz, Ph.D., RN, FAAN, Associate Professor of Clinical Pediatrics, USC Keck School of Medicine, Department of Pediatrics, and Director of Nursing Training, USC University Center of Excellence in Developmental Disabilities, Childrens Hospital Los Angeles, 3250 Wilshire Boulevard, Suite 500, Mailstop #53, Los Angeles, California 90010.

Dr. Betz has worked with children, adolescents, and families for more than 30 years in a variety of roles as a clinician, educator, administrator, and researcher. She has served as the editor-in-chief of the *Journal of Pediatric Nursing*, the official journal of the Society of Pediatric Nursing and Pediatric Endocrinology Nursing Society, since the mid-1980s. She has published extensively on topics pertaining to pediatric nursing, developmental disabilities, and health care transition planning for adolescents with special health care needs. Her textbook *Pediatric Nursing Reference* (Mosby, 2008) is in its sixth edition; this textbook and others she has authored have been translated into three languages. Dr. Betz has been the principal investigator for a number of extramurally funded federal and state grants and has served on a number of regional, state-level, and national professional committees representing the interests of pediatric nurses and adolescents with special health care needs and disabilities. She also served as one of the organizers and founding members of the Society of Pediatric Nursing, a national pediatric nursing association founded nearly 2 decades ago. She is a fellow of the American Academy of Nursing of the American Nurses Association and was formerly the Chair of the Child and Family Expert Panel. In 2008, Dr. Betz received the Margaret S. Miles Service Award from the Society of Pediatric Nurses for her service and contribution to pediatric nursing.

Wendy M. Nehring, Ph.D., RN, FAAN, FAAIDD, Dean and Professor, College of Nursing, East Tennessee State University, Box 70617, Johnson City, Tennessee 37614.

Dr. Nehring joined East Tennessee State University in 2009. Previously, she held administrative and faculty positions at Rutgers, The State University of New Jersey, Southern Illinois University at Edwardsville, and the University of Illinois at Chicago, and a faculty position at Illinois Wesleyan University. She received her doctorate in nursing science from the University of Illinois at Chicago, her master's degree in pediatric nursing from the University of Wisconsin-Madison, and her bachelor's degree in nursing from Illinois Wesleyan University. Dr. Nehring is nationally and internationally known in the field of intellectual and developmental disabilities. She wrote one of the only history books on nursing in the field of intellectual and developmental disabilities. She and her colleagues revised the

Scope and Standards of Practice in this specialty in 2004 for American Nurses Publishing and the American Association on Mental Retardation. Dr. Nehring is also the editor of a core curriculum for nurses and health professionals specializing in the field of intellectual and developmental disabilities (Jones & Bartlett, 2005), an evidence-based practice book on specific health promotion topics and the research that was conducted on these topics with persons with intellectual and developmental disabilities (American Association on Mental Retardation, 2005). She also co-edited a book with Cecily L. Betz on the health concerns of adolescents with special health care needs and disabilities making the transition into adulthood (Paul H. Brookes Publishing Co., 2007). She has written, presented, and consulted widely on this nursing specialty, as well as received internal and external funding for her research on people with Down syndrome and neural tube defects. Dr. Nehring is a fellow of the American Academy of Nursing and the American Association on Intellectual and Developmental Disabilities (AAIDD). In 2009, she received the Leadership Award from the AAIDD.

Contributors

Sarah H. Ailey, Ph.D., RN-BC
Assistant Professor
Rush University College of Nursing
600 South Paulina #1080
Chicago, IL 60623

Lee Barks, Ph.D., ARNP
Postdoctoral Fellow
Veterans Administration Office of
 Academic Affairs
Wesley Chapel, FL

**Sandie M. Bass-Ringdahl,
 Ph.D., CCC-A**
Assistant Professor
The University of Iowa
Wendell Johnson Speech and Hearing
 Center, 125C
Iowa City, IA 52242

Jean E. Beatson, RN, M.S., Ed.D.
Research Assistant Professor
University of Vermont
UHC RE 477, Room 4318
1 South Prospect Street
Burlington, VT 05401

Joni Bosch, Ph.D.
Family Nurse Practitioner
University of Iowa Center for
 Disabilities and Development and
 Medical Genetics
200 Hawkins Drive
Iowa City, IA 52242

Pamela P. DiNapoli, Ph.D., RN
Associate Professor
University of New Hampshire
247 Hewitt Hall
Durham, NH 03824

Janice S. Dorman, M.S., Ph.D.
Professor and Associate Dean for
 Scientific and International Affairs
University of Pittsburgh School of
 Nursing
3500 Victoria Street
Pittsburgh, PA 15261

Sandra A. Faux, M.N., Ph.D.
Associate Professor
Rush University College of Nursing
600 South Paulina, 1036A AAF
Chicago, IL 60612

J. Carolyn Graff, Ph.D.
Associate Professor
University of Tennessee Health
 Science Center
711 Jefferson Avenue
Memphis, TN 38015

Dalice L. Hertzberg, M.S.N., FNP-C
Senior Instructor
JFK Partners, Department of
 Pediatrics, School of Medicine
University of Colorado Denver
Campus Mail Stop F541, Education 2
 North
13120 East 19th Avenue
Aurora, CO 80045

**Martha Wilson Jones, M.S.N., RN,
 CPNP**
Developmental Pediatrics, Children's
 Hospital of The King's Daughters
Instructor of Pediatrics, Eastern
 Virginia Medical School
Children's Specialty Group
601 Children's Lane
Norfolk, VA 23507

Marilyn J. Krajicek, Ed.D. RN, FAAN
Professor
University of Colorado Denver College of Nursing
13120 East 19th Avenue
Aurora, CO 80045

Rebecca Kronk, M.S.N., CRNP, Ph.D.
Assistant Professor
University of Pittsburgh School of Nursing
Children's Hospital of Pittsburgh of UPMC
3420 Fifth Avenue
2nd Floor, Children's Hospital Office Building
Pittsburgh, PA 15213

Felissa R. Lashley, Ph.D., RN, FAAN, FACMG
Dean Emerita and Professor Emerita
School of Nursing
Southern Illinois University Edwardsville
Past Dean and Professor Emerita
College of Nursing
Rutgers, The State University of New Jersey
Newark, NJ 07102

Tanya Melich-Munyan, B.S.N., RN
Community/Public Health Supervisor, Faculty Practice
Rush University College of Nursing
600 South Paulina Street
Armour Academic Building, Room 1080
Chicago, IL 60612

Elaine Morgan, B.S.N., RN. P.N.P, CRRN
Children's Hospital of The King's Daughters
601 Children's Lane
Norfolk, VA 23507

Teresa A. Savage, Ph.D., RN
Assistant Professor, Research
University of Illinois at Chicago College of Nursing
845 South Damen, Room 841
Chicago, IL 60612

Kathryn Smith, M.N., RN
Associate Director for Administration
USC University Center of Excellence in Developmental Disabilities
Childrens Hospital Los Angeles
4650 Sunset Boulevard, MS # 53
Los Angeles, CA 90027

Mary Theresa Urbano, Ph.D., M.P.H., RN
Clinical Professor of Pediatrics
Vanderbilt University
230 Appleton Place
Nashville, TN 37203

Preface

The purpose of this book is to provide the reader with comprehensive information about the care of individuals with intellectual and developmental disabilities (IDD) across the life span. This book addresses a number of areas related to nursing and health care for individuals with IDD and provides comprehensive coverage for nursing and health care professionals working in school, employment, and community settings.

Thematic areas address the biopsychosocial concerns of individuals with IDD using interdisciplinary and life span frameworks. The chapters include content on developmental disabilities historical perspective and systems of care and developmental concerns from infancy to old age. The remaining chapters address topics pertaining to ethical and legal issues, continuum of nursing care, and general nursing considerations that can be applied widely to the care of individuals with IDD. Chapters on specific disabilities include intellectual disability, Down syndrome, cerebral palsy, dual diagnosis, autism, fragile X, genetics, and sensory problems. Other chapters provide the needed supporting evidence enabling the professional to address the range of needs presented by individuals with IDD.

This textbook addresses a need for a nursing and health-related textbook that has been unmet for nearly a decade. It is intended to provide nurses and other professional audiences such as physical therapists, occupational therapists, social workers, psychologists, and speech and language specialists who work with individuals with IDD with the comprehensive health-related content needed to address their needs for ongoing services. Readers may apply the information presented in the myriad of health care and community settings in which individuals with IDD reside. This book provides readers with the content, resources, and tools to better understand the meaning and scope of nursing practice based upon an interdisciplinary model of care and evidence. The information provided will increase the knowledge and skills of readers in addressing the unique biopsychosocial needs of individuals with IDD across the life span.

Our experience with working with individuals with IDD and their families has taught and sensitized us to their comprehensive needs for services. Living with an IDD changes everything for the individual who has the disability and his or her entire family. Learning to live with IDD means that parents need to become experts in the management of their child's condition beginning in infancy until the time the child can begin to assume responsibility for self-management.

We want to enhance the awareness of our colleagues to what life is like when learning to live with IDD by incorporating throughout the book the theme of family-centered care. Living with IDD means learning to do things differently from what other individuals who are typically developing do. Having an IDD may mean learning to use assistive technology such as a gastrostomy tube and/or a speech augmentation device. In addition, living with an IDD means not only learning the daily and ongoing treatment regimen but also ensuring that the individual can adapt these skills in work, school, and community settings. Nurses who work in the developmental disabilities field are expected to apply nursing knowledge and skills in a myriad of settings that are considered to be atypical for health care professionals.

Our challenge and purpose in writing this book is to provide our colleagues with the range of topical content on IDD written by recognized experts to improve the quality of services provided. It is our hope that this text will be a resource for our colleagues to provide care that is evidence-based and results in the improvement of outcomes for individuals with IDD and their families.

To my beloved brother, Craig L. Betz,
whose love of life and others
was and continues to be
a great inspiration;
and to my dear husband, Robert Nini,
whose gift of charity and kindness to others
is ever a reminder
of what really matters
—CLB

To Felissa Lashley, Marilyn Krajicek,
and Kay Engelhardt,
who shared their passion with me
for persons with intellectual
and developmental disabilities
—WMN

CHAPTER 1

Historical Perspective and Emerging Trends

Wendy M. Nehring

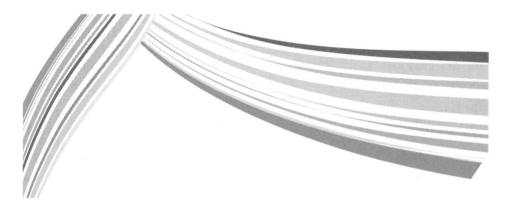

T he field of intellectual and developmental disabilities (IDD) has always involved multiple disciplines, and nursing's role was integral in the history of this field. In this chapter, the impact of nursing on this field, as well as on the lives of individuals with IDD and their families, is illustrated through three foci: nursing care, nursing education, and public policy and nursing leadership. Before these foci are addressed, a discussion of issues that influenced the field is presented.

INFLUENCING ISSUES

The field of IDD is influenced by terminology and classification systems, federal legislation, medical and health care advances, and public opinion. This section explores each of these areas, starting from the 19th century.

Terminology and Classification Systems

The terminology used to describe a person with a cognitive and adaptive behavior deficit has changed over time, and often has been viewed negatively. In the 19th and early 20th century, *idiots* and *imbeciles* were the terms used most often to describe people with cognitive and adaptive behavior deficits. In 1877, William W. Ireland first described this population in medical terms and focused on etiology in his book, *On Idiocy and Imbecility*. He focused on idiocy and subclassified this condition into the following 10 conditions: genetous idiocy, microcephalic idiocy, eclampsia idiocy, epileptic idiocy, hydrocephalic idiocy, paralytic idiocy, cretinism, traumatic idiocy, inflammatory idiocy, and idiocy by deprivation.

Kerlin (1877) also thought that there were etiologic causes for cognitive and adaptive behavior deficits. He defined three classifications of "mental defectives," as he called them: superior grades (highest level of functioning), orphaned idiots and imbeciles, and lower grades (lowest level of functioning). Kerlin felt that people with superior grades could live independently with appropriate education, but that those with the lower grades needed "medical treatment, exercise, and basic life skills" (Kerlin, 1877, p. 19). In 1892, Down identified 27 types of "idiots," with one category related to ethnicity. However, he abandoned that idea soon after his classification was published (Kanner, 1967).

At the turn of the 20th century, Laird (1902), a nurse, wrote that idiocy and imbecility were categories of mental enfeeblement, which in turn was one of three classes of insanity. The other two classes of insanity were mental depression and mental exaltation. In 1903, the Association of Medical Officers of American Institutions for Idiotic and Feebleminded Persons (which would be renamed as the American Association on Mental Deficiency and is now the American Association on Intellectual and Developmental Disabilities) used the term *feeblemindedness* to describe individuals with cognitive deficits (Sloan & Stevens, 1976).

In 1912, Goddard produced a classification system that was based on the results of a standardized intelligence test, the Simon-Binet test. In 1921, the Association of Medical Officers of American Institutions for Idiotic and Feebleminded Persons published the first definition and classification manual with the National Committee for Mental Hygiene (as cited in Luckasson et al., 2002). Then in 1925, Morgan called for an individualized approach that did not include categories—an idea that was realized about 70 years later (Luckasson et al., 2002).

In 1934, the term *feeblemindedness* was changed to *mental deficiency*—a condition that was further classified into *idiot, imbecile,* and *moron,* similar to the previous century. These categories were based on scores from standardized intelligence tests (*1934 Proceedings of the American Association on Mental Deficiency Annual Meeting,* as cited in Sloan & Stevens, 1976). Then in 1941, Doll wrote that mental deficiency was not a result of intelligence only, but was also influenced by personality and motor skills. However, this view was not widely adopted until adaptive behavior and intelligence became the focus of the term's definition in a 1959 manual by the American Association on Mental Deficiency (Heber, 1959). Prior to that, in 1952, the American Psychiatric Association published the first edition of the *Diagnostic and Statistical Manual of Mental Disorders.* In this manual, mental deficiency was divided into three categories—mild, moderate, and severe—based on standardized intelligence scores.

By the 1960s, the term *mental retardation* was used with more frequency. Over the next 20 years, additional terms were used, including *developmental disabilities, behavioral disorders, emotional disorders, mentally handicapped,* and *learning disabilities.* Interestingly, the origin of the term *developmental disabilities* was actually influenced by U.S. politics. President Richard Nixon would not reauthorize legislation that affected people with "mental retardation" because that was the term used by President John F. Kennedy in his legislative actions. Thus, in order to continue funding for programs for this population, a new term had to be coined (Nehring, 1999). The other terms arose to describe specific conditions, but less stigmatized labels.

The term *intellectual disabilities* is now used more widely (Schalock et al., 2008). The 11th edition of the American Association on Intellectual and Developmental Disabilities' classification text (AAIDD, formerly known as the American Association on Mental Retardation and the American Association on Mental Deficiency) describes intellectual disability rather than mental retardation (Wehmeyer et al., 2008). Since the 9th edition of the text (Luckasson et al., 1992), mental retardation (or now, intellectual disability) has not been classified by levels of intelligence, but rather by the levels of support needed to provide an individual's optimal environment. Thus, terms used to describe individuals with cognitive and adaptive behavior deficits often changed as they became too pejorative. Even today, *disability* connotes a negative term. However, it may be difficult to find an appropriate term without a negative connotation because the condition does refer to a change from typical development.

Classification systems have followed the knowledge of the etiologies of IDD at different points in time. Certainly, genetic and environmental causes exist—some of which can be prevented. For an in-depth discussion of these terminology and classification issues, see Luckasson and Reeve (2001), MacMillan and Reschly (1997), and Odom, Horner, Snell, and Blacher (2007).

Federal Legislation

The field of IDD has been influenced by a number of public laws, federal legislation, and court cases. Three seminal public laws were enacted in the late 20th century. First, the Education for All Handicapped Children Act of 1975 (PL 94-142) provided for free appropriate public education for all children 3–21 years old. Provisions were made for individualized education programs, due process, assignment to the least restrictive environment, and protection from being assigned to an inappropriate educational setting based on incorrect classification.

In 1986, the Education of the Handicapped Act Amendments of 1986 (PL 99-457) was enacted to provide mandated educational programs for any child 3–5 years old (Part B) and optional funding for early intervention services for any child between the ages of birth to 3 years (Part H). An individualized family service plan was a provision under Part H. The third law, the Americans with Disabilities Act of 1990 (PL 101-336), was signed into law in 1991. Heralded as the greatest civil rights act since the 1960s, this law addressed employment; public accommodations; discrimination by public entities; and transportation, communications, and architectural barriers.

The Social Security Act of 1935 (PL 74-271) and its revisions, along with Section 504 of the Rehabilitation Act of 1973 (PL 93-112), have been very influential in providing for the financial well-being of people with IDD. With each revision to these pieces of legislation, advocates for persons with IDD must be diligent to make sure any changes are not detrimental to people receiving Supplemental Security Income (SSI) benefits.

Four significant court cases have further positively altered the lives of persons with IDD in the 20th century. *Pennsylvania Association for Retarded Children v. Commonwealth of Pennsylvania* (1971) and *Mills v. Board of Education* (1972) were the seminal court cases that led to the drafting and passage of the Education of All Handicapped Children Act of 1975 (PL 94-142). These court cases provided for the mandate that all children in Pennsylvania and Washington, DC, respectively, should have access to free appropriate public education in the least restrictive setting and when necessary, the opportunity for due process. Also in 1970, *Wyatt v. Stickney* (later *Wyatt v. Aderholt*) in Alabama argued the right of individuals with intellectual disabilities to be provided humane care. This case lasted 33 years, but in those years, this case led to assuring appropriate standards of care and rehabilitation for individuals with IDD and mental illness in facilities. Deinstitutionalization also resulted which has had positive and negative consequences (Braddock & Heller, 1985). The final case was *Pennhurst State School v. Halderman* (1981) in Pennsylvania, which further supported deinstitutionalization, appropriate housing in community settings, and appropriate education. Unfortunately, the outcome of this case was not upheld by the Supreme Court in that same year.

Medical and Health Care Advances

Over the past century, many notable medical and health care advances have taken place, including the development of dietary supplements (e.g., folic acid) to prevent birth defects; advances in fetal surgery; genetic engineering techniques; newborn screening techniques; and the development of immunizations, gene therapies, and new medications (e.g., antibiotics, psychopharmaceuticals, sulfa drugs). Knowledge of the causes of IDD has also greatly increased, resulting in significant improvements in prenatal and postnatal care, birth delivery, treatment of prematurity, and comprehensive health assessment (including secondary conditions and mental health concerns) across the life span. Advances in equipment have further aided in health assessment, mobility, transportation, and additional accommodations. A detailed discussion of these advances can be found in Nehring and Betz (2007).

Public Opinion

Public opinion and stigma has influenced the lives of people with IDD and their families across time. From the late 1800s to about 1970, segregation of this population was the norm. The number of persons with IDD who resided in institutions in the United States was at its highest level of 193,200 in 1967 (Scheerenberger, 1981). With the movement towards deinstitutionalization beginning in the 1970s, community placements became more common. However, developmental centers (formerly known as institutions) still exist because not enough community settings provide the necessary care and supports to persons with IDD who have complex medical and behavioral needs.

Over the years, public opinion of IDD has changed. Schools and social programs include children with a variety of acute and chronic conditions, such as IDD. Books, television, and movies have featured people with IDD of all ages, which has helped to improve understanding of IDD. Terminology continues to change as this understanding has grown. Individuals with IDD (i.e., self-advocates) also have spoken out about derogatory language; they have encouraged the removal of labels in order to be viewed as people first.

NURSING CARE AND PRACTICE

This section presents a synopsis of the history of nursing care and practice in the field of IDD, beginning with the 19th century in the United States. For a comprehensive review of the history of this nursing specialty, see Nehring (1999).

Early Nursing Care in the 19th Century

Nursing care in the beginning of the 19th century was not yet formalized; institution-based training was not available for either general nursing or the specific nursing care of persons with IDD. As a result, until the 1920s, nursing care in institutions was often provided by housekeepers, other patients with a higher level of functioning, former patients, or slaves. This practice existed until the 1920s because of the high number of educated nurses who did not want to work in such settings (Anonymous, 1876, as cited in Goodnow, 1949; Barrus, 1908). The highest quality and most humane care was given by religious orders (Griffin & Griffin, 1969).

Early responsibilities for nurses working in institutions were not highly sophisticated and were similar to those of a present-day nursing assistant. As listed in 1840, the mental health nurse primarily provided for the patient's safety, gave comfort and personal hygiene to the patients, ambulated the patients, provided amusements (i.e., games and exercises), and prevented the escape of any patient (Russell, 1945). By the end of the century, after formalized training had begun for nurses, the responsibilities also included electricity treatments, massage, and charting (Howe, 1896). It was not until the turn of the century that standards of care were instituted for nurses; Linda Richards was instrumental in starting this movement in 1899 (Anonymous, 1876, as cited in Goodnow, 1949).

The Eugenics Period

The early decades of the 20th century were identified as the eugenics period—a time when our country attempted to determine who was considered "normal" and who was not. During this time of immigration, Darwin's theory of evolution and the concept of the survival of the fittest, in addition to Galton's research on heredity and intelligence led to his concept of "nature versus nurture" and helped to set the stage for eugenics. Nurses were told by their instructors to be role models in both their presence and teaching; they were held to the highest moral standards and refrained from alcohol use (Bradley, 1914).

Even with these high expectations, nurses were considered to be the servants of the physicians and often performed the duties of a housekeeper on the floors of the institution. Nurses who cared for people with IDD worked a day shift of 14 hours or a night shift of 10 hours, with a 6.5-day workweek (Santos & Stainbrook, 1949). The role of the nurse continued to involve the responsibilities from the 19th century, in addition to providing written and verbal reports, toileting, hydrotherapy, physical assessments, feeding, and admission of patients (Mabon, 1910; Purcell, 1911). By the end of the 1920s, the mental health nurse earned between $75 and $100 per month, which included the nurse's meals and housing—less than what a nurse working in a general hospital or in the community earned (Mabon, 1910; Tucker, 1916).

A Period of Mental Hygiene and Growth of Institutions (1930–1959)

Health professionals gained much knowledge about mental health during World War I, which ushered in a period of mental hygiene. In the 1930s, *mental illness* and *mental retardation* became two distinct diagnoses, so the care of patients with these conditions diverged for the first time. Different institutions were built for patients with these diagnoses in a continuing effort to separate persons with IDD from the general population (Nehring, 2003).

As a result of this distinction, nursing authors spoke specifically about the care of patients with IDD, particularly children (Jeans & Rand, 1936; Sloan & Stevens,

1976). For the first time in the literature, public health nurses wrote about children who remained in their homes, rather than being sent to the institution after birth. Prior writing by nurses focused on institutional nursing care. In such cases, public health nurses provided preventive health care, education to parents about communicable diseases, well-child care, and appropriate moral behavior (Flory, 1957; Sloan & Stevens, 1976). At that time, much was written about the role of nurses in case finding and providing referrals for appropriate evaluation and diagnosis. As a result, these responsibilities were also carried out by public health nurses and nurses working in developmental diagnostic clinics (Nehring, 2004b). Often, however, public health and school nurses also assisted parents in completing the application for admission to an institution by the time the child was school age; a practice that persisted through the 1950s (Corcoran, 1947; Jeans & Rand, 1936; Julian & Mischke, 1980).

The responsibilities of nurses working in institutions included many of the same functions as in earlier years, but with less attention to providing amusements and preventing patients from escape. Now, nurses provided more therapeutic interventions that required critical thinking skills, although housekeeping functions were still prevalent (Dick, 1941). Nurses also recorded daily vital signs; height, weight, and immunizations were recorded on an annual basis. Nursing notes began to appear by the end of the 1950s (Central Wisconsin Center, 1994; Grand Junction Regional Center, 1994). In addition, nurses in the institutions provided some continuing education to nurses in the community; this allowed community nurses to better assist the parents of children with IDD who remained at home, including providing information about a child's diagnosis and how best to provide daily care (Julian & Mischke, 1980).

By the mid-1930s, the workday decreased to 8 hours per day (Wallace, 1948); nevertheless, nurses began leaving the institutions. Those who remained were usually assigned a full wing of the institution, which resulted in a nurse-to-patient ratio of 1:400. Nurses thus had only minimal time to administer medications and give needed treatments (Corcoran, 1947; Fitzsimmons, 1944). Devine (1983) stated that the nursing care in the institution that she worked in during the early 1950s was basically nonexistent. In the 1940s, the salary of the staff nurse had increased to $150 to $200 per month (Lincoln State School & Colony, 1996b), but African American nurses earned less than Caucasian nurses (Noll, 1995).

The Kennedy Years and the Pivotal Decade of the 1960s

The efforts of President Kennedy during his years in the White House—and thereafter by members of his family—positively altered the care, evaluation, definitions, and attitudes surrounding persons with IDD. Although humanitarian attempts had been made in previous years, the steps that Kennedy put into place revolutionized services provided to people with IDD in the 1960s, including the nursing care that was provided. Nevertheless, the conditions in institutions were not often made safe or hygienic until after media exposure at the Willowbrook institution, such as reported by Geraldo Rivera and Burton Blatt in 1972 (Devine, 1983).

Throughout the 1960s, the nursing role expanded. Nurses recorded vital signs, height and weight, intake and output, restraint use, isolation care, medications, and range-of-motion exercises. Often, a weekly summary was recorded with brief daily nursing notes describing assessment data, interventions given (e.g., restraint use, medications, isolation care, range-of-motion exercises), nursing care goals, positioning, concerns regarding activities of daily living, and developmental issues. Care plans were also written (Central Wisconsin Center, 1994) and medications were given in abundance. Ellibee (1960) reported that she gave 162 patients 22,000 doses of various medications in 1 month in 1960. Nurses also began to supervise members of the health care team, such as licensed practical nurses, nursing assistants and other individuals performing tasks related to the patient's health (Patterson & Rowland, 1970). However, nurses often delivered care to groups of patients at a time, rather than to one individual at a time (Teague, 1966), but this would eventually change.

Funding became available to assist in the improvement of care, which included building on the knowledge base provided in initial nursing education programs. Nurses in this specialty were now instructed to have appropriate knowledge of typical and atypical development, genetics, embryology, microbiology, nutrition, psychology, and prevention screening (Murray & Barnard, 1966).

Some nurses wrote about their efforts in programming and research in the institutional setting. An active treatment model was initiated that replaced the medical model. Programs implemented by nurses included aversive therapy (Slamar & Kachoyeanos, 1969), operant therapy (Barnard, 1968), and sensory-motor training (Pothier, 1968). Patricia McNelly, who was Director of the Nursing at the Central Wisconsin Colony and Training School in 1965, initiated a research pilot study that investigated team nursing with a unit of four children thereby providing more individualized nursing care in a more home-like setting. This program was ahead of its time in normalizing institutional nursing care (Miller, 1979).

Nurses working in the community also initiated training programs for families and wrote seminal guides for the public health nurse. Programs were delivered on such topics as case management (Belfint & Sylvester, 1962), developmental assessment (Paulus, 1966), feeding and positioning (Haynes, 1968), home training (Dittmann, 1961; Steele, 1966), parent education (McCarthy & Chisholm, 1966), and parent support (Fackler, 1966). The guides for public health nurses written during the 1960s were considered classic writings in this field; for a number of years, they were mandatory additions to the public health bag carried by every public health nurse, particularly the guides by Haynes (1967), Holtgrewe (1964), and Borlick (1961).

The Past Four Decades

Beginning in the 1970s, the modern era for the field of IDD began. Miller (1979) wrote that the medical model for care was banished in this decade and replaced by the developmental model which focused on all aspects of a person, not just their illness. In the medical model, IDD is viewed as an illness. Some felt that the new model also represented a social focus with attention given to needed social supports rather than individual limitations (Luckasson et al., 1992; Nehring, 2003), which has been echoed in the recent editions of the AAIDD definition and classification book (e.g., Luckasson et al., 2002).

Nurses working in institutional settings (now referred to as developmental centers) provided quality care equivalent to that in any other health care setting. Nurses continued to provide programming for their patients on such topics as behavioral modification (Knapp, O'Neil, & Allen, 1974), behavioral therapy (Etters,

1975), elimination of rumination (Libby & Phillips, 1978), and therapeutic handling (Pothier, 1971).

The expansion of nursing roles in the community provided access to persons with IDD of all ages. Nurses had opportunities to care for people with IDD as they worked in hospitals, University Affiliated Programs or Facilities (now University Centers of Excellence in Developmental Disabilities), interdisciplinary specialty clinics, colleges and schools of nursing, elementary and secondary schools, group homes, health maintenance organizations, and federal agencies (Worthy, 1975). Responsibilities in these settings included prevention of IDD, case finding, use of developmental screening tools, counseling, genetic counseling, developing and implementing infant programs, participating in early intervention programs, developing and providing specific programs in such areas as sex education and behavior modification, and providing community follow-up (Godfrey, 1975; Krajicek & Roberts, 1976). Specialty roles further emerged with the birth of the clinical nurse specialist in mental retardation in 1978 (Bumbalo, 1978), the genetics nurse in the late 1970s (Cohen, 1979; Horan, 1977), and the early intervention nurse in the 1980s (Coyner, 1986).

Today, developmental centers still exist in many states. People with IDD who reside in these settings often have multiple and complex primary and secondary diagnoses; they may be older, be nonambulatory, have behavior problems, and/or have uncontrollable seizures. However, most nursing care provided to these patients takes place in the community.

Nursing care continued to evolve in the 1990s. Morse wrote the following:

> Developmental disabilities nursing is the subspecialty of nursing practice that deals with assisting the individual with developmental disabilities to attain/maintain an optimal level of wellness across the life span. Individuals served by the developmental disabilities nurse have disorders that reflect a variety of health, cognitive, communication, social adaptation, sensory, perceptual, gross motor, and fine motor strengths and limitations. These are manifested over time and affect the family as well as the individual. (1994, p. 26)

This definition remains the same in the 21st century. It is essential that nurses recruit and mentor future nurses for the continuation of the IDD specialty. The specialty must keep expanding to survive and should include nurses (e.g., those who care for medically complex premature infants) who do not label themselves as an IDD nurse but who care for individuals with IDD (Kelly, 2006).

NURSING EDUCATION ACROSS TIME

This section explores nursing education in the field of IDD. Similar to general nursing in the United States, formalized education for "asylum nursing" (which included the care of persons with IDD) began in the late 19th century. However, the depth and quality of the training was not as good as general nursing until the late 1920s, when basic education and training for nurses in all specialties was combined (Haydon, 1928; Nehring, 2005).

Formalized education for IDD nurses began in the last quarter of the 19th century by physicians. The first school for asylum nurses was started in 1882 by Dr. Edward Cowles at the McLean Asylum in Somerville, Massachusetts (Cowles, 1887). Nursing students were taught basic nursing skills and learned about injury and illness. The philosophy and theory of "mental nursing" was taught in the second year. Each year of the 2-year program of study lasted 8 months and consisted of 30 lectures. Applicants to the early nursing programs had to be unmarried, be between 20 and 35 years of age, and have good morals (Russell, 1945). They received a stipend of $15–$35 per month. Besides the classroom time, nursing students had to work 12–15.5 hours per day, 6.5 days per week (Tucker, 1916).

During the first three decades of the 20th century, nurses received training for the care of persons with IDD in asylums, general hospitals, institutions, and mental hospitals. The curricula during this time were similar to the general nursing curriculum with the addition of training in hydrotherapy (Lincoln State School & Colony, 1996a).

By the end of the 1930s, the education of all nurses took place in the general hospital (Haydon, 1928), although Presbyterian Hospital in Chicago was the first general hospital to affiliate with a mental hospital in 1909 (Goodnow, 1949). The National League for Nursing Practice (1926) published a revised curriculum guide for all nursing programs in the United States; this curriculum included lectures on psychology and psychiatry. The psychology lectures included content on IQ, mental age, mental testing, theories of intelligence, and problems of the "mental deviate." The psychiatry lectures included content on feeblemindedness and idiocy, colonies and institutions, legislation and state responsibilities, diagnoses, mental testing, etiology, care and education, and grades and types.

The specific education of nurses in IDD and the care of patients with IDD changed little until the late 1960s. With the influence of the Kennedy presidency and a focus on the population of persons with IDD, nurse educators began to arrange for clinical experiences in settings where persons with IDD resided, such as institutions (Lange & Whitney, 1966; Pennington, 1968). A postgraduate program developed by Kathryn Barnard at the University of Washington in 1965 was attended by several future nurse leaders in the field (e.g., Marilyn Krajicek, Marcene Powell Erickson, Sally O'Neil, Mary Seidel, Elizabeth Worthy). Continuing to lead the field, Brandt and Magyary at the University of Washington implemented a graduate nursing program in early intervention for the clinical nurse specialist in 1989. Then, beginning in the 1990s, the Maternal and Child Health Bureau provided funding for the education of pediatric nurse practitioners to assume leadership roles in the care of children with special health care needs, including children with IDD. A program headed by Marilyn Krajicek at the School of Nursing at the University of Colorado Health Sciences Center has existed since this funding initiative began; it is the foremost nursing graduate program in the United States for the specialization of IDD nursing (Nehring, 1999, 2003).

The University Affiliated Programs or Facilities (now University Centers for Excellence in Developmental Disabilities), initiated by President Kennedy, provides fellowships for interdisciplinary learning in this field, including nursing, if the program is funded by the Maternal and Child Health Bureau's Leadership in Neurodevelopmental and Related Disabilities program (Nehring, 2004a). In these university settings, a nurse is identified as a liaison for this interdisciplinary effort to serve as a reference and role model for the nursing student interested in the field.

Continuing education for nurses on topics related to the care of persons with IDD began to appear by the late 1950s. The most notable programs were the in-service trainings provided by Una Haynes during the 1960s and 1970s related to the developmental and physical assessment of infants. Live babies were used for the demonstrations and hands-on learning. Over 17,000 nurses attended these in-service trainings over the years. In 1978, a working group of nursing leaders in the field wrote the booklet *Guidelines for Continuing Education in Developmental Disabilities* (Haynes et al., 1978), which was later revised as *Continuing Education Needs for Nurses Caring for Children with Special Health Care Needs* in 1996 (Austin & Donohoe, 1996).

In 1958, the Children's Bureau offered the first of six national workshops for nurses working with persons with IDD. This initial workshop was attended by 14 nurses and covered the role of public health nurses who worked in developmental diagnostic clinics and the role of the nurse in the diagnostic process (O'Neil & Newcomer, 1974).

Today, efforts by nursing leaders and national organizations to provide in-service trainings, publications, and Internet educational sources have maintained a modest level and will most likely never reach the degree of offerings and attention as witnessed in the late 1960s-1970s. Continuing efforts, such as the inclusion of genetic content and new genetic discoveries, environmental influences, and health promotion, are necessary to maintain the knowledge base for new and practicing nurses in the future (Boisseau & Barrett, 2008; Graff, 2007; Graff, Murphy, Ekvall, & Gagnon, 2006).

ISSUES OF POLICY AND LEADERSHIP

The final section of this chapter focuses on the issues influencing policy and leadership for nurses in the field of IDD. Issues such as maintaining standards of care, manpower, participation in organizations and federal agencies, and nursing education opportunities will influence this nursing specialization in the future.

Standards of Care

Nurses have been leaders in the interdisciplinary field of IDD in writing standards of practice. The first set of standards, *Standards for State Residential Institutions for the Mentally Retarded*, was published by the American Association on Mental Deficiency in 1964 (Leboiteux, 1964). Currently, there are two specific sets of standards that apply to this nursing specialization: *Aspirational Standards of Developmental Disabilities Nursing Practice* (Willis, 2008) and *Intellectual and Developmental Disabilities Nursing: Scope & Standards of Practice* (Nehring et al., 2004). These standards were written by nurses from the primary professional organizations for IDD nurses: the Developmental Disabilities Nurses Association (DDNA) and AAIDD.

The nursing division of AAIDD wanted the earlier version of their standards (Nehring et al., 1998) to be co-published with the American Nurses Association (ANA). However, this could not occur until the ANA formally recognized their specialty of nursing. The formal recognition finally occurred in 1997, despite the many years that nurses already worked in caring for patients with IDD.

Two other sets of standards include information about the care of persons with IDD: *Genetics/Genomics Nursing: Scope & Standards of Practice* (International Society of Nurses in Genetics, 2005) and *School Nursing: Scope & Standards of Practice* (National Association of School Nurses, 2005). It is important that nursing leaders in this specialty field continue the revisions of these documents, although this may be affected by the next issue of manpower.

Manpower

The issue of manpower always has been present in the field of IDD nursing. Historically, most nurses in this specialty have been employed in institutions (i.e., developmental centers). As these settings have closed across the country, nurses have been displaced. In some instances, they have been allowed to transfer to other state facilities serving persons with IDD and/or mental illness. For many of these nurses, however, the distance to travel to the other facilities was too far. Also, few or no opportunities exist for these nurses to move to the community settings into which the patients were being transferred, which allowed for little continuity of care. This resulted in these nurses either seeking employment in other areas of nursing or leaving nursing altogether (Nehring, 2003).

Now, with managed care, many community settings (e.g., specialized clinics, diagnostic clinics, early intervention programs, public health agencies) have been eliminated or diluted enough so that their original purpose in serving patients with IDD has been lost. As patients with IDD are integrated into mainstream society, it is important that education efforts continue, both in pre-service and in-service training, to inform nurses about the definition, epidemiology, classification, etiology, specific conditions, and care that must be provided to patients with IDD. It is also essential that nurses who specialize in this field achieve graduate degrees with the intention of taking leadership roles to continue to influence nurses, other disciplines, and the public in the necessary care and treatment needed for persons with IDD (Nehring, 2004a).

Organizations and Federal Agencies

After World War II, support groups for parents of children with IDD emerged. The first was the United Cerebral Palsy Association in 1946, followed by Arc of the United States (initially called Parents and Friends of Mentally Retarded Children) in 1950, and then the March of Dimes Foundation (originally called the National Foundation for Infantile Paralysis) in 1958 (Nehring, 1999). Una Haynes was an original member of the United Cerebral Palsy Association's Committee on Nursing (Haynes, 1963). Nurse consultants were also employed by the Arc of the United States. In addition, other groups, such as the National Down Syndrome Congress, formed interdisciplinary professional committees to advise them on issues and included nursing representation (Nehring, 2003). Nurses should continue to be actively involved in these support groups—if not at the national level, then at least on the local level.

Federal agencies, specifically the former Children's Bureau and the U.S. Public Health Service (the former Mental Retardation Branch of the Division of Chronic Diseases and the former Division of Neurological Diseases and Stroke), employed nurse consultants in the past. Such positions no longer exist, but there is nursing representation at the state level in the agencies that oversees state-supported services for persons with IDD (Nehring, 2003). State representation by nurses should remain to oversee the nursing care delivered in state-funded agencies. Nurses also are asked to consult periodically with federal agencies or committees, such as the President's Committee for Persons with Intellectual Disabilities.

As mentioned previously, two major organizations exist for nurses who care for persons with IDD: AAIDD (an interdisciplinary organization) and DDNA. The membership for DDNA is much greater than that of AAIDD because it is entirely nurse centered. Another organization, the American Association on Health and Disability, was formed as a result of the Surgeon General's conference in 2001 (U. S. Public Health Service, 2001). Although the organization is focused on physicians and dentists, nurses can apply for associate membership.

The membership of nurses in AAIDD—and in fact, the membership of all health professionals—has decreased significantly over the past decade. This decrease is most likely because of the increasing number of new organizations—often for specific purposes or populations, such as autism—that have drawn members away from AAIDD. The economy may also be driving the decrease in numbers, as nurses cut down on their memberships due to rising costs. Even so, it is imperative that nurses become active in their specialty organizations. The organizations will not continue to be viable and meet the needs of their memberships nor the constituents that they serve if they have no members. For many organizations, this situation is reaching a crisis level.

Educational Opportunities

The time spent in the basic pre-licensure nursing curriculum on the conditions and care of persons with IDD is limited. The information has been restricted primarily to a course on pediatric nursing and occasionally one on public health nursing (Nehring, 2004a). Pediatric nursing courses have been greatly decreased in length in some schools and totally eliminated in others.

The number of nursing leaders in the IDD field is also diminishing, especially those employed as nurse educators and researchers. As a result, not only will opportunities for this educational content further decrease but also there will be fewer role models for recruitment to the field, fewer faculty who can appropriately chair doctoral dissertations and capstone projects, and fewer publications from nurses about their roles and the evidence-based care that they provide. Nurses should therefore take measures to advocate for this specialization and encourage current nurses to seek graduate degrees, conduct research, and publish. The field of IDD nursing may be expanded by networking across borders and describing this specialization around the world (Nehring, 1999, 2003, 2004a). However, such an approach would require an understanding of the meaning of IDD for other cultures and sensitivity to providing appropriate evidence-based care (Nehring, 2007). In addition, the development and implementation of web-based instruction can be addressed, including the advent of virtual patient case studies (Hahn & Willis, 2004; Sanders et al., 2007; Sanders et al., 2008).

CONCLUSION

The future for IDD nursing may look bleak, but it does not need to be. However, much needs to be achieved to prolong the life of this specialty, which will require the infusion of new nurses, the use of new models of care (i.e., models that do not adversely label people), new roles and accessible settings to deliver care, an increased knowledge base and a continued legacy of nursing publications and scholarly efforts, knowledge of and ability to use new technology, continuing supportive legislation, and leadership opportunities. The field has been stigmatized, but as people with IDD are further integrated, as well as provided with improved access to and delivery of health care, it is important to incorporate the lessons of history to the future of nursing in the care of persons with IDD and their families.

REFERENCES

American Psychiatric Association. (1952). *Diagnostic and statistical manual of mental disorders.* Washington, DC: Author.

Americans with Disabilities Act of 1990, PL 101-336, 42 U.S.C. §§ 201 *et seq.*

Austin, J.R.D., & Donohoe, M.L. (1996). *Continuing education needs for nurses caring for children with special health care needs.* Washington, DC: Health Resources and Services Administration, Maternal and Child Health Bureau and Georgetown University Child Development Center.

Barnard, K. (1968). Teaching the retarded child is a family affair. *American Journal of Nursing, 68,* 305–311.

Barrus, C. (1908). *Nursing the insane.* New York: Macmillan.

Belfint, E.K., & Sylvester, L.W. (1962). Delaware's program for mentally retarded children. *Nursing Outlook, 10,* 442–444.

Boisseau, J., & Barrett, R. (2008). Nurse practitioner knowledge and attitudes regarding developmental disabilities health screening and health promotion. *International Journal of Nursing in Intellectual and Developmental Disabilities, 4*(1).

Borlick, M.M. (1961). *Guide for public health nurses working with children from the developmental point of view.* Washington, DC: U.S. Department of Health, Education, and Welfare, Children's Bureau.

Braddock, D., & Heller, T. (1985). The closure of mental retardation institutions II: Implications. *Mental Retardation, 23,* 222–229.

Bradley, E.B. (1914). The problem of the feeble-minded. *American Journal of Nursing, 14,* 628–631.

Bumbalo, J.A. (1978). The clinical nurse specialist. In K.E. Allen, V.A. Holm, & R.L. Schiefelbusch (Eds.), *Early intervention—a team approach* (pp. 124–145). Baltimore: University Park Press.

Central Wisconsin Center (1994). [Charting documentation.] Unpublished raw data. Madison, WI: Author.

Cohen, F.L. (1979). Genetic knowledge possessed by American nurses and nursing students. *Journal of Advanced Nursing, 4,* 493–501.

Corcoran, M.E. (1947). Observations and suggestions for improving the care of mental defectives. *American Journal of Mental Defectives, 51,* 599–605.

Cowles, E. (1887). Nursing-reform for the insane. *American Journal of Insanity, 44,* 176–191.

Coyner, A. (1986). The nurse as primary interventionist for high risk and disabled infants: A personal perspective. In K.E. Barnard (Ed.), *Early intervention. Concerns of a career in nursing: Proceedings of a symposium in honor of Camille L. Cook* (pp. 36–50). Washington, DC: National Center for Clinical Infant Programs.

Devine, P. (1983). Mental retardation: An early subspecialty in psychiatric nursing. *Journal of Psychiatric Nursing & Mental Health Services, 21,* 21–30.

Dick, K.R. (1941). Nursing in a state hospital. *American Journal of Nursing, 41,* 401–407.

Dittmann, L.L. (1961). *The nurse in home training programs for the retarded child.* Washington, DC: U.S. Department of Health, Education, and Welfare, Children's Bureau and Social Security Administration, U.S. Government Printing Office.

Doll, E.A. (1941). The essentials of an inclusive concept of mental deficiency. *American Journal of Mental Deficiency, 46,* 214–219.

Education for All Handicapped Children Act of 1975, PL 94-142, 20 U.S.C. §§ 1400 *et seq.*

Education of the Handicapped Act Amendments of 1986, PL 99-457, 20 U.S.C. §§ 1400 *et seq.*

Ellibee, E. (1960). *Annual report 1959–1960.* Unpublished document. Madison, WI: Central Wisconsin Colony and Training School.

Etters, L.E. (1975). Adolescent retardates in a therapy group. *American Journal of Nursing, 75,* 1174–1175.

Fackler, E. (1966). Community organization in culturally deprived areas. *Mental Retardation, 4,* 12–14.

Fitzsimmons, L.W. (1944). Facts and trends in psychiatric nursing. *American Journal of Nursing, 44,* 732–735.

Flory, M.C. (1957). Helping parents train a retarded child. *Nursing Outlook, 5,* 426–427.

Goddard, H. (1912). *The Kallikak family: A study in the heredity of feeble-mindedness.* New York: Macmillan.

Godfrey, A.B. (1975). Sensory-motor stimulation: A specialized program. *American Journal of Nursing, 75,* 56–62.

Goodnow, M. (1949). *Nursing history* (8th ed.). Philadelphia: W.B. Saunders.

Graff, J.C. (2007). Integrating genetics and genomics into developmental disabilities nursing practice. *International Journal of Nursing in Intellectual and Developmental Disabilities, 3*(2).

Graff, J.C., Murphy, L., Ekvall, S., & Gagnon, M. (2006). In-home toxic chemical exposures and children with intellectual and developmental disabilities. *Pediatric Nursing, 32,* 596–603.

Grand Junction Regional Center. (1994). Charting documentation. Unpublished data. Grand Junction, CO: Author.

Griffin, G. J., & Griffin, J. K. (1969). *Jensen's history and trends of professional nursing* (6th ed.). St. Louis: Mosby.

Hahn, J.E., & Willis, M.A. (2004). Multimedia web-based courseware in intellectual and developmental disabilities nursing: From concept to development. *International Journal of Nursing in Intellectual and Developmental Disabilities, 1*(1).

Haydon, E.M. (1928). Teaching and supervision of mental nursing. *American Journal of Nursing, 28,* 499–501.

Haynes, U. (1963). *The role of nursing in programs for patients with cerebral palsy and related disorders.* New York: United Cerebral Palsy Association.

Haynes, U. (1967). *A developmental approach to casefinding among infants and young children.* Washington, DC: U.S. Department of Health, Education, and Welfare, Children's Bureau.

Haynes, U. (1968). Nursing approaches in cerebral dysfunction: 16,000 nurses ask for help. *American Journal of Nursing, 68,* 2170–2176.

Haynes, U., Bumbalo, J., Cook, C., Haar, D., Krajicek, M., & Slamar, C.F. (1978). *Guidelines for continuing education in developmental disabilities.* Kansas City, MO: American Nurses Association.

Heber, R. (1959). A manual on terminology and classification in mental retardation. *American Journal of Mental Deficiency, 64* (Suppl.), 1–111.

Holtgrewe, M.M. (1964). *A guide for public health nurses working with mentally retarded children.* Washington, DC: U.S. Government Printing Office.

Horan, M. (1977). Genetic counseling: Helping the family. *Journal of Obstetrical, Gynecological, and Neonatal Nursing, 6,* 25–29.

Howe, D.E. (1896). Training schools for attendants. *Journal of Psycho-Asthenics, 1,* 75–84.

International Society of Nurses in Genetics. (2005). *Genetics/genomics nursing: Scope and standards of practice.* Silver Spring, MD: American Nurses Association.

Ireland, W.W. (1877). *On idiocy and imbecility.* London: J & A Churchill.

Jeans, P.C., & Rand, W. (1936). *Essentials of pediatrics* (3rd ed.). Philadelphia: J.B. Lippincott.

Julian, D., & Mischke, K. (1980). Nursing and mental retardation: An Oregon perspective 1900–1979. *Oregon Nurse, 12,* 10–15.

Kanner, L. (1967). Medicine in the history of mental retardation 1800–1965. *American Journal of Mental Deficiency, 72,* 165–189.

Kelly, M.M. (2006). The medically complex premature infant in primary care. *Journal of Pediatric Health Care, 20,* 367–373.

Kerlin, I.N. (1877). The organization of establishments for idiotic and imbecile classes. *Proceedings of the Association of Medical Officers of American Institutions for Idiotic and Feeble-Minded Persons,* 19–28.

Knapp, M.E., O'Neil, S.M., & Allen, K.E. (1974). Teaching Suzi to walk by behavior modification of motor skills. *Nursing Forum, 13,* 158–183.

Krajicek, M.J., & Roberts, P. (1976). Nursing. In R.B. Johnston & P.R. Magrab (Eds.), *Developmental disorders: Assessment, treatment, education* (pp. 363–374). Baltimore: University Park Press.

Laird, S.L. (1902). Nursing of the insane. *American Journal of Nursing, 2,* 170–180.

Lange, S., & Whitney, L. (1966). Teaching mental retardation nursing: The faculty learn. *Nursing Outlook, 14,* 58–63.

Leboiteux, F. (1964). Standards for state residential institutions for the mentally retarded. *Journal of Mental Deficiency, 68* (Suppl.), 1–101.

Libby, D.G., & Phillips, E. (1978). Eliminating rumination behavior in a profoundly retarded adolescent: An exploratory study. *Mental Retardation, 16,* 57.

Lincoln State School & Colony. (1996a). *Lectures from the training school at the Lincoln State School & Colony, 1912–1918. Lincoln State School & Colony, Record Series 254.55.* Chicago: Illinois State Archives.

Lincoln State School & Colony. (1996b). *Nurses' salaries from the Lincoln State School & Colony. Lincoln State School & Colony Record Series 254.1–254.54.* Chicago: Illinois State Archives.

Luckasson, R., Borthwick-Duffy, S., Buntinx, W.H.E., Coulter, D.L., Craig, E.M., Reeve, A., et al. (2002). *Mental retardation: Definition, classification, and systems of supports* (10th ed.). Washington, DC: American Association on Mental Retardation.

Luckasson, R., Coulter, D.L., Polloway, E.A., Reiss, S., Schalock, R.L., Snell, M., et al. (1992). *Mental retardation: Definition, classification, and systems of supports* (9th ed.). Washington, DC: American Association on Mental Retardation.

Luckasson, R., & Reeve, A. (2001). Naming, defining, and classifying in mental retardation. *Mental Retardation, 39,* 47–82.

Mabon, W. (1910). The nursing care of the insane. *American Journal of Nursing, 10,* 887–896.

MacMillan, D.L., & Reschly, D.J. (1997). Issues of definition and classification. In W.E. MacLean, Jr. (Ed.). *Ellis' handbook of mental deficiency, psychological theory and research* (3rd ed., pp. 47–74). Mahwah, NJ: Lawrence Erlbaum Associates.

McCarthy, K.A., & Chisholm, M.M. (1966). Group education with mothers of retarded children. *Nursing Clinics of North America, 1,* 703–713.

Miller, J.A. (1979). *A history of nursing at Central Wisconsin Center for the developmentally disabled.* Unpublished manuscript. Chicago: University of Illinois at Chicago.

Mills v. Board of Education, 348 F. Supp. 868 (D.D.C. 1972).

Morgan, J.J.B. (1925). *The psychology of the unadjusted school child.* New York: Macmillan.

Morse, J.S. (1994). An overview of developmental disabilities nursing. In S.P. Roth & J.S. Morse (Eds.), *A life-span approach to nursing care for individuals with developmental disabilities* (pp. 19–58). Baltimore: Paul H. Brookes Publishing Co.

Murray, B.L., & Barnard, K.E. (1966). The nursing specialist in mental retardation. *Nursing Clinics in North America, 1,* 631–640.

National Association of School Nurses. (2005). *School nursing: Scope & standards of practice.* Silver Spring, MD: American Nurses Association.

National League for Nursing Practice. (1926). Revision of the standard curriculum: Psychology. *American Journal of Nursing, 26,* 140–146.

Nehring, W.M. (1999). *A history of nursing in the field of mental retardation and developmental disabilities.* Washington, DC: American Association on Mental Retardation.

Nehring, W.M. (2003). History of the roles of nurses caring for persons with mental retardation. *Nursing Clinics of North America, 38,* 351–372.

Nehring, W.M. (2004a). Directions for the future of intellectual and developmental disabilities as a nursing specialty. *International Journal of Nursing in Intellectual and Developmental Disabilities, 1*(1).

Nehring, W.M. (2004b). Formal health care at the community level: The Child Development Clinics of the 1950s and 1960s. In S. Noll & J.W. Trent Jr. (Eds.), *Mental retardation in America: A historical reader* (pp. 371–383). New York: New York University Press.

Nehring, W.M. (2005). History of nursing and health professionals in intellectual and developmental disabilities. In W.M. Nehring (Ed.), *Core curriculum for specializing in intellectual and developmental disability: A resource for nurses and other health care professionals* (pp. 3–24). Boston: Jones & Bartlett.

Nehring, W.M. (2007). Cultural considerations for children with intellectual and developmental disabilities. *Journal of Pediatric Nursing, 22,* 93–102.

Nehring, W.M., & Betz, C.L. (2007). General health. In S.L. Odom, R.H. Horner, M.E. Snell, & J. Blacher (Eds.), *Handbook of de-*

velopmental disabilities (pp. 79–97). New York: Guilford Press.

Nehring, W.M., Roth, S.P., Natvig, D., Betz, C.L., Savage, T., & Krajicek, M. (2004). Intellectual and developmental disabilities nursing: Scope & standards of practice. Silver Spring, MD: American Nurses Association.

Nehring, W.M., Roth, S.P., Natvig, D., Morse, J.S., Savage, T., & Krajicek, M. (1998). Statement on the scope and standards for the nurse who specializes in developmental disabilities and/or mental retardation. Washington, DC: American Association on Mental Retardation and the American Nurses Association.

Noll, S. (1995). Feeble-minded in our midst: Institutions for the mentally retarded in the South, 1900–1940s. Chapel Hill, NC: University of North Carolina Press.

Odom, S.L., Horner, R.H., Snell, M.E., & Blacher, J. (2007). The construct of developmental disabilities. In S.L. Odom, R.H. Horner, M.E. Snell, & J. Blacher (Eds.), Handbook of developmental disabilities (pp. 3–14). New York: Guilford Press.

O'Neil, S.M., & Newcomer, B. (Eds.). (1974, March). Sixth national workshop for nurses in mental retardation: Summary of proceedings. Cincinnati, OH: University of Cincinnati.

Patterson, E.C., & Rowland, G.T. (1970). Toward a theory of mental retardation nursing: An education model. American Journal of Nursing, 70, 531–535.

Paulus, A.C. (1966). A tool for the assessment of the retarded child. Nursing Clinics of North America, 1, 659–668.

Pennhurst State School v. Halderman, Civil Action Nos. 79-1404, 79-1408, 79-1414, 79-1415, 79-1489, U. S. Third Circuit Court of Appeals (1981).

Pennington, M. (1968). Nursing students work with the mentally retarded. Nursing Outlook, 16, 38–39.

Pennsylvania Association for Retarded Children v. Commonwealth of Pennsylvania, 343 F. Supp. 279 (D. Pa. 1971).

Pothier, P.C. (1968). Implementing a training program with a severely retarded young child in a home setting. ANA Clinical Sessions (pp. 332–357). New York: Appleton-Century-Crofts.

Pothier, P.C. (1971). Therapeutic handling of the severely handicapped child. American Journal of Nursing, 71, 321–324.

Purcell, M. (1911). Nursing care of the insane. American Journal of Nursing, 11, 430–433.

Rehabilitation Act of 1973, PL 93-112, 29 U.S.C. §§ 701 et seq.

Russell, W.L. (1945). The New York Hospital: A history of the psychiatric service 1771–1936. New York: Columbia University Press.

Sanders, C.L., Kleinert, H.L., Free, T., King, P., Slusher, I., & Boyd, S. (2008). Developmental disabilities: Improving competence in care using virtual patients. Journal of Nursing Education, 47, 66–73.

Sanders, C.L., Kleinert, H.L., Free, T., Slusher, I., Clevenger, K., Johnson, S., et al. (2007). Caring for children with intellectual and developmental disabilities: Virtual patient instruction improves students' knowledge and comfort level. Journal of Pediatric Nursing, 22, 457–466.

Santos, E.H., & Stainbrook, E. (1949). A history of psychiatric nursing in the nineteenth century. Part I. Journal of the History of Medicine, 4, 48–60.

Schalock, R. L., Luckasson, R. A., Shogren, K. A., Borthwick-Duffy, S., Bradley, V., Buntinx, W. H., et al. (2008). The renaming of mental retardation: Understanding the change to the term intellectual disability. Intellectual and Developmental Disabilities, 45, 116–124.

Scheerenberger, R.C. (1981). Deinstitutionalization: Trends and difficulties. In R.H. Bruninks, C.E. Mayers, B.B. Sigford, & K.C. Lakin (Eds.), Deinstitutionalization and community adjustment of mentally retarded people (pp. 3–13). Washington, DC: American Association on Mental Deficiency.

Slamar, C.F., & Kachoyeanos, M.K. (1969). Nursing therapy in a combined treatment approach to rumination. ANA Clinical Sessions (pp. 185–195). New York: Appleton-Century-Crofts.

Sloan, W., & Stevens, H.A. (1976). A century of concern: A history of the American Association on Mental Deficiency 1876-1976. Washington, DC: American Association on Mental Deficiency.

Social Security Act of 1935, PL 74-271, 42 U.S.C. §§ 301 et seq.

Steele, S. (1966). The role of the public health nurse in the discharge of the handicapped child in the community. *Nursing Clinics of North America, 1,* 153–162.

Teague, B.E. (1966). Implementing changes in the traditional institutional environment of the mentally retarded. *Nursing Clinics of North America, 1,* 651–658.

Tucker, K. (1916). Nursing care of the insane in the United States. *American Journal of Nursing, 16,* 198–202.

U.S. Public Health Service. (2001). *Closing the gap: A national blueprint for improving the health of individuals with mental retardation. Report of the Surgeon General's conference on health disparities and mental retardation.* Rockville, MD: U.S. Department of Health and Human Services, Public Health Service, Office of the Surgeon General.

Wallace, A.M. (1948). Progress and problems in maternal and child health. *Nursing Outlook, 6,* 278–281.

Wehmeyer, M.L., Buntinx, W.H.E., Lachapelle, Y., Luckasson, R.A., Schalock, R.L., & Verdugo, M.A. (2008). The intellectual disability construct and its relation to human functioning. *Intellectual and Developmental Disabilities, 48,* 311–318.

Willis, M.A. (2008). *Aspirational standards of developmental disabilities nursing practice.* Orlando, FL: Developmental Disabilities Nurses Association.

Worthy, E.J. (1975). Symposium on the child with developmental disabilities. *Nursing Clinics of North America, 10,* 307–308.

Wyatt v. Stickney, 344 F. Supp 373 (N.D. Ala. 1972).

CHAPTER 2

Theoretical Models Guiding Care

Pamela P. DiNapoli

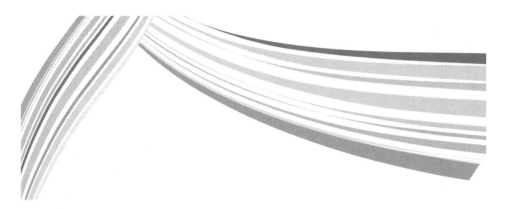

In the United States, it is estimated that 13.9% of children have special health care needs, and that 21.8% of households with children include at least one child with a special health care need (U.S. Department of Health and Human Services, 2008). Children with special health care needs (CSHCN), as defined by the Maternal Child Health Bureau (MCHB), are "all children who have, or are at increased risk for, chronic physical, developmental, behavioral, or emotional conditions and who also require health and related services of a type or amount beyond that required by children generally" (McPherson et al., 1998, p. 138). This definition encompasses many terminologies, including *disabled* (a diverse group of severe chronic conditions that are due to mental and/or physical impairments) (Centers for Disease Control and Prevention, n.d.), *handicapped, exceptional,* and *special needs.* The term *CSHCN* reflects an evolution in society's understanding of the unique needs of this population.

Since the 1980s, there have been innumerable scientific and technological advances in health care, including changes that have had a significant impact on the care of CSHCN. Even the term *CSHCN* reflects a recognition of the unique needs of this population and an evolution of thinking beyond the categorization of children according to a medical model of simple or complex diagnoses.

To ensure quality outcomes for patient care, nurses need to consider the theoretical models that will guide their care and services for individuals with special health care needs. Theoretical models may emphasize the individual from a developmental or functional perspective, stress family participation and the individual's functioning within a daily social context, or focus on health-related quality-of-life objective and subjective health outcomes (Bjorck-Akesson, Granlund, & Simeonsson, 2000). Theoretical models also may provide a frame of reference about a phenomenon, a way of understanding a situation, or possible solutions to a practical problem. The models of care proposed in this chapter are specific to individuals with intellectual and developmental disabilities (IDD) as defined in Chapter 1. There is no best theoretical model; each model influences an individual perception and helps achieve consistency in outcomes (Fawcett, 2005).

Historically, theoretical models that focused on body functions were used to guide care as they measured objective dimensions, such as mobility and activities of daily living. More recently, health-related quality-of-life outcomes have gained popularity in planning care because of their inclusion of both objective and subjective dimensions. The latter component tends to be more valued by children and their parents, whereas the former is typically more informative for the service provider's needs (Guyatt, 1997). Ever-changing trends in care may challenge the provider's philosophy of care. Thus, the purpose of this chapter is to offer perspectives from theoretical models that can guide nursing care of individuals with special health care needs (with an emphasis on IDD) to promote optimal outcomes.

The following theoretical models may be adopted by providers of care to individuals and families impacted by IDD across the life span. The frameworks discussed in this chapter are loosely categorized as social norms (i.e., self-advocacy and normalization), systems of care (i.e., inclusion and medical home), and holistic models of care (i.e., family-centered care and person-focused care). Each of the frameworks considers care from differing perspectives and is also presented from a historical perspective. Newer frameworks, such as interdisciplinary services, holistic patient-centered care, and lifestage-specific models of care, are also discussed. These framework models are summarized in Table 2.1.

SOCIAL NORMS FRAMEWORKS

Two types of social norms frameworks are discussed in this section: self-advocacy and normalization.

Self-Advocacy

Self-advocacy started as a civil rights movement by people with IDD who were rebelling against being underestimated, being deprived of choices, and being treated as children (Shapiro, 1993). The self-advocacy movement began in 1973 by a small group of activists in Salem, Oregon, who are credited with formulating the phrase "We are people first" (Perske, 1996). In 1974, this self-advocate group became known as People First and began discussing housing, business, and equality in society as alternatives to life in institutions (Lehr & Taylor, 1986). According to Lehr and Taylor,

> Self-advocacy means being able to speak for yourself, to make decisions for yourself, to know what your rights are and how to "stick up" for yourself when your rights are being violated or diminished. It also means being able to help others who cannot speak for themselves. (1986, p. 3)

Self-advocacy is based on the principle that all individuals, regardless of their developmental stage or cognitive abilities, are capable of learning self-advocacy skills. Self-advocacy refers to the ability to use good coping strategies, to identify and use resources, and to be empowered. It shifts the role of the health care provider from an authoritarian professional to that of a consultant on health care issues. The goal of self-advocacy is to enhance advocacy skills (which should be

Table 2.1. Theoretical models guiding care

Theory	Central concepts	Roots
Self-advocacy	Health care provider serves consultative role versus authoritarian one	People First movement
Normalization	Availability of equal choice	Normalization principles
Inclusion	Fostering social skills in a least restrictive environment	Education for All Handicapped Children Act (PL 94-142)
Medical home	Accessible, continuous, comprehensive, family-centered, coordinated, compassionate, and culturally effective	American Academy of Pediatrics Medical Home Initiative
Family-centered care	Significant family members are included in establishing objectives to meet the health care needs of the child	Maternity care
Interdisciplinary services	Collaboration among and between professionals, families, and the child	Institute of Medicine's Crossing the Quality Chasm
Holistic patient-centered care	Incorporates all aspects of the individual's mind, body, and spirit	Philosophy of holism
Lifestage-specific models of care	Successful acquisition of developmental tasks	Human development

started as early as possible) through such simple strategies as offering choices to children with disabilities at a very young age (e.g., having the child with a disability involved in their own individualized education program and transition plan processes). Knowing self-advocacy skills is particularly important during the transition from adolescence to adulthood, as this transition involves leaving secondary school programs for work responsibilities, enrolling in a postsecondary program for additional education or job training, achieving financial independence, and/or moving out from the parent's home to another type of independent or supported living arrangement. Self-advocacy skills are crucial to living a self-determined life. Researchers have demonstrated that self-determination, or the free choice of a person's own actions, is associated with a better quality of life (Wehmeyer & Schwartz, 1998).

The ASSERT model (Kling, 2000) depicts the steps to achieving self-advocacy:

- **A**wareness of the disability
- **S**tate the disability
- **S**tate the strengths and weaknesses
- **E**valuate problems and solutions
- **R**ole play solutions
- **T**ry it in the real setting

The ASSERT model allows for self-determination related to both small and sentinel aspects of living. For most people, self-determination tends to be attained over more minor aspects of life at an earlier developmental stage than the more major aspects. For example, a child may be self-determined in regard to his bedtime and playtime (minor aspect), but not in relation to his educational options (major aspect). By contrast, an older adolescent has a greater degree of self-determination over the educational and vocational alternatives affecting future plans. Thus, normative development in regard to self-determination can be described as a trend of increasing self-determination with age, in both the extent and degree of personal control exerted (Smith, Morgan, & Davidson, 2005).

The barriers to self-determination as identified by the Alliance for Self-Determination (n.d.) continue to be based on the perspective of society, which views disability as a medical rather than a sociopolitical problem. From a medical model perspective, a disability is described as a deficiency that must be cured, whereas from a sociopolitical perspective, it is explained as a difference for which accommodations can be made. When based on the medical model perspective, a disability would preclude self-determination because the agent of cure is considered to be a professional rather than the individual. Viewing a disability from a sociopolitical perspective serves to remove barriers to self-determination and creates access to supports and services.

To achieve self-determination, individuals with IDD need to achieve control of their lives with adequate supports and services, which can be partially realized by being a self-advocate. To become self-advocates, people with special health care needs should be given leadership roles in the development of policies, programs, and practices that directly affect their life choices. These leadership roles may include participation on advisory committees, in-service trainings, or family-to-family support services. Taking leadership roles offers opportunities for successes and failures with the goal of improving quality of life as determined by the individual, regardless of whether it is consistent with the wishes of the medical team or family (Center for Self-Determination, n.d.).

Normalization

Normalization is a concept that has influenced care and evolved over time. In 1969, Nirje defined normalization as "making available to all intellectually disabled people [sic] patterns of life and conditions of everyday living, which are as close as possible to the regular circumstances and ways of life of society" (p. 19). He proposed eight planks of normalization (Perske, 2004):

1. Having a normal rhythm of the day
2. Having a normal routine of life
3. Having a normal rhythm of the year
4. Having normal developmental experiences of the life cycle
5. Valuing individual choices
6. Living in a bisexual world
7. Applying normal economic standards
8. Living, learning, and recreating in facilities similar to those others in the community enjoy

In subsequent iterations of the definition, the term *social role valorization* was coined by psychologist Wolf Wolfensberger (1983), creator of the group Citizen Advocacy. Here normalization was equated with social value, based upon the perspective that those individuals viewed as having little social value were normalized negatively. In Wolfensberger's definition of normalization, the role of the provider is to advocate for or change the perception of the individual's social value.

Normalization has also been used to characterize a family's response to the diagnosis of chronic illness in a child, which has been referred to as the *family management style* (Knafl & Deatrick, 1986; Deatrick, Knafl, & Murphy-Moore, 1999).

This characterization describes the processes by which family members construct lives as close to "normal" as possible. The framework examines family life within the context of the illness to strengthen family attributes that will contribute to positive outcomes for all family members across the life span (Knafl & Deatrick, 2003). The attributes of normalization were first defined in 1986 and revised in 1999 by Knafl and Deatrick to include the following (Knafl & Deatrick, 2002, p. 49):

1. Acknowledging the condition and its potential threat to lifestyle

2. Adopting an interpretative lens that serves to reconstruct the reality of the child and family and engaging in parenting behaviors and family routines consistent with this interpretative lens

3. Engaging in parenting behaviors and family routines that are consistent with normalization

4. Developing treatment regimens that are consistent with normalcy

5. Interpreting with others based on a view of the child and family as normal

The outcome of normalization is managing illness-related demands in a way that sustains usual patterns of family and child functioning.

Another definition of normalization is delineated for children with chronic conditions, such as those growing up with congenital conditions wherein disability is considered as a different life experience. In this view, normalization refers to the acceptance of reality as a way of preventing the disability from dominating the life experience as "deficit-oriented" (Van Staa, Jedelooa, Latour, & Trappenburg, 2008). Although Knafl and Deatrick (2002) conceptualized normalcy as a contextual phenomeon, Van Staa et al. (2008) examined normalcy from the perspective of the individual. Their definition is characterized by the perspective "I am like everyone else; my illness is something else" (Van Staa et al., p. S103). Rather than a family management perspective, their definition of normalization is an adaptation strategy.

SYSTEMS OF CARE FRAMEWORKS

Two types of systems of care frameworks are discussed in this section: inclusion and the medical home model.

Inclusion

An important part of disability history involves inclusion as a guiding principle of care. Since the Rehabilitation Act of 1973 (PL 93-112) was passed by Congress, inclusion has gained increasing attention, particularly as it relates to education. The Rehabilitation Act of 1973 was also supported by federal mandates passed over the years, starting with the Education for All Handicapped Child Act of 1975 (PL 94-142) through the passing of the Individuals with Disabilities Education Improvement Act of 2004 (PL 108-446).

Theoretical arguments for inclusion are rooted in the fostering of social skills for people with IDD. Inclusion also provides unintended benefits for individuals without disabilities, such as greater awareness of differences and social membership. The goals of inclusion are community membership, integrated education, and social acceptance (Downing & Peckham-Hardin, 2007).

Medical Home Model

The most common recommendations by the American Academy of Pediatrics (AAP) for best practices regarding the primary health care of CSHCN are those identified in the AAP's policy statement on the medical home. In the AAP definition, "a *medical home* is defined as primary care that is accessible, continuous, comprehensive, family-centered, coordinated, compassionate, and culturally effective" (AAP, 2007). Cooley and McAllister (2004) highlighted the motivation to be improved quality of life for both the child and family. Guidance for the implementation of a medical home model has been made available by the AAP (see http://www.medicalhome info.org). Several studies (e.g., Starfield & Shi, 2004; Strickland et al., 2004) have demonstrated that the medical home model has positive outcomes for children.

Likewise, research findings suggest that the medical home model benefits disability care coordination organizations (DCCO) for adult consumers with disabilities. DCCOs are community nursing organizations that are based on a philosophy of care that is similar in part to the medical home model, but extends to include a social service–nursing partnership to ensure continuity of care across the life span (adolescence to elderly). These programs are designed primarily for Medicaid beneficiaries with disabilities and have produced outcomes similar to those of the medical home model, including improved access to care and increased quality of life in a cost-effective way (Palsbo, Mastal, & O'Donnell, 2006).

HOLISTIC FRAMEWORKS

The hallmark philosophy of holism is often cited as a fundamental difference between the provision of nursing care and medical care, in which the provision of care is centered around the client's physical condition rather than individual needs. Holistic care is also different from lifestage-specific models of care because it does not focus on the achievement of tasks such as autonomy or ego identity (Harder, 2002). The holistic frameworks of family-centered care and youth-centered care are discussed in this section.

Family-Centered Care

Family-centered care is an approach to the planning, delivery, and evaluation of health care; its cornerstone is active participation between families and professionals. Family-centered care helps support the family's relationship with the child's health care providers and recognizes the importance of the family's customs and values in the child's care. The vision of family-centered care was first proposed in 1960, relating to the field of maternity nursing, and it continues to evolve and be relevant today (Dokken & Ahmann, 2006). The essential element of family-centered care requires that the family and the provider partner together to meet the needs of the child. The hallmark of the partnership is a therapeutic relationship that fosters mutual goal setting and systematic planning to meet family needs. Simply stated, when care is truly family-centered, the provider

- Spends enough time with the family
- Listens carefully to the parent
- Makes the parent feel like a partner in the child's care

- Is sensitive to the family's values and customs
- Provides the specific information that the parent needs (Luciano, 1972, p. 41)

To ensure quality outcomes using a family-centered care approach, the following six core outcomes have been identified (Maternal Child Health Bureau, n.d.):

1. All children with special health care needs receive coordinated ongoing comprehensive care within a medical home.
2. All families of children with special health care needs have adequate private and/or public insurance to pay for the services they need.
3. All children are screened early and continuously for special health care needs.
4. Services for children with special health care needs and their families are organized in ways that families can use them easily.
5. Families of children with special health care needs are partners in decision making at all levels and are satisfied with the services they receive.
6. All youth with special health care needs receive the services necessary to make appropriate transitions to adult health care, work, and independence.

The Society of Pediatric Nurses (SPN) has also played a major role in the evolution of family-centered care concept. In 2003, Linda Lewandowski, then President of SPN, published *A Guide to Family-Centered Care* with the American Nurses Association (Lewandowski & Tesler, 2003), which proposed eight evidence-based elements of family-centered care:

1. Family at the center
2. Family-professional collaboration
3. Family-professional communication
4. Diversity of families
5. Coping differences and support
6. Family-centered peer support
7. Specialized service and support systems
8. Holistic perspective of family-centered care (Curry, 2008, p. 1)

This guide was used to shape the AAP's policy statement on family-centered care and the pediatrician's role (AAP, 2003) and the SPN's *Position Statement on Family-Centered Care Content in the Nursing Curriculum* (Curry, 2008, p. 1).

Youth-Centered Care

A subset of family-centered care and one endorsed by self-advocacy theory is the use of youth-centered care. Kids as Self Advocates, a national grassroots coalition of youth with disabilities advocating for youth, funded in part by MCHB and Administration on Developmental Disabilities, calls for youth-centered care characterized by information that can be understood by all people with disabilities, including youth (Kids as Self Advocates, n.d.).

OTHER, NEWER, SELECTED FRAMEWORKS

While systems of care frameworks, social norms frameworks, and, to a lesser degree, holistic models of care frameworks, are well documented in literature and supported by outcomes evaluation, there are newer models of care that continue to be developed and tested. Both interdisciplinary services and holistic patient-centered care models are supported by the Institute of Medicine as promising practices for improving patient outcomes (Greiner & Knebel, 2003). This section discusses these promising models, as well as an ecological model of care that supports lifestage development.

Interdisciplinary Services

The cornerstone of interdisciplinary services is collaboration among and between professionals, the family, and the child to ensure that individualized supports and services are identified and provided to support the child's special health care needs. The successful interdisciplinary team will consider the child from a biopsychosocial perspective. Communication and problem solving are based upon a broadening of professional perspectives using assessment tools and measures across disciplines rather than those that are discipline specific. As discussed in Chapter 1, interdisciplinary services were initiated during President John F. Kennedy's administration with the development of the University Affiliated Programs (now known as the University Centers for Excellence in Developmental Disabilities), which were designed originally to provide interdisciplinary services to individuals with mental retardation. Since then, the MCHB has funded interdisciplinary training programs for more than 30 years.

In 1996, the Institute of Medicine launched an initiative called Crossing the Quality Chasm to improve the quality of the nation's health care system. Central to this effort were recommendations on preparing the public in support of an interdisciplinary workforce. As recognized in the report (Committee on Quality of Health Care in America, Institute of Medicine, 2001), one of the barriers to quality care outcomes for CSHCN (e.g., resource utilization, quality of life, care coordination, clinical, financial outcomes) is poorly integrated services, particularly for children with complex needs. Care derived from an interdisciplinary perspective is characterized by integration and synthesis of information from numerous disciplines. It contributes to quality care by creating a model of care that is more comprehensive in nature and addresses the biopsychosocial needs of the child and family.

Interdisciplinary care has been linked to improved clinical outcomes as measured by decreased hospitalizations, emergency department use, and complications. Unfortunately, this interdisciplinary care is often only delivered in specialty clinics within tertiary care centers, which typically are not accessible to the majority of families. In addition, the primary care physician may be excluded from these teams, thus leaving primary care needs largely unmet (Sadof & Nazarian, 2007).

Holistic Patient–Centered Care

One model of holistic care focused on the total patient is the patient-centered care model (sometimes also referred to as the person-centered care model). The patient-centered care model is an integrated model that incorporates all aspects of the individual's mind, body, and spirit, requiring both an interactive and interpersonal relationship with the child and family (Romeo, 2000). For example, it emphasizes the role of the provider in manipulating the environment using music, sensory, or kinesthetic modalities to achieve patient outcomes. The model is based upon the nursing philosophy that the central concern of nurses is caring and heal-ing the child and family using a family-centered care approach (Dorn, 2004).

Lifestage–Specific Models of Care

Lifestage-specific models of care focus on the achievement of specific developmen-tal tasks as outcomes of care. This type of model offers support to the child or ado-lescent with special health care needs to meet specific developmental tasks. For example, the identity-focused cultural ecological intervention model (Youngblood & Spencer, 2002) is an ecological model that describes supports necessary for stu-dents to successfully achieve normative developmental milestones, such as iden-tity formation. The major concepts of this framework involve assessment of the adolescent based on

1. Special risk factors

2. Net effects of supports versus experienced stressors

3. Reactive coping strategies employed

4. Emergent identities manifested (Youngblood & Spencer, 2002, p. 96)

The framework suggests that a positive outcome for a child with special health care needs is successful transition through developmental phases. For example, an emergent identity that would signify successful transition would be an evolving sense of self. Applied specifically to educational processes, the model is similar to the self-advocacy and self-determinism models. However, an important compo-nent of this model is the adolescent's perspective. Based on the adolescent's per-spective of concepts identified above, maximizing "fit" between students' perspec-tives, resources, and desired outcomes increases the likelihood of achieving success (Youngblood & Spencer, 2002).

CONCLUSION

The goal of this chapter was to provide nurses caring for individuals with IDD knowledge that will enable them to frame their care to ensure quality patient out-comes. A theoretical model should provide a lens with which a perspective can be viewed. Nurses often adopt a perspective that is consistent with their philosophy of caring. The frameworks of social norms, systems of care, and holistic models of care were discussed. Newer frameworks, such as interdisciplinary services, holis-tic patient-centered care models, and lifestage-specific models of care, were also discussed. Nurses are encouraged to reflect on their personal philosophy of care and reconcile this with proposed models of care.

REFERENCES

Alliance for Self Determination. (2009). *Alliance for self determination*. Retrieved on June 28, 2009, from http://alliancefor selfdetermination.com.

American Academy of Pediatrics. (2003). Organizational principles to guide and define the child health care system and/or improve the health of all children. *Pediatrics, 112*, 1545–1547.

American Academy of Pediatrics. (2007). *Children's health topics: Medical home*. Retrieved on November 8, 2008, from http://www.aap.org/healthtopics/medicalhome.cfm.

Bjorck-Akesson, E., Granlund, M., & Simeonsson, R.J. (2000). Assessment philosophies and practices in Sweden. In Guralnick, M.J. (Ed.), *Interdisciplinary clinical assessment of young children with developmental disabilities* (pp. 391–411). Baltimore: Paul H. Brookes Publishing Co.

Center for Self-Determination. (2009). *Center for self-determination*. Retrieved on August 10, 2009, from http://www.centerfor self-determination.com.

Centers for Disease Control and Prevention. (n.d.). *Developmental disabilities: Topic home*. Retrieved on January 9, 2009, from http://www.cdc.gov/ncbddd/dd/default.htm.

Committee on Quality of Health Care in America, Institute of Medicine. (2001). *Crossing the quality chasm: A new health system for the 21st century*. Washington, DC: National Academies Press.

Cooley, W.C., & McAllister, J. (2004). Building medical homes: Improvement strategies in primary care for children with special health care needs. *Pediatrics, 113*, 1499–1506.

Curry, J.M. (2008). *Position statement on family-centered care content in the nursing education curriculum*. Retrieved June 28, 2009, from http://www.pedsnurses.org/component/option,com_docman/Itemid,222/task,cat_view/gid,49/.

Deatrick, J., Knafl, K., & Murphy-Moore, C. (1999). Clarifying the concept of normalization. *Image: Journal of Nursing Scholarship, 31*, 209–214.

Dokken, D., & Ahmann, E. (2006). The many roles of family members in "family-centered care"—Part 1. *Pediatric Nursing, 32*, 562–565.

Dorn, S. (2004). Caring-healing inquiry for holistic nursing practice: Model for research and evidence-based practice. *Topics in Advanced Practice Nursing eJournal, 4(4)*.

Downing, J.E., & Peckham-Hardin, K.D. (2007). Inclusive education: What makes a high quality education for students with moderate severe disabilities? *Research & Practice for Persons with Severe Disabilities, 32*, 16–30.

Education for All Handicapped Children Act of 1975, PL 94-142, 20 U.S.C. §§ 1400 *et seq*.

Fawcett, J. (2005). *Contemporary nursing knowledge*. Philadelphia: F.A. Davis.

Greiner, A.C., & Knebel, E. (Eds.). (2003). *Health professions education: A bridge to quality*. Washington, DC: National Academies Press.

Guyatt, G.H. (1997). Measuring health-related quality of life: General issues. *Canadian Respiratory Journal, 4*, 123–130.

Harder, A.F. (2002). *The developmental stage of Erik Erikson*. Retrieved on January 9, 2009, from http://www.learningplaceon line.com/stages/organize/Erikson.htm.

Individuals with Disabilities Education Improvement Act of 2004, PL 108-446, 20 U.S.C. §§ 1400 *et seq*.

Kids as Self Advocates. (n.d.). *KASA: Kids as self advocates, a project of family voice*. Retrieved on January 9, 2009, from http://www.fvkasa.org.

Kling, B. (2000). Assert yourself: Helping students of all ages develop self-advocacy skills. *TEACHING Exceptional Children, 32ii*, 66–70.

Knafl, K., & Deatrick, J. (1986). How families manage chronic conditions: An analysis of the concept of normalization. *Research in Nursing & Health, 9*, 215–222.

Knafl, K., & Deatrick, J. (2002). The challenge of normalization for families of children with chronic conditions. *Pediatric Nursing, 28*, 49–53, 56.

Knafl, K., & Deatrick, J. (2003). Further refinement of the family management style framework. *Journal of Family Nursing, 9*, 232–256.

Lehr, S., & Taylor, S.J. (1986). Self-determination for people with developmental disabilities and autism: Two self-advocates' perspectives. *Focus on Autism and Other Developmental Disabilities, 14,* 133–139.

Lewandowski, L., & Tesler, M.D. (Eds.). (2003). *Family-centered care: Putting it into action: The SPN/ANA guide to family-centered care.* Washington, DC: Society of Pediatric Nurses/American Nurses Association.

Luciano, K.B. (1972). Components of planned family-centered care. *Nursing Clinics of North America, 7,* 41–52.

Maternal Child Health Bureau. (n.d.). *Achieving and measuring success: A national agenda for children with special health care needs.* Retrieved on November 1, 2008, from http://mchb.hrsa.gov/programs/special needs/measuresuccess.htm.

McPherson, M., Arango, P., Fox, H., Lauver, C., McManus, M., Newacheck, P., et al. (1998). A new definition of children with special health care needs. *Pediatrics, 102,* 137–140.

Nirje, B. (1969). The normalization principle and its human management implications. In R. B. Kugel & W. Wolfensberger (Eds.), *Changing patterns in residential services for the mentally retarded* (pp. 179-196). Washington, DC: President's Committee on Mental Retardation.

Palsbo, S.E., Mastal, M.F., & O'Donnell, L.T. (2006). Disability care coordination organizations: Improving health and function in people with disabilities. *Lippincott's Case Management, 11,* 255–264.

Perske, R. (1996). The battle for Richard Lapointe's life. *Mental Retardation, 34,* 323–327.

Perske, R. (2004). Nirje's eight planks. *Mental Retardation, 42,* 147–150.

Rehabilitation Act of 1973, PL 93-112, 29 U.S.C. §§ 701 *et seq.*

Romeo, J. (2000). Comprehensive versus holistic care: Case studies of chronic disease. *Journal of Holistic Nursing, 18,* 352–361.

Sadof, M.D., & Nazarian, B.L. (2007). Caring for children who have special health-care needs. *Pediatrics in Review, 28,* e36–e42.

Shapiro, J. (1993). No pity: People with disabilities forging a new civil rights movement. New York: Random House.

Smith, R.B., Morgan, M., & Davidson, J. (2005). Does the daily choice making of adults with intellectual disability meet the normalisation principle? *Journal of Intellectual & Developmental Disability, 30,* 226–235.

Starfield, B., & Shi, L. (2004). The medical home, access to care, and insurance: A review of evidence. *Pediatrics, 113,* 1493–1498.

Strickland, B., McPherson, M., Weissman, G., van Dyck, P., Huang, Z.J., & Newacheck, P. (2004). Access to the medical home: Results of the National Survey of Children with Special Health Care Needs. *Pediatrics, 113,* 1485–1492.

U.S. Department of Health and Human Services, Health Resources and Services Administration, Maternal and Child Health Bureau. *The National Survey of Children with Special Health Care Needs Chartbook 2005–2006.* Rockville, MD: U.S. Department of Health and Human Services, 2008.

Van Staa, A.L,. Jedeloo, S., Latour, J., & Trappenburg, M. (2008). A normal life with an unhealthy body: Self-identity in adolescents growing up with chronic illness. *Pediatrics, 121,* S103.

Wehmeyer, M.L., & Schwartz, M. (1998). The relationship between self-determination and quality of life for adults with mental retardation. *Education and Training in Mental Retardation and Developmental Disabilities, 33,* 3–12.

Wolfensberger, W. (1983). Social role valorization: A proposed new term for the principle of normalization. *Mental Retardation, 21,* 234–239.

Youngblood, J., & Spencer, M.B. (2002). Integrating normative identity processes and academic support requirements for special needs adolescents: The application of an Identity-focused Cultural Ecological (ICE) Perspective. *Applied Developmental Science, 6,* 95–108.

CHAPTER 3

Systems of Care for Individuals with Intellectual and Developmental Disabilities

Cecily L. Betz

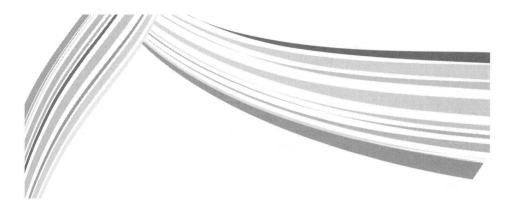

Individuals with intellectual and developmental disabilities (IDD) will require services and supports from a number of agencies throughout their life span. Access to the varied service agencies for individuals with IDD begins at diagnosis with a referral to the early intervention system and support programs for parents. Later, adult referrals will be made to services systems that will enable individuals with IDD to live as independently and productively as fully included members of the community.

This chapter presents information on the range of service agencies that individuals with IDD use across the life span. Content on the systems of care is presented based on a life-span approach beginning with infancy and extending through the senior years. The role of the nurse in facilitating access to these services through care coordination and referral is discussed as well.

INFANTS AND TODDLERS

It is estimated that 4% of infants and toddlers have a disability or developmental delay (U.S. Census Bureau, 2002). Although, other estimates vary upwards from nearly 6% to approximately 13% depending on the methods used to gather the data (Rosenberg, Zhang, & Robinson, 2008; Simpson, Colpe, & Greenspan, 2003). Low enrollment rates and delays in program enrollments have created barriers for infants and toddlers with disabilities and developmental delays who are eligible to receive needed early intervention services (Bailey, Hebbeler, Scarborough, Spiker, & Mallik, 2004; Hebbeler et al., 2007; Rosenberg et al., 2008). It is essential that infants who are diagnosed with a disability, or present with the diagnostic criteria and environmental circumstances considered to be at risk for a disability, are referred promptly to an early intervention program. Children who are referred earlier rather than later for early intervention services have demonstrable better developmental outcomes (Guralnick, 1997).

Early Intervention

Infants with IDD or who are at risk for disabilities are referred to early intervention programs upon discharge from neonatal intensive care units. The purpose of early intervention programs is to provide infants and toddlers from birth to 3 years of age and their families with the services and supports needed to facilitate their acquisition of developmental competencies and milestones. According to the Individuals with Disabilities Education Act (IDEA) of 2004 (PL 108-446), an infant or toddler who is eligible for services

> [Is] a child under the age of 3 years who (a) is experiencing developmental delays in one of more of the areas of cognitive development, physical development, communication development, social or emotional development and adaptive development, or (b) has a diagnosed physical or mental condition that has a high probability of resulting in developmental delay. (Part C, § 632 (5) (A))

In addition, some states, such as California, provide early intervention services to children who are considered to be at risk for IDD.

A child's eligibility for services is determined by an interdisciplinary team of health care professionals that may include occupational and physical therapists, nursing specialists, developmental pediatricians, speech and language specialists, audiologists, and social workers. The composition of the team will be dependent upon the needs of the infant or toddler to be assessed.

After eligibility has been determined, each infant enrolled into an early intervention program receives an individualized family service plan (IFSP) that delineates the services the infant requires based on the infant's and family's needs. The evidence-based services that an infant or toddler may receive under IDEA to prevent additional developmental impairments are specified in the IFSP. These evidence-based services, which are provided in a developmental center of the child's home, include occupational therapy, physical therapy, speech and language services, family support services, psychological counseling, audiology, and assistive technology. Other services include case management and medical diagnostic testing. Early intervention programs also are required to provide a school readiness component that includes language and preliteracy instruction (Federal Register, 2006).

A child's IFSP includes identification of outcomes the child is expected to achieve based on the plan of care. The IFSP is evaluated by the early intervention team on an annual basis to monitor and evaluate the child's achievement of expected results. In anticipation of the child's transition into a preschool program, a transition plan is developed as a means of facilitating a smooth transfer (Federal Register, 2006).

Title V Programs for Children with Special Health Care Needs

The Title V Programs for Children with Special Health Care Needs (CSHCN) are publicly funded programs for low-income children and youth who need specialized services from an interdisciplinary team of health care members to address their comprehensive needs for services. Eligibility criteria vary from state to state, but the federal definition of CSHCN includes "children who have, or are at increased risk for, chronic physical, developmental, behavioral, or emotional conditions and who also require health and related services of a type or amount beyond that required by children generally" (McPherson et al., 1998, p. 138). Depending upon state eligibility guidelines, the upper age limit for the programs varies from 18 to 21 years.

Services provided to CSHCN include:

1. Diagnostic evaluations

2. Treatment services that include medical services, inpatient hospitalization, case management services, diagnostic and laboratory tests, durable equipment, among others

3. Long-term occupational and physical therapy, nursing, and social work services (Health Resources and Services Administration, n.d.)

State Child Health Insurance Program

The State Child Health Insurance Program (SCHIP) is a jointly funded health insurance program by the federal and state governments for eligible children. Although the eligibility rules vary according to each state, the basic guidelines are designed to provide insurance coverage for children and youth up to 19 years of age whose family income exceeds the limits of income eligibility for the Medicaid program. Children are eligible for the SCHIP if they are uninsured and their families' income is less than $32,500 per year (for a family of four). The basic benefit plan includes coverage for pediatric care including immunizations, hospitalizations, and emergency room visits. Other services covered by many states are dental and vision care and medical equipment (Insure Kids Now!, n.d.).

Medicaid Program

The Medicaid program is a federally funded health insurance program for three categories of beneficiaries:

1. Categorically needy

2. Medically needy

3. Special groups

These categories of beneficiaries include both children and adults. Eligible groups of children and families per beneficiary categories are listed in Table 3.1. The services available for eligible children are inpatient hospitalizations, outpatient services, physician/nurse practitioner services, durable equipment, early and periodic screening, diagnosis and treatment (EPSDT), and laboratory and diagnostic tests (Centers for Medicaid and Medicare Services, 2005).

The EPSDT service offers preventive and comprehensive care, including screening services, for children and youth younger than 21 years. Health screen-

Table 3.1.   Categories of Medicaid beneficiaries

Category	Benefits
Categorically needy	Families eligible for Aid to Families with Dependent Children
	Pregnant women whose income is at and below 133% the federal poverty level and their children younger than 6 years of age
	Children between the ages of 6 and 19 years of age whose family income is up to 100% of federal poverty level
	Relatives or legal guardians who care for children younger than 18 years of age (19 years if high school student)
	Supplemental Security Income (SSI) beneficiary
	Individuals in institutional placements with monthly income at 300% of SSI income guidelines
Medically needy (varies by state)	Full-time students younger than age limits (between 19 and 21 years of age)
	Relative or legal guardians who care for children younger than 18 years of age (19 years if high school student)
	Blind individuals
	Individuals who meet SSI criteria for disability
	Individuals age 65 years and older
Special groups	Qualified Medicare beneficiaries whose income is 100% of federal poverty level and have resources at or less than SSI standards
	Qualified working individuals with disabilities whose income is 200% of federal poverty level and have resources not more than twice than SSI standards
	Working individuals with disabilities whose income and resources are not qualifying for SSI benefits

Source: Centers for Medicare and Medicaid Services (2005).

ing services offered are physical, developmental and mental health assessments; diagnostic and laboratory testing including screening for lead toxicity (for suspected children only); immunizations; health education; vision and hearing services; dental services; and other services for conditions diagnosed during EPSDT screenings.

SCHOOL-AGE CHILDREN

Most children with IDD will be enrolled in special education programs to receive the services, supports, and accommodations needed to learn in school. Each child in special education will have an individualized education program (IEP) developed based upon the identification of their needs during the planning process by a team of educational specialists. The IEP is developed every 3 years by the IEP team and evaluated on an annual basis. Members of the IEP team include the educational and related services personnel who will be responsible for implementing it and the parents. School-age children may or may not be part of the IEP team depending on the preferences of the child. Members will attend an IEP meeting to finalize the plan that will provide the basis for educational services for the next 3 years.

The range of services includes those that assist the child academically, such as supplemental assistance for reading, writing, and math. The child's needs for academic support may include the need for a one-on-one school aide who assists the student with note taking and mobility on the school campus. Students may require the assistance of related services personnel, such as a school nurse or health aide to perform medically related procedures at school (e.g., catheterization, gastrostomy feedings, administration of medications). Other related services made available to students with IDD include physical therapy and occupational therapy, audiology, speech and language, and nutrition services. Life skills and social skills training and transportation services to and from school—and in some cases, to after-school programs—may be included in the student's IEP (Betz, 2007; Betz & Sowden, 2007; Federal Register, 2006).

After-school and recreational programs offer students with IDD the opportunities to learn important social and recreational skills. Very often, as the research has demonstrated, students with IDD have few friendships with peers outside of school, as well as limited recreational interests or pursuits (Bauminger et al., 2008; Johnson, 2009; Parkes et al., 2008). After-school programs provide supervised activities to assist students with IDD in developing these important extracurricular skills that support children in learning to become more independent, self-reliant, and productive. Through these programs, children learn in supportive settings how to interact appropriately with others by recognizing social cues, such as facial expressions indicating emotion; rules of conduct, such as responding appropriately to the statements made by peers; listening attentively to others; learning to appropriately share information about themselves to others; and engaging in prosocial behaviors. In addition, students learn to develop recreational interests and pursuits that bring pleasure, generate new interests, and develop additional skills and knowledge.

ADOLESCENTS AND YOUNG ADULTS

The adolescent and young adult period represent a dramatic shift in the philosophy, purpose, and type of services provided. Whereas services from birth to school-age years were provided based on a family-centered approach acknowledging the dependency and developmental competency skill-building needs of the children served, services for adolescents and young adults are predicated on fostering the independence, autonomy, and self-sufficiency needed for approaching adulthood. As such, preparation for the transition to adulthood is focused on ensuring the adolescent and young adult are referred to the adult system of health care and prepared for postsecondary education, vocational programs, and job training programs. This section presents information on these service systems.

Health Care

This is a critical time for youth and young adults whose eligibility for pediatric health insurance plans is about to terminate, whether the individual is enrolled in public or private health insurance plan options. All youth who are enrolled in public health insurance programs—whether it be Title V Programs for CSHCN, SCHIP, or Medicaid—need to confer with program staff or the service coordinator of their specialized health care team to plan their transition to an adult health insurance plan to receive health care services. Depending on the state, the age of eligibility termination occurs between 18 and 21 years of age for Title V Programs for CSHCN. For SCHIP, eligibility terminates at 19 years of age. Redetermination for Medicaid services is conducted at 18 years of age (Health Resources and Services Administration, n.d.; 2000; Insure Kids Now!, n.d.).

For those youth and young adults who want to explore public health insurance options, income and disability eligibility is necessary. Income eligibility is assessed based upon the income and asset resources of the individual with IDD.

For youth with private health insurance, the process for transfer from pediatric to adult health care providers may be different, particularly if the student plans to enroll in a 2- or 4-year college or university. Students who are covered by private insurance are likely covered as a dependent on a parent's health insurance plan. Students with IDD who are full-time college students, dependent on their parents' resources, and not married often can continue to be covered by their parents' health insurance plan until 23 or sometimes 25 years of age. An option following termination from the parents' policy is to enroll in the Consolidated Omnibus Reconciliation Bill Act (COBRA; United States Department of Labor, 2008a) program, which requires the beneficiary to pay for the full cost of the insurance premium. An additional 29 months of insurance coverage is available through COBRA. The challenge of COBRA is the expense of the program; the cost of paying health insurance premiums is high, sometimes amounting to more than $1,000 per month.

Employment Resources for Youth and Young Adults

Important employment resources to introduce youth with IDD to the world of work are vocational rehabilitation (VR), the Workforce Investment Agencies (WIA) youth programs, Job Corps, and Americorps. These programs offer job training opportunities for youth to explore career interests, have supervised work-based experiences, learn job skills, acquire interpersonal skills needed to interact appropriately in employment settings, and learn work-related codes of conduct.

VR services are available to eligible youth with IDD in high school settings beginning at age 16. The VR services for youth include career assessment, job training and placement, job skills training, and payment for work-related supplies and equipment such as uniforms, safety glasses, tools, and computer equipment. VR rehabilitation specialists can be contacted through the high school setting and be invited by the student and/or parent (as stated in IDEA) to attend the youth's IEP and participate as a member of the IEP team. As a member of the IEP team, the rehabilitation specialist can respond to the youth's need for employment opportunities by providing recommendations based on the youth's career interests, needs, and preferences as identified during the IEP planning process. VR services for adults are discussed later in the chapter (Betz, 2007; Betz & Nehring, 2007; Rehabilitation Services Agency [RSA], 2006).

WIA youth programs are offered throughout the year. Comprehensive services are offered to youth to obtain employment experience, develop job skills, learn interpersonal skills needed for work environments, complete requirements needed for high school graduation or a general equivalency diploma (GED), and function in a developmentally appropriate manner. The available work-related services include paid and unpaid work experience, skill training, summer employment jobs, and payment for the expenses of work uniforms and supplies. The educational services that can be provided to youth are tutoring, classroom instruction, and alternative high school instruction to obtain the GED. Supportive services to assist students in acquiring social skills are counseling and guidance, leadership training, linkage to an adult mentor, and 12-month follow-up services after exit from the program (National Collaborative on Workforce and Disability, 2002, 2005).

WIA services are available for high-risk and low-income eligible youth, including youth with IDD. WIA youth programs are required to provide WIA services to at least 10% of youth with disabilities, including youth with IDD. Income eligibility is not required, as youth with disabilities are considered eligible based on their disability status and not parental income. Anyone can make a referral; self-referral is acceptable as well. WIA programs are located in communities across the United States. WIA program locations can be found in the community services section of the yellow pages or via the Internet (National Collaborative on Workforce and Disability, 2002, 2005).

Job Corps

The Job Corps is a vocational training program for eligible low-income 16- to 24-year-old adolescents and young adults. This program provides training in the occupational fields of electronics, surveying, welding, carpentry, culinary arts, landscaping, construction, facilities management, and clerical services. Other program benefits for participants are health insurance coverage, living accommodations on the program campus, monthly allowance, and assistance with obtaining a GED. Following completion of the program, career counseling and follow-up services are offered for 12 months. Additional information on the Job Corps program can be accessed at www.jobcorps.org (United States Department of Labor, 2008b).

Americorps

Americorps, known as the "domestic version of the Peace Corps," was established during the President William Clinton's administration. It is a federally supported community service program providing tutorial services, literacy training, and mentorship programs for at-risk groups of children and adults. This service program is designed for eligible young adult volunteers, ages 18–24, including youth with disabilities. In exchange for 10 months and 1,700 hours of community service, the volunteer receives a living allowance, living accommodations (depending on program), health insurance, training, and a $4,275 education award to help pay for college or vocational training. Additional information can be accessed at www.americorps.org (Americorps, 2008).

Income Assistance

The Social Security Administration (SSA) has two disability programs that provide income assistance to individuals with disabilities, including IDD: Supplemental Security Income (SSI), wherein low-income beneficiaries receive assistance if they have a disability; and Social Security Disability Insurance (SSDI), which provides benefits to previously employed individuals with disabilities who have paid Social Security taxes. Children are more likely to be enrolled in SSI than SSDI if they are under the age of 18 years. The SSI eligibility criteria are

1. The child must be under 18 years of age (or 22 years if attending school).

2. The child has medically verifiable physical/mental condition(s) resulting in marked and severe functional limitations.

3. The condition is expected to last at least 1 year or result in death.

Enrollment in the adult SSI program requires an eligibility determination process discussed later in the chapter (SSA, 2007).

In the past, outdated SSA regulations were considered to be a disincentive to work because the individual risked losing health insurance coverage if not enrolled in the SSI program. SSA has made substantial progress in developing work incentive programs to enable an individual to both work and collect SSI income supplementation with the recognition that the transition to work is fraught with challenges for individuals with disabilities, including IDD. A summary of the work incentive programs is listed in Table 3.2.

Postsecondary Education

Today, there are many more opportunities for students with IDD to enroll in postsecondary programs. New programs enable students with IDD to enroll in 4-year colleges and/or universities based upon the philosophical belief that these students should be as fully included in 4-year university programs as they are in secondary programs. This postsecondary trend is in the seminal stages of development; it is anticipated that as time progresses many more students with IDD will be enrolled in inclusive 4-year university/college classes and programs (Hart, Grigal, Sax, Martinez, & Will, 2006).

An important resource for students with IDD on all postsecondary campuses, 2-year community colleges, and 4-year colleges and universities are disability support services (DSS). This campus resource provides students with IDD with an array of supports, services, and accommodations (as documented in the 504 Plan) needed to participate and learn in these academic environments.

The type of services and resources available for students include priority registration, which enables the scheduling of classes at times or in locations that are accommodating to the student's needs. For example, a student with cerebral palsy may benefit from having classes scheduled together in the morning to accommodate for limited energy levels and in close proximity to accommodate the limitations imposed by mobility challenges. Accommodations for classroom learning include the use of interpreters, signers, and notetakers, as well as modifications with course assignments and testing (e.g., longer periods of time for test taking; writing a paper rather than giving an oral presentation). Other services that may be offered are housing assistance, peer support programs, mobility assistance to travel about the campus, and disability parking permits (Getzel & Wehman, 2005; University of Washington, 2007).

There is variability in the range of services offered by DSS on different college campuses. It is essential that prospective students include DSS as part of their exploration process in determining their choice for attendance. Choice of college program may be predicated in part by the provided DSS services and programs for students with IDD.

Students with verifiable disabilities are eligible for DSS. Verification of a disability by a licensed professional is necessary. Some Section 504 plans that specify academic accommodations needed to learn (e.g., notetakers) developed in secondary school settings may not be transferable to postsecondary settings; administrators may require the development of a new Section 504 plan (Betz & Nehring, 2007).

Table 3.2.   Employment supports programs provided by the Social Security Administration (SSA)

Program	Requirements
Student Earned Income Exclusion	Enrolled in grades 7–12 for a minimum of 12 hours a week
	Enrolled in college or university for a minimum of 8 hours per week
	Enrolled in a vocational or technical training program for minimum of 12 hours per week (15 hours if practicum included)
	Less than 22 years of age
	Exceptions made for students who require in home training/education
	Can earn up to $1,550 per month but not more than $6,240 per year (2008 figures) and still receive same level of SSI monthly benefits
	Level of monthly and annual income is not counted against SSI benefits
Earned Income Exclusion	First $65 of earned income is not counted against SSI benefit
	Over $65 of earned income, the SSI benefit is reduced $1 for every $2 earned income
	$20 general income exclusion is applied for individuals who have unearned income
Impairment-Related Work Expenses	Disability-related supplies and expenses needed for work and daily living can be deducted from earned gross income
	Deductible expenses include medical equipment (i.e., wheelchair, respirator), medical supplies, safety equipment, van modifications, mileage to and from work, attendant care in the work setting or to prepare for work, prosthesis
	Amount of SSI income the beneficiary receives is based on deducting impairment-related expenses from earned income
Plan for Achieving Self-Support (PASS)	Used to develop a time-limited plan to save income to achieve career or occupational goal
	Examples of income savings to achieve career or occupational goal: major equipment purchase, start a business, and fund career or vocational training
	Income set aside for PASS plan not calculated in determining SSI payment
Ticket to Work	Designed to give beneficiary choice in the selection of employment service provider
	Beneficiary receives "ticket" enabling the individual to obtain employment services and support from provider of their choice—either the state Vocational Rehabilitation agency or Network Employment–approved provider
1619A	Beneficiary can continue to collect SSI benefits while earning at the substantial gainful activity (SGA)
	SSI benefit will decrease as earned income increases
1619B	Beneficiary can continue to receive Medicaid benefits while income exceeds SGA
	Requires Medicaid benefits to continue working

Source: Social Security Administration (n.d.).

ADULTS

Adulthood is a period of significant personal and community changes as the social structures associated with childhood and adolescence such as school, community programs, and child-oriented, publicly-funded programs are no longer available. The organization of adult services is considerably different from those for children and youth as they are not conveniently located in one setting (Betz, 2007; Betz & Nehring, 2007; RSA, 2006). The adult, unless the individual has a conservator, will be expected to behave more independently and to make their own decisions about services that meet their needs. This section will provide an overview of employment, community living, health services, and income support and housing programs available for adults.

Employment

A number of employment options are available for adults with IDD, including VR, WIA, and employment agencies that provide job placement and job training services to prospective workers. WIA and VR have similar yet different employment programs and services available for adults compared to those previously described for youth (National Collaborative on Workforce and Disability, 2002, 2005; RSA, 2006; Workforce Development Act of 1998 [PL 105-220]).

Adults interested in obtaining VR services can apply directly at the local VR office or by mail or fax. VR is required to notify the consumer of eligibility status within 60 days of application submission. If VR services are over capacity, then the prospective beneficiary is put on a waitlist until services are available. During the interim period, while eligibility is being determined, the applicant can access a limited number of VR agency services, such as using the VR databases to search for a job.

Once eligibility has been determined, then an individualized plan for employment (IPE) is formulated by the rehabilitation specialist with the consumer. The IPE specifies the blueprint for determining what services, programs, supplies, and equipment the beneficiary will need to obtain their employment goal. The goal of any IPE is the acquisition of employment. The IPE may specify the need for vocational training, enrollment in a college program, purchase of equipment and supplies needed for the job, assistance with finding a job, and the provision of on-the-job training or job coaches (Betz, 2007; Betz & Nehring, 2007; RSA, 2006).

Community Living

Throughout the country, there are networks of federally funded agencies and independent living centers (ILCs) whose purpose is to assist individuals with disabilities to live independently as productive members of the community. ILCs are grassroots organizations that are managed and staffed by individuals with disabilities. Each ILC will vary in terms of the services offered, as these organizations are dependent on extramural funding for program development and/or research. For example, an ILC may offer a job training program in computer programming that is funded by a private foundation and not available at other ILCs (RSA, 2007).

The core services offered by ILCs are

1. Advocacy and legislative monitoring to inform clients of current and pending legislation that may have direct impact on their lives

2. Housing services to assist consumers to locate affordable housing

3. A registry listing of attendants who have been screened as competent to provide in-home services to individuals with disabilities, as well as referral services enabling consumers to interview and hire individuals for attendant care

4. Clearinghouse services to provide disability-related information about and referrals to community-based agencies

5. Peer counseling services for consumers by ILC counselors who have disabilities themselves on a wide range of topics of personal concern related to employment (RSA, 2007)

Supplemental Security Income

The SSI program is an income assistance program for eligible low-income adults with disabilities. All beneficiaries who are enrolled in the program receive monthly income assistance of cash. The funds are designed to assist the unemployed person with a disability with the monthly living expenses as incurred for rent, food, transportation, and household necessities. Disability eligibility will be determined by the local disability determination services (DDS) office, a nationwide system of agencies contracted by the SSA to ascertain the eligibility of individuals with IDD. DDS conducts a paper review of the individual's eligibility for SSI using adult enrollment criteria. Youth and young adults who are deemed eligible for SSI are automatically considered eligible for Medicaid. SSI eligibility determination for adults is of a higher standard than for children. All children who receive SSI and reach 18 years of age, or age 22 if still in school, must be redetermined for eligibility for the adult program (SSA, 2007).

More recently, SSI initiatives have been instituted to assist individuals in making the transition from SSI to employment (see Table 3.2). In the past, individuals who received SSI were hesitant to disenroll from the program for fear of losing their health insurance.

U.S. Department of Housing and Urban Development

The federal government provides housing assistance to low-income individuals and families. This program is known as Section 8 housing. Through this subsidy program, eligible beneficiaries, including individuals with IDD, pay no more than 30% of their income for rent. The remaining portion of the rental costs are paid by the U.S. Department of Housing and Urban Development (HUD) to the apartment owner according to the fair market rent cap. Beneficiaries may choose to rent an apartment in a government-subsidized apartment project or use the voucher to rent an apartment in the private sector. The demand for housing by eligible low-income individuals far exceeds the available supply, sometimes resulting in prolonged waiting periods of upward to 5 years. Individuals with disabilities receive preferential treatment for their waiting periods for housing, although the waiting period still may be 1 year or more (HUD, 2006).

Medicaid

As Table 3.1 indicates, there are several categories of Medicaid eligibility for low-income individuals, including those with IDD. In addition to the package of services available for children described above, home health care services and skilled nursing facilities admissions are available for individuals 21 years and older (Centers for Medicare and Medicaid Services, 2005).

Medicare Program

Medicare is a federal health insurance program for individuals 65 years and older, individuals enrolled in SSDI, and individuals that have end-stage renal disease. Senior citizens are eligible for Medicare parts A (hospitalization), B (medical care), and C (medications).There are no eligibility requirements for parts A and B, but eligibility for part C is dependent on the individual's annual expenditures for medications (Centers for Medicare and Medicaid Services, 2005).

CONCLUSION

This chapter has presented content on the systems of care that individuals with IDD would likely utilize across their life span. It is important for nurses who provide care to individuals with IDD to be knowledgeable about available services from the various systems of care. Quality of life for individuals with IDD will be enhanced by having access to systems whose services and supports promote achievement of developmental competencies thus enabling them to function more independently and live inclusively in the community.

REFERENCES

Americorps. (2008). *Americorps*. Retrieved on July 8, 2008, from http://www.americorps.org.

Bailey, D.B., Hebbler, K., Scarborough, A., Spiker, D., & Mallik, S. (2004). First experiences with early intervention: A national perspective [electronic versions]. *Pediatrics, 113*, 887–896.

Bauminger, N., Solomon, M., Aviezer, A., Heung, K., Gazit, L., Brown, J., et al. (2008). Children with autism and their friends: A multidimensional study of friendship in high-functioning autism spectrum disorder. *Journal of Abnormal Child Psychology, 36*, 135–150.

Betz, C.L. (2007). Facilitating the transition of adolescents with developmental disabilities: Nursing practice issues and care. *Journal of Pediatric Nursing, 22*, 103–115.

Betz, C.L., & Nehring, W.M. (2007). *Promoting health care transition planning for adolescents with special health care needs and disabilities*. Baltimore: Paul H. Brookes Publishing Co.

Betz, C.L., & Sowden, L. (2007). *Pediatric nursing reference* (6th ed.). St. Louis: Mosby Elsevier.

Centers for Medicare and Medicaid Services. (2005). *Medicaid-at-a-glance: 2005: A Medicaid information source*. Retrieved on September 17, 2009, from http://www.cms.hhs.gov/MedicaidEligibility/Downloads/MedicaidataGlance05.pdf. Baltimore: Centers for Medicare and Medicaid Services.

Centers for Medicaid and Medicare Services. (2008). *State Children's Health Insurance Program*. Retrieved on July 17, 2008, from http://www.cms.hhs.gov/LowCostHealthInsFamChild/.

Federal Register. (2006). *Assistance to states for the education of children with disabilities and preschool grants for children with disabilities*. Retrieved on July 14, 2008, from http://www.ed.gov/legislation/FedRegister/finrule/2006-3/081406a.html.

Getzel, E.E., & Wehman, P. (Eds.). (2005). *Going to College: Expanding opportunities for people with disabilities*. Baltimore: Paul H. Brookes Publishing Co.

Guralnick, M.J. (Ed.). (1997). *The effectiveness of early intervention*. Baltimore: Paul H. Brookes Publishing Co.

Hart, D., Grigal, M., Sax, C., Martinez, D., & Will, M. (2006). Postsecondary education options for students with intellectual disabilities. *Research to Practice, 45*, 1–4.

Health Resources and Services Administration. (n.d.). *Maternal and Child Health Services Title V Block Grant*. Retrieved on July 1, 2008, from http://mchb.hrsa.gov/programs/.

Health Resources and Services Administration (2000). *Understanding Title V of Social Security Act*. Retrieved on July 1, 2008, from ftp://ftp.hrsa.gov/mchb/titlevtoday/UnderstandingTitleV.pdf.

Hebbeler, K., Spiker, D., Bailey, D., Scarborough, A., Mallik, S. et al. (2007). Early intervention for infants and toddlers with disabilities and their families: Participants, services, and outcomes. Menlo Park, CA: SRI International. Retrieved on June 25, 2009, from http://www.sri.com/neils/pdfs/NEILS_Final_Report_02_07.pdf.

Individuals with Disabilities Education Improvement Act of 2004, PL 108-446, 20 U.S.C. §§ 1400 *et seq.*

Insure Kids Now! (n.d.). *Questions and answers*. Retrieved on July 17, 2008, from http://www.insurekidsnow.gov/.

Johnson, C.C. (2009). The benefits of physical activity for youth with developmental disabilities: A systematic review. *American Journal of Health Promotion, 23*, 157–167.

McPherson, M., Arango, P., Fox, H., Lauver, C., McManus, M., Newacheck, P.W., et al. (1998). A new definition of children with special health care needs. *Pediatrics, 102*, 137–140.

National Collaborative on Workforce and Disability. (2002). *How young people can benefit from one-stops*. Retrieved on July 10, 2008, from http://www.ncwd-youth.info/resources_&_Publications/information_Briefs/issue3.html.

National Collaborative on Workforce and Disability. (2005). *The right connections: Navigating the workforce development system*. Retrieved on July 10, 2008, from http://www.ncwd-youth.info/resources_&_Publications/information_Briefs/issue13.html.

Parkes, J., White-Koning, M., Dickinson, H.O., Thyen, U., Arnaud, C., Beckung, E., et al. (2008). Psychological problems in children with cerebral palsy: A cross-sectional European study. *Journal of Child Psychology & Psychiatry & Allied Disciplines, 49*, 405–413.

Rehabilitation Services Agency. (2006). *Vocational rehabilitation state grants.* Retrieved on July 05, 2008, from http://www.ed.gov/programs/rsabvrs/index.html.

Rehabilitation Services Agency. (2007). *Centers for independent living.* Retrieved on July 5, 2008, from http://www.ed.gov/programs/cil/index.html.

Rosenberg, S.A., Zhang, D., & Robinson, C.C. (2008). Prevalence of developmental delays and participation in early intervention services for young children. [electronic version], *Pediatrics, 121,* e1503–1509.

Simpson, G.A., Colpe, L., & Greenspan, S.I. (2003). Measuring functional developmental delay in infants and young children: Prevalence rates from the NHIS-D. *Paediatric & Perinatal Epidemiology, 17,* 68–80.

Social Security Administration. (n.d.). *Ticket to work.* Retrieved on July 7, 2008, from http://www.yourtickettowork.com/.

Social Security Administration. (2007). *2007 Red Book: A summary guide to employment support for individuals with disabilities under the Social Security Disability Insurance and Supplemental Security Income programs.* Baltimore: Social Security Administration, Office of Disability and Income Security Programs.

U.S. Census Bureau. (2002). *Disability Status of Children Under 15 Years Old.* Survey of Income and Program Participation. Retrieved on June 25, 2009, from http://www.census.gov/hhes/www/disability/sipp/disab02/ds02t7.pdf.

United States Department of Housing and Urban Development. (2006). *Section 8 assistance.* Retrieved on July 10, 2008, from http://www.hud.gov/progdesc/pih indx.cfm.

United States Department of Labor. (2008a). *Health plans and benefits: Continuation of coverage—COBRA.* Retrieved on July 18, 2008, from http://www.dol.gov/dol/topic/health-plans/cobra.htm.

United States Department of Labor. (2008b). *Job Corps.* Retrieved on July 7, 2008, from http://jobcorps.dol.gov/.

University of Washington. (2007). *Disability resources for students.* Retrieved on July 10, 2008, from http://www.washington.edu/students/drs/.

Workforce Development Act of 1998. PL 105-220. 29 U.S.C. §§ 794 *et seq.*

CHAPTER 4

Developmental Transitions for Children with Intellectual and Developmental Disabilities

Prenatal to School-Age Period

Marilyn J. Krajicek and Dalice L. Hertzberg

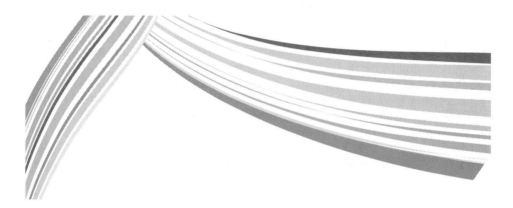

For children with intellectual and developmental disabilities (IDD) and their families, early childhood is a period of challenges and rapid transformation. IDD can result from a variety of causes present at or near birth, including birth defects, prematurity, infection, and trauma. The presence of these conditions may complicate and prevent attainment of early growth and developmental milestones for the child and result in lifelong disability and functional outcomes, such as cognitive deficits, mobility problems, and chronic illness. This chapter discusses the types of developmental transitions that can be achieved from the prenatal to school-age period to facilitate growth and learning in children with IDD.

PRENATAL/PERINATAL PERIOD

Fertilization to implantation represents the most vulnerable period for the potential fetus. This period lasts 5–7 days from the time of the woman's ovulation and fertilization by the male. A prenatal insult at this time usually results in failure of implantation and loss of the pregnancy. During the first few weeks of pregnancy, the fetus is very susceptible to teratogens (environmental substances that alter the developing fetus) because this is the period of most rapid differentiation of cells that form the basis for organs. A prenatal insult during this time often results in congenital malformations with enduring effects. If the malformation is very severe, spontaneous abortion may occur.

Genetic conditions account for about one third of IDDs (Dykens, Hodapp, & Finucane, 2000) and more causative genetic syndromes are identified each year. Genetic syndromes causing IDD are often, but not always, noticeable at or shortly after birth. For example, the typical physical features of Down syndrome are generally recognized very early, whereas Prader-Willi syndrome and fragile X syndrome are not diagnosed until behavioral symptoms emerge in preschool or later. In general, genetic conditions that result in specific physical anomalies are more likely to be identified in the neonatal period. Less common genetic conditions, or those for which a clinical syndrome has not yet been identified, may go undiagnosed for many years. For more information about genetic mechanisms, see Chapter 10.

In the United States, birth defects occur in approximately 3% of all births. Birth defects are conditions affecting the body structure, resulting in long-term health or functional disorders that are present at birth (Bhasin, Brochsin, Avchen, & Braun, 2006). Usually caused by chromosomal abnormalities, birth defects may also be caused by teratogens. Recognition of environmental teratogens is increasing. Lead and other heavy metals, such as mercury, have long been implicated as potent neurotoxins for the fetus and the brain of the young child. More recently, polychlorinated biphenyls (found in striped bass and fresh water fish) and phthalates have been identified as toxins. Phthalates, which are used in plastics, including some baby bottles and water bottles, are potent endocrine disruptors affecting the developing nervous, endocrine, and immune systems. Other substances found in the environment that may be unknowingly ingested during pregnancy include pesticides, fungicides, and herbicides that remain on food or enter the community water supply.

With each of these substances, the timing of the exposure during pregnancy and the size of the dose affect the amount of damage to the fetus. The mother's health is also a factor: Women with poor health or nutrition may be more vulnerable. Chronic exposure to teratogens may be more harmful to the fetus than a single episode. Potentially toxic chemicals are found in the air, water, soil, household cleaning products, and consumer products ranging from carpets to cosmetics and even food and food packaging (Greater Boston Physicians for Social Responsibility, 2000).

The father's age, occupation (i.e., exposure to toxins), and health habits (e.g., smoking) can affect fetal development and the health and mental health of the child into adulthood. A father's occupational exposure to chemicals (e.g., those used in semiconductors) and fumigants (e.g., those used in flour manufacturing) may cause birth problems as disparate as congenital anomalies and low birthweight (Lin, Wang, Hsieh, Chang, & Chen, 2008; Milham & Ossiander, 2008). Older age of fathers has been linked with congenital heart disease, Down syndrome, and other disorders. Younger age of fathers at time of conception has been associated with neural tube defects, although there is less research in this area than in maternal factors (Yang et al., 2007).

Maternal infections, a well-known cause of neural damage in the fetus, are associated with prematurity. Recent studies suggest that the fetal response to perinatal chorioamnionitis, a subclinical infection, in the mother may result in periventricular leukomalacia, a particularly devastating cause of cerebral palsy, as well as an increased risk for bronchopulmonary dysplasia (Bashiri, Burstein, & Mazor, 2006). The TORCH infections (i.e., toxoplasmosis, other [human immunodeficiency virus, syphilis], rubella, cytomegalovirus, and herpes simplex infections) although identified for years, are not yet eradicated. Maternal group B *Streptococcus* infection causes neonatal sepsis, resulting in death or neurologic damage (Gilbert, 2007).

Other maternal factors influencing the fetus include disease or chronic conditions, medications, use of illicit drugs, and nutritional status. Maternal diseases that affect fetal neurological development include type I diabetes, epilepsy, hypertension, thyroid disease, and autoimmune conditions, such as systemic lupus erythmatosis. Maternal obesity has been implicated in increased rates of stillbirth and pregnancy complications. Prescription medications—particularly chemotherapy for cancer, antiepileptic drugs, and some drugs for hypertension—increase the risk of birth anomalies (Davies, 2008).

Family Adaptation

Prenatal screening is initially performed at 14–20 weeks of gestation, when the triple or quadruple screen is performed. Ultrasound may detect nuchal translucency or open spine. These prenatal screening tests are performed routinely on all pregnant women. Prenatal diagnosis is performed when an adverse result comes up on a screening test, such as an elevated alpha-fetoprotein level. Prenatal diagnosis may present a major ethical dilemma for the mother or parents: The decision must be made to continue the pregnancy, terminate, or opt for a prenatal intervention. Women and couples who are opposed to abortion may decline prenatal diagnosis, whereas others may wish additional information to better prepare both emotionally and medically for the birth. Women who are classified as having a high-risk pregnancy due to age (very young or old), history of fetal loss, or a pre-existing medical condition are most likely to undergo the more advanced methods of prenatal diagnosis—amniocentesis or chorionic villus sampling.

Concerns exist among clinicians and families that obstetricians frequently fail to provide unbiased information to prospective parents (Dixon, 2008). Genetic counselors can present families with a realistic picture of the possibilities and encourage families to make their own decisions. Nurses are in a unique position to support families in information seeking and decision making.

Developmental Risks and Concerns

Perinatal causes of IDD (e.g., prematurity, intrauterine growth retardation, hypoxia) are now believed to be a result of prenatal factors (e.g., maternal infections or chronic illness, placental disease, environmental or genetic factors). Although birth asphyxia due to perinatal causes remains a cause of neurodevelopmental disabilities, it is not as common as was previously believed (Keogh & Badawi, 2006). Mechanical or operative delivery, made necessary by threats to the fetus or mother (e.g., deceleration of fetal heartbeat, prolonged labor, infection, or preeclampsia), may cause trauma. Multiple births frequently lead to cesarean section because of the risk of prematurity and fetal distress. Other delivery problems, such as premature separation of the placenta from the uterus, abnormal placement of the placenta, and umbilical cord prolapse, may have their beginnings in prenatal factors such as preeclampsia, collagen vascular diseases, older maternal age, and chorioamnionitis (Gilbert, 2007).

The first task of the newborn infant is to establish independent physiologic function—a complex and challenging process that illness, trauma, and prematurity hamper. Then, the newborn must establish a relationship with a nurturing caregiver. Neurologic and sensory systems (e.g., vision, hearing, smell, taste, alertness) are innately primed to elicit and respond to attention from the mother. The infant's neurologic immaturity combined with limited time for bonding and maternal contact compromise attachment. Frequent medical and nursing interventions further stress the neonate, increasing vulnerability to illness.

For the process of attachment to be successful, the mother—and later the father as well—must be able to correctly interpret the infant's behavior and respond appropriately. Barriers to bonding for the parents include recent loss or bereavement, mental illness, relationship problems, lack of support, or financial stress. Other factors such as prior removal of a child from the home, unwanted pregnancy, extreme immaturity, or poor experiences with one's own parents may require referral to a social worker or mental health professional (Davies & Richards, 2008; Odent, 2008).

For preterm infants, particularly those who are low birth weight or very low birth weight, the developmental tasks of birth are complicated by marked immaturity of all organ systems. This immaturity places the neonate at increased risk for intraventricular hemorrhage, hydrocephalus, neonatal seizures, and infection—all of which are threats to typical development. Immature lungs place the neonate at risk for respiratory distress and long-term pulmonary problems, such as bronchopulmonary dysplasia. Other organ problems commonly occurring in premature infants include necrotizing enterocolitis from ischemia of the intestines, cardiovascular problems from a patent ductus arteriosus or other cardiac anomalies, renal problems, and life-threatening sepsis from a fragile immune system.

The neonatal intensive care unit (NICU) provides lifesaving medical and nursing care for infants who are born prematurely with congenital conditions and/ or birth trauma. While NICU care has saved the lives of many children, enabling infants weighing as little as 800 g to survive, some of these children encounter significant complications that lead to lifelong neurodevelopmental disabilities (Rais-Bahrami & Short, 2004). Premature infants are more likely to experience developmental delays, more frequent infections, require special education, and have more difficulty with work and family relationships (Taylor, Klein, Drotar, Schlucter, & Hack, 2006). The NICU environment provides unique stressors to the premature infant, with continuous bright light, a high level of noise, frequent interruptions for procedures or tests, frequent painful procedures, and reduced opportunity for positive touch and soothing. Parents may not be able to visit frequently, and when they do visit, medical technology may interfere with holding, touching, and other sensory stimuli. The premature infant's physiologic immaturity often interferes with parental bonding, as overstimulation may be poorly tolerated and result in physiologic stress reactions in the neonate. Self-protective behavior exhibited by the premature infant may be interpreted as lack of interest in the parent and lead to withdrawal on the part of the parents. Finally, families may not be emotionally prepared for the stresses of early delivery and an ill newborn.

Family Challenges and Adaptation

Families experiencing a preterm birth, or the birth of a child with congenital anomalies, may be overwhelmed by the barrage of information and the highly technical environment of the NICU. This event represents a crisis for the family; it may result in feelings of guilt for the infant's condition, as well as shock and grief for the loss of the expected child. The family must cope with an event for which they have no prior experience and integrate the significant lifestyle changes necessary to provide the intensive and technical care the premature infant requires. Some families have difficulty adapting and coping; they may withdraw from the infant and the NICU. Very young mothers, single mothers, or families lacking a support system are most likely to have trouble adapting to the demands of a critically ill or premature infant and to caring for the infant at home.

The way in which a distressing diagnosis is presented can significantly influence the family's response to the news and aid them in their subsequent information seeking and coping. The American Academy of Pediatrics recommends the formation of a parent–physician (or provider) partnership, using responsive communication skills to meet the informational and emotional needs of the family. Addressing the family's fears and concerns in a private setting is a critical component of communication (Levetown & Committee on Bioethics, 2008).

Since the 1980s, numerous theories have been promoted to address the response of the family to the birth of a child with lifelong medical needs. The concept of *chronic sorrow* proposes that families go through a period of grieving the expected child and then adapting to the needs of the actual child (Olshansky, 1962). A resurgence of grief may occur when the child fails to achieve specific developmental milestones, such as walking independently or graduating from high school. Although there are many similarities among the ways families adjust to a difficult diagnosis, coping abilities are based on a variety of factors unique to each family: formal and informal networks of support, support within the family, communication within the family, past experiences, ethnicity and culture, and available resources including finances, personal beliefs, and faith (Howland, 2007).

Developmental care in the NICU is carried out primarily by nursing staff but also by other medical staff. Developmental care focuses on minimizing the effects of NICU routines and invasive procedures to promote the optimal development of the premature neonate. Because neurologic development interacts significantly with the environment, recent research suggests that the stressful NICU environment contributes to poorer outcomes in premature infants (Gibbins, Hoath, Coughlin, Gibbins, & Franck, 2008). Family-centered care includes families as team members, intrinsic to the care and development of the child. Nurses are important proponents of family-centered care because they are in the ideal position to teach families how to care for their neonate, to advocate for families, and to enable families to advocate for themselves and their child.

INFANCY: FROM NICU TO HOME

Premature infants are discharged from the NICU when stable. A number of conditions arise from prematurity and cause medical fragility in infancy, such as chronic lung disease or bronchopulmonary dysplasia (BPD), static encephalopathy, seizure disorders, neurosensory disorders (e.g., hearing and vision problems), and feeding problems. Depending on the infant's condition, care after discharge may range from medical monitoring for growth to dependence on medical technology, such as oxygen supplementation, tube feeding, or respiratory ventilator dependence. Parents may need to provide most of this technical care at home. Medically fragile infants are more vulnerable to infections and other complications, and use a disproportionate amount of medical care dollars.

BPD ranges in severity from mild to severe; it is most likely due to arrested pulmonary alveolar development in the lung. Premature infants with very low birth weights develop BPD. Risk factors for BPD include prematurity, chorioamnionitis in utero, maternal smoking, patent ductus arteriosus, and genetic factors (Lavoie, Pham, & Jang, 2008). Infants with BPD require long-term care and monitoring for delays in growth and development and treatment of chronic lung disease. Prevention of lung infection (e.g., respiratory syncytial virus) is critical. Incidence of retinopathy of prematurity, a complication of oxygen therapy, has decreased with better treatment (Capper-Michel, 2004; Taylor et al., 2006).

Intraventricular hemorrhage, most common in infants who weigh less than 1,000 g at birth, is a major cause of long-term neurologic injury. In its most severe form, periventricular leukomalacia may occur, damaging the white matter of the brain around the ventricles and causing cerebral palsy. Infants who require a shunt show lower than normal intellectual scores at age 18–22 months (Adams-Chapman & Stoll, 2007). Hypoxic-ischemic injury occurs when inadequate oxygen limits blood flow to the brain, possibly resulting in seizures or cerebral palsy. Other organ damage to the heart, lungs, and kidneys may result if ischemia is severe.

Feeding problems may result from prematurity and neurologic damage. An immature and poorly coordinated suck-swallow pattern initially necessitates nasogastric tube feedings. Infants who fail to achieve normal oral function need feeding and nutrition support indefinitely. Premature infants may develop dysphagia—the inability to coordinate swallowing and breathing—which requires surgical placement of a gastrostomy feeding tube and long-term tube feeding.

Developmental Strengths and Risks

The neonatal period lasts from birth to 1 month of age. Infancy, from 1 month to 1 year of age, is a time of rapid growth and development. Infants whose start in life is challenged by prematurity, illness, trauma, congenital anomalies, or genetic conditions have a more difficult time achieving developmental milestones. Delays may manifest in any domain of development. IDD tend to emerge as variations in a specific domain or domains. An example is autism, which presents as delays in communication and social areas of development.

Implementation of close developmental surveillance in early childhood is critical to early detection of developmental delays. In addition to early intervention, close monitoring of weight gain, head circumference, and growth is important, using growth charts to plot trends in length, weight, and head circumference. (Growth charts are also available for children with Down syndrome and other special populations.) Infants with feeding problems may have growth problems, such as failure to thrive. Feeding problems may be physiologically based, such as in premature infants with poorly coordinated suck–swallow patterns. Very young mothers without support systems may need frequent coaching in feeding irritable infants or those with conditions that affect feeding, such as cerebral palsy or cleft palate.

Table 4.1. Common ages of presentation for developmental abnormalities in a premature infant

Year 1	Cerebral palsy
	Severe sensory abnormalities
	Significant visual compromise
	Severe hearing loss
Year 2	Speech and language difficulties
	Early cognitive delays
	Subtle visual and hearing difficulties
Years 3–5	Fine motor difficulties
	Difficulties in regulation of behavior
	Hyporesponsive or hyperresponsive behavior (i.e., attention-deficit/hyperactivity disorder)
	Motor and behavioral "immaturity"
Years 6–8	Learning disabilities
	Sensory processing problems
	Visual-motor difficulties
	Minor degrees of compromised motor coordination

This table was published in *Encounters with children: Pediatric behavior and development, 4th edition,* Dixon, S.D. & Vaucher, Y.E., p.189, Copyright Mosby Elsevier (2006). Reprinted by permission.

One of the earliest warning signs of neurological, visual, and/or cognitive concerns is the inability of the infant to visually attend to and follow a person or object as they move. An infant at 3–4 months of age with appropriate visual and cognitive abilities will become alert if an interesting object is placed before him: The infant will try to grab the object and manipulate it. Similarly, the infant will turn his or her head to locate a sound, demonstrating intact hearing. An infant who shows little interest in the environment is likely to have neurologic problems.

Motor disorders manifest during infancy as asymmetrical posture or movements, such as using the right hand exclusively to reach for objects. Infants who experienced insults to the brain may show low muscle tone for the first few months of life then develop increased tone and spasticity later on, which is a cardinal sign of cerebral palsy. Fine and gross motor abilities develop in response to environmental stimuli; therefore, allowing a child to explore the environment safely will encourage development. Primitive reflexes, such as the asymmetric tonic neck reflex, are present at term birth and disappear as the brain matures, usually by 12 months of age. In cerebral palsy and other brain disorders, these reflexes may persist past 1 year of age and interfere with voluntary movement.

Speech develops from crying and vocalization at birth to cooing and babbling by about 4 months of age. The infant who vocalizes and babbles but then stops making sounds other than crying as he or she matures through infancy may have hearing loss or another developmental concern (Dixon, 2006a). Table 4.1 provides a summary of the common ages for developmental abnormalities to occur.

Transition Issues: Discharge from the NICU

The home environment is very beneficial for the infant and family. Since the 1980s, Medicaid waivers have been available in all states, which allow funding for infants who are technology dependent to receive care in the home instead of an institutional setting. Katie Beckett, a child who was ventilator dependent, lived in the hospital until her mother, Julie Beckett, advocated for her daughter to be cared for in the home. As a result of her efforts, and the efforts of other parents and professional advocates, Medicaid rules were changed to allow home care for children with significant disabilities and care needs (Hummel & Cronin, 2004).

Specially trained discharge nurses or nurse case managers coordinate the discharge process. Prior to discharge, health insurance coverage is evaluated to determine the services that will be available to the family in the home. It is necessary to obtain prior authorization for home nursing services and durable medical equipment, as well as to establish medical necessity with the insurance company, for the care and equipment. Parents are taught the technical care that their infant will need at home to survive. Discharge planning is often easier when the family lives in an urban area rather than in a faraway rural area or another state. Community agency referrals are made to Child Find and the early intervention system. Refer to Chapter 6 for additional information.

Family Adaptation and Coping

Discharge can be frightening for parents, particularly if they must learn and administer tube feedings, oxygen, or other medical technology. Families must be able to provide a stable, safe home environment and be able to take on the major burden of care for their infant. While home nursing care is often necessary, it is usually intermittent, as funding rarely allows 24-hour home nursing care. Parents must be knowledgeable about the technology the child uses, how to troubleshoot the technology, and how to respond to unexpected events. An emergency plan is critical for mechanical failure, sudden illness, or natural disaster. Spare equipment must be available, including an alternative power source, as well as the contact information for all medical and service providers. The public service utilities need to be contacted; in case of a power failure, they will restore power first to the home of an infant who is dependent on technology. Emergency response staff is also notified, so that staff can have the appropriate size of equipment for a premature infant available in case of an emergency call. Ideally, a respite source is available to provide care when parents or their other children become ill, or when parents need some "time off" (Hummel & Cronin, 2004).

Parents bringing their child home for the first time after the NICU may be overwhelmed by the amount of care and equipment necessary. The infant's around-the-clock care needs can be exhausting for both parents. If home nursing care is required, the family must adapt to the invasion of privacy that the care necessitates. While discharge planning and community referrals seek to assist families, the sheer amount of effort necessary to provide a safe environment for the infant often results in stress. Caring for the child is not the only stressor—parents may miss work beyond the usual maternity leave, jeopardizing jobs and finances. The effects of stress are cumulative, altering existing and expected family roles and relationships, and possibly resulting in illness or discord. Mothers tend to bear the brunt of these effects because they often are the primary caregivers, but fathers are also affected. Single-parent families may have a more difficult time, even if grandparents or siblings are able to step in and help. Guilt and/or blame on the part of the parents may lead to relationship problems and separation if not resolved (Howland, 2007).

Family support and education is crucial. Although professional counseling is important, only other parents who have gone through the same challenges can relate to the day-to-day experience of caring for a premature infant or child with IDD. Parent support groups may have a general focus, such as information and support for all ages of individuals with IDD, or they may specialize in a particular aspect of raising a child with IDD, such as special education and school services. Family Voices (http://www.familyvoices.org) is one such organization, offering information on health care funding and advocating for families with insurers and government agencies. Support groups may be formed around a specific diagnosis and provide information to members about all aspects of raising a child and living with the condition.

Early Intervention

Infants who are discharged from the NICU are at risk for IDD. As a result, they and their families require an array of community services for support from various agencies. One important source of publicly provided services is the early intervention system. The Education of the Handicapped Amendments of 1986 (PL 99-457) established early intervention as a comprehensive program of developmental assessment, therapies to promote speech and language, motor skills, social skills, and education for all children with IDD from birth to 3 years. Part C of the Individuals with Disabilities Education Improvement Act (IDEA) of 2004 (PL 108-446) is the section of the law that mandates the state-based early intervention program. The goals were to promote development of young children at risk for or diagnosed with disabling conditions, to reduce the need for special education later on, and to promote independent living when the child reached adulthood (Wrightslaw, 2008). Although eligibility requirements vary slightly from state to state due to individual states' definitions of developmental delay, the law specifies the services that must be available at no cost to families.

As part of the law, an individualized family service plan (IFSP) is formulated, which specifies the needed services as well as coordination of those services for the family. The IFSP encompasses the family as well as the infant, because research has demonstrated that culturally sensitive family support and education, focused on promoting the infant's development, results in much better developmental outcomes for the child. Particularly in this crucial early stage of development, the family provides the environment the infant needs to grow and develop. When the environment is enriched through parent training in methods to stimulate and teach their child with special needs, developmental declines can be prevented (Guralnick & Conlon, 2007).

Part C of IDEA provides for case finding, that is a Child Find system to identify infants who qualify for services due to diagnosis of a congenital or genetically based condition (i.e., Down syndrome) or who are at risk for developmental problems due to prematurity or early illness. Young children who demonstrate developmental delays prior to age 3 years are also candidates for Child Find, and may receive a free screening to determine eligibility for early intervention. Once a child receiving services through early intervention reaches age 3 years, Part C provides for a transition process to the next level of service, Part B of IDEA, which offers educational programming for preschool through high school.

TODDLERHOOD: EARLY INTERVENTION TO PRESCHOOL

Toddlers, or children 1–3 years of age, are active explorers. Neurologic maturation enables potty training between 2 and 3 years of age, when the toddler shows increasing muscle control and interest in staying dry. Stranger anxiety appears at about 8–9 months and may continue through the second year. The tantrums of the "terrible twos" are most frequent between 18 months and 2 years. Limit-testing behavior (e.g., a 2-year-old girl runs to the edge of the playground, then stops and looks back at her mother, but refuses to come to the mother's call) is a declaration of independence. At this age, self-regulation skills emerge, such as falling asleep at night and staying asleep, self-feeding, increasing speech, and communication skills (Stein, 2006a). The beginnings of autonomy bring about negativism, as the toddler attempts to take control of the environment. Frustration in learning new tasks leads to outbursts. A parent's response to outbursts not only affects the immediate outcome, but has long-term implications for the child's ability to self-regulate and express emotions productively. Discipline during this period seeks to set limits on the child for societal and safety reasons; however, at the same time, the child is testing these limits (Stein, 2006a).

Common Conditions

Increasing social abilities make the toddler period key to early identification of autism spectrum disorders. A toddler who does not make eye contact, point to objects, understand directions, and/or communicate and interact with parents may have autism or another developmental or behavioral disorder. Screening tools exist for young children with autism, but they tend to have a low specificity. Diagnosis of autism is best accomplished by an interdisciplinary team of developmental professionals, including, at a minimum, a pediatrician, a child psychologist, and a speech-language pathologist. The team may also include a developmental behavioral pediatrician, occupational therapist, and/or early childhood special education teacher. For more information on autism, see Chapter 15.

Speech and language disorders become more obvious as a toddler matures; they may have one or more causes. Hearing problems, cognitive delay, oral-motor delays, or neuroprocessing disorders may result in communication problems. Lack of environmental stimulation may also be implicated in speech disorders. Stuttering may emerge during this period. By 2 years of age, the toddler should have a fairly large expressive vocabulary of about 75 words, be able to put together two-word sentences, be able to label many familiar objects (e.g., body parts), and be able to comprehend basic one-step requests and common nouns (Dixon, 2006b; Stein, 2006a). Any child who is unable to communicate at the expected level requires a speech and language evaluation or referral to Child Find.

Motor development progresses rapidly. Although toddlers tend to be clumsy and fall with their efforts to walk, limb use is generally symmetrical (Dixon & Hennessy, 2006a). Children who are not progressing in their fine and gross motor skills should have a developmental evaluation through Child Find and visit an occupational or physical therapist skilled with children. Toddlers who were born prematurely may be delayed but will catch up; they may not follow the usual developmental sequence exactly. Table 4.2 lists warning signs for fine and gross motor development during the toddler period.

Table 4.2.   Warning signs for fine and gross motor development: age 6 months to 3 years

Age	Fine motor development	Gross motor development	Possible causes
6–12 months	Does not reach for objects, rake objects, reach across midline Does not transfer objects from hand to hand No self-feeding or hand-to-mouth behavior By 10 months, no pincer grasp-and-release skill	By 6–8 months, no or poor head control By 7 months, unable to roll prone to supine By 9 months, unable to roll supine to prone By 10 months, no unsupported sitting Asymmetrical limb use	Central nervous system disorders (e.g., cerebral palsy) Mental retardation Infant depression Autism spectrum disorders Nonspecific developmental delay Neural tube defects (e.g., spina bifida) Visual disorders
12–24 months	Not using spoon or cup Unable to grasp pencil, make a mark on paper Unable to stack 7 blocks	By 18 months, no independent steps By 2 years, unable to run Asymmetric limb movement, limping Refusal to bear weight Frequent falling forward instead of backward	Central nervous system disorders (e.g., cerebral palsy) Congenital hip dysplasia (walking) Limb length discrepancy Osteomyelitis Septic arthropathy
24–36 months	Unable to imitate drawing circle Difficulty stacking 10 blocks	By 3 years, unable to stand on one foot, jump, or hop Unable to throw and catch ball with extended arms Unable to scoot a riding toy with feet Persistent toe walking Loss of proximal motor abilities	Central nervous system disorders (e.g., cerebral palsy) Muscular dystrophies

Sources: Dixon and Hennessy (2006a, 2006b).

Behavioral Concerns

Young children with existing IDD are at risk for behavioral and/or psychiatric disorders. Hearing impairments affect speech and communication and may result in aggressive behavior to communicate wants and needs. Toddlers who were born prematurely show a high rate of attention-deficit/hyperactivity disorder (ADHD) as they age and enter group settings, such as child care (Wolraich, 2006). The toddler who is constantly in movement, unable to attend to anything, and often described as "bouncing off the walls" may be diagnosed with ADHD; however, most children are diagnosed during preschool or school age (Cormier, 2008). Care must be taken, however, to distinguish typical toddler exuberance from actual inability to maintain attention. Young children who experience frequent hospitalizations and therapies experience a great deal of stress and often lack coping skills. Separation from parents exacerbates these stressors. Families may overprotect their child; in doing so, they may limit the child's environmental exploration and opportunity to practice responses to situations.

A child's behavior changes can be a sign of family stress. Parental conflict, loss, divorce, or other major changes in circumstance may affect the young child. Toddlers may regress developmentally, such as in feeding or toileting, may withdraw, or may become more aggressive with siblings or other children. Regression in these hard-won behaviors is particularly difficult for parents to manage in addition to the family stresses. Families will often require support and assistance to work through these stages (Stein, 2006a).

Typical toddler behavior is challenging, so toddlers with particularly demanding behavior, especially those with preexisting health or developmental problems, are at risk for child abuse. Young children, because of their dependence and vulnerability, are the age group at greatest risk for abuse. IDD may result from maltreatment, such as a shaking injury that results in global damage to the brain. Young children with IDD and chronic health conditions, particularly those with behavioral or mental health disorders, are at even greater risk. While current statistics are believed to underrepresent children with IDD, about 7.3% of the 872,000 children who experienced abuse in 2004 were identified as having an IDD or chronic health condition. Furthermore, experts contend that social services workers lack experience with children with IDD, contributing to underrepresentation in statistics (Hibbard, Desch, Committee on Child Abuse and Neglect, & Council on Children with Disabilities, 2007).

Researchers have suggested that children in special education programs are more likely to be injured than children in regular classrooms (Ramirez, Peek-Asa, & Kraus, 2004). Young children with hearing or vision disorders may be unable to detect warning sirens or flashing lights. Children with mobility disorders who are unable to move independently must rely on others to move them out of harm's way, in case of fire or other emergency.

Psychiatric disorders occur more frequently in children with IDD than in the general population. Early symptoms may include lack of attachment or inability to attach to a significant parent figure, unrelenting tantrums, and/or withdrawal and regression of developmental milestones. Disorders such as bipolar disorder, depression, schizophrenia, and anxiety disorders may show early symptoms. When psychiatric disorders co-occur with IDD, the child is said to have a dual diagnosis. Children exhibiting major behavioral symptoms out of proportion to the situation or their development are best referred to the mental health system. For more information on dual diagnosis, refer to Chapter 14.

Family Challenges and Adaptation

Young children with IDD who are medically fragile generally become more physiologically stable as they pass through infancy and toddlerhood. As a result, families are more likely to consider part-time child care settings, both to enhance the child's development and to provide some respite for themselves. Families may have difficulty finding child care programs in their area that are equipped to serve children with IDD and special health care needs. While the Americans with Disabilities Act (ADA) of 1990 (PL 101-336) mandates inclusion in all public programs, including child care, there are some exceptions to the law, usually based on the center's income and ability to make extensive changes (Child Care Law Center, 2007). There are a number of federal and state resources for centers to aid them in providing inclusive child care. Many early intervention programs offer center-based programs, which provide child care and interventions for several hours a day or week.

The task of caring for a young child with IDD who is dependent on technology is often challenging. Care needs may span 24 hours a day, 7 days a week, and require constant vigilance. Families may experience isolation, sleep deprivation, and anxiety over changes in the child's condition. Relationships may be strained as a result of family members' changed roles. Siblings may receive less attention or may be enlisted to provide care. Financial concerns are often a source of worry (Rehm & Bradley, 2005). Despite these challenges, most families adapt, even single-parent families. Periodic nursing care or home-based therapies can provide a brief break for the parent or caregiver; however, in most cases, the parent must be present for these interventions.

Respite is very important for families; it allows parents and siblings time together and gives caregivers time for rest and restoration. Some formal programs exist, but in the absence of formal respite, informal arrangements between parents and friends or family members often suffice (Macdonald & Callery, 2008). Community agencies may link trained volunteers with families, or offer a respite "night out" for parents, where they may register to drop their child off at a center and then go out to dinner.

Transition Issues: Early Intervention to Part B Programs

IDEA legislation provides for development of a transition plan from Part C (early intervention) programs to Part B (preschool and school-age special education programs). While early intervention programs are very family focused, with a great deal of autonomy and control for the family, Part B programs are child focused and school based. Early intervention legislation was designed to promote development of young children with IDD, and those who are at risk for developing IDD, while the purpose of Part B of IDEA is to provide free appropriate public education in the least restrictive environment. Eligibility requirements for Part B of IDEA are different than the requirements for Part C, and most states require an evaluation for eligibility before the child transitions. Since most school systems operate on a 9-month schedule, children who turn 3 over the summer may not receive a timely assessment or individualized education program (IEP) planning meeting, and thus may experience interruption in services. The fact that Part C may be administered by one of several state programs but Part B programs are always administered by the State Department of Education also complicates matters of eligibility (U.S. Government Accountability Office, 2005).

PRESCHOOL TO KINDERGARTEN

The preschool period is one of rapidly expanding language and social development leading to reciprocal play. The preschooler begins to take initiative in social interactions and may involve other children in group play. The child may begin to use toys in a representative way, act out a story or a fantasy, or engage in imaginative solitary play as well as organized group play. An active imagination contributes to "magical" thinking, which ascribes human motivation to objects and animals. Awareness of gender emerges, followed by more gender-specific behavior and dress. Progress in fine and gross motor skills allows the child to engage in vigorous play and physical activity as well as fine motor activities, such as drawing or painting.

Increasing control over behavior and impulsivity is displayed in the pre-schooler's abilities to stand in line with other children, to sit still at a table, and to take turns. Taking the initiative in a situation may easily cross over into aggressive behavior as the child strives to learn how to manage feelings and impulses. If a child begins to have a serious, ongoing problem with aggression, intervention is often required and referral to a mental health provider may be necessary.

Common Conditions

As children grow and develop, more is expected of them with regard to behavior and learning, so IDDs are more likely to be recognized. The preschooler with com-munication difficulties or who is socially immature becomes obviously different from his or her peers. Cognitive disorders, except the most severe and global, tend to manifest and be identified during this period. Rapid growth may result in toe walking from tight Achilles tendons in children with cerebral palsy. Preschoolers who were born prematurely or diagnosed with BPD become more physiologically stable; children with milder BPD may progress to reactive airway disease, whereas those who were more severely affected must strive to achieve developmental milestones while tethered to oxygen tubing. Both growth and development are af-fected in preschoolers with feeding problems. Loss of motor milestones, particu-larly in males, may lead to suspicions of muscular dystrophy, which first appears at around 3–5 years of age with proximal muscle weakness. For term infants who were hypotonic and had feeding difficulties at birth, then present with hyperpha-gia and rapid weight gain to obesity in the preschool years, a genetic workup for Prader-Willi syndrome is indicated.

Behavioral Disorders

Preschool is often the setting where young children begin to learn the skills, rules, and routines they will need when they enter elementary school, as well as the so-cial skills they will need to get along. Young children who were premature are more likely to be diagnosed with ADHD (McGrath et al., 2005). While attention problems may be identified in younger children, actual diagnosis rarely occurs be-fore the preschool years. Young children with sensory processing disorders may be unable to tolerate noise, crowds, or excessive stimulation and thus may act out. Children with IDD or those who are at risk for developmental problems and who exhibit challenging behavior are best referred to a developmental evaluation cen-ter or to a pediatrician trained in developmental/behavioral pediatrics. If autism is suspected, referral to a specialized team experienced in the diagnosis and treat-ment of autism is indicated. Any child who is suspected of developmental delay may be referred to Child Find for evaluation and possible placement in a special education program.

Accommodations and Adaptation

Young children (3–4 years of age) who have been identified with IDD are eligible for federal and state subsidized preschool programs under IDEA and the local school system. If a child did not receive transition services into Part B of IDEA, or if the delay or disability was recognized after age 3 years, a Child Find develop-mental evaluation must be performed to qualify the child for services. In order to

Table 4.3.   School-based services provided under IDEA

Speech-language pathology and audiology
Psychology
Physical therapy
Occupational therapy
Recreation and therapeutic recreation
Early identification and assessment of disabilities
Rehabilitation and other counseling
Orientation and mobility services for children with visual problems
Medical (solely for diagnostic or evaluation purposes)
School health
School-based social work services
Parent counseling and training
Transportation to and from school

Sources: Guralnick and Conlon (2007); Wrightslaw (2008).

receive these services, a child must have an IEP, which specifies the services and supports that are necessary for learning. For a list of school-based services that are available under IDEA, please see Table 4.3.

Private preschool programs under ADA are required to serve children with IDD and chronic conditions. While they are not required by law to participate in the IEP and the services offered through the IEP, it is very much to their advantage to do so. Most private programs lack the resources of the school district and can benefit greatly from the recommendations and interventions of the school district professionals on behalf of the child's IEP. Physical and occupational therapists, speech and language pathologists, psychologists, and special educators are some of the professionals who provide services through the IEP.

Head Start is a national school readiness program serving disadvantaged children, ages 3 and 4, and families. Started in 1965, Head Start provides comprehensive services, including health, nutrition, education, and family support at no cost to qualifying families. In 1995, Early Head Start was implemented to extend comprehensive health and education services to children from birth to 3 years of age. The Office of Head Start provides grant funding to community nonprofit agencies to offer programs in low-income communities. Children with IDD are fully included in Head Start programs and receive an IEP. A transition plan assists the child and family in moving from Head Start to the public education system (National Head Start Association, 2007).

In order for children with IDD to be included in child care or preschool programs, adaptations to programs, staffing, physical space, and/or attitudes of teachers may be required. Additional training or education of child care providers may be necessary. The support of an inclusion consultant can also be very helpful. Some health procedures may need to be delegated and supervised by a registered nurse. State nurse practice acts and child care licensing regulations can offer guidance as to which procedures can be safely delegated in a child care setting.

Family Challenges and Adaptation

By the time a child with a disability reaches 4 or 5 years of age, families have established a routine to manage the child's needs and balance work, day-to-day tasks, and the rest of the family's priorities. Progress in the child's development gives hope and contributes to positive coping. A support system is in place, often composed of family members, neighbors and friends, professionals, and/or parents of other children with disabilities. Marital relationships that were strong to begin with usually continue to strengthen as the family accepts the child with a disability as an intrinsic family member. Stability is easier to achieve if the child's condition is stable and nonprogressive rather than changing or worsening.

Siblings must adjust to the many changes the child with an IDD causes in a family. Siblings may receive less attention, may lose out on privileges (e.g., parents cannot attend an important sporting event that the sibling is participating in), may experience stress, and may even be on the receiving end of challenging behavior. Some siblings may be recruited as caregivers and may provide highly technical care at times (e.g., the 10-year-old sister of a young child who was ventilator dependent was able to do suctioning and tracheostomy care when necessary). Often, siblings take the same joy in their brother's or sister's accomplishments as the parents and experience a great deal of stress if the child with a disability is hospitalized or very ill (Giallo & Gavidia-Payne, 2006).

Researchers (Dykens, 2005; Stoneman, 2005) suggest that siblings who experience difficulty adjusting are from families who lack resources and that a sibling's coping mirrors difficulties in family functioning. Coping difficulties may manifest as behavioral problems (e.g., ADHD), school problems, falling grades, or emotional disorders. While little cultural data exists, Lobato, Kao, and Plante (2005) suggest that disparities of health care, resources, and other services among Latino families who have a child with a disability may result in an increased level of internalizing behavioral issues in siblings. Siblings who experience problems with adjustment may benefit from professional intervention and family counseling (Giallo & Gavidia-Payne, 2006).

Transition from Preschool to Kindergarten

Preschoolers with disabilities face a number of changes as they enter kindergarten. Children may be coming from preschool-age child care centers, from public school programs a few days a week, from small playgroups or family child care homes, or from Head Start programs. Expectations for behavior, self-regulation, attention, and social interaction are greater, and the time in class is usually longer. Classes are often larger and more structured, with longer periods in which the child is expected to sit still, pay attention, or get along with other children.

Preparations for the transition to kindergarten include sharing records between programs, educating parents on the process, and preparing the child for the kindergarten experience. While a preschool IEP may provide information about the child's strengths and needs, most school systems require an evaluation prior to kindergarten to determine the best placement for the child. Most school systems offer options with regard to placement, such as a fully integrated or inclusive classroom, a homeroom specifically for children with disabilities with participation in some integrated classes; or a segregated setting specifically for children with severe disabilities or challenging behavior. Most systems also offer some home services for children who cannot be accommodated in the school setting. Families who have prepared ahead of time, becoming knowledgeable about teachers and placement options in their district, will be able to better facilitate the transition (Maine Parent Federation, 2002).

Options other than the traditional public school system exist. Parents may place their child in an out-of-district school; however, they may need to prove that the necessary programs are not available in the home district. Private schools, which generally offer smaller class sizes and more individualized attention, may be an option. The school district must provide some special education services to children placed in private schools according to parent's preference. Another option is home schooling, which can provide a more tailored educational program; this is particularly useful for those children who do not tolerate groups or distractions well. However, social interaction is limited and requires a well-educated, motivated parent who can stay home with the child. If the state recognizes home schooling as the same as a private school, then the school district must provide special education services. However, if the state does not recognize home schooling as a "legitimate" placement, then children with disabilities who are home schooled will not receive special education services (Chapman, 2008).

SCHOOL AGE: ELEMENTARY TO MIDDLE SCHOOL

School age, or middle childhood, is considered to be 6–11 years of age. The 6-year-old child is faced with the need to sit still and attend school for even longer periods of time. According to Stein (2006b), "This age marks the beginning of a lifetime of obligations and adherence to schedules and routines imposed outside the familiar family environment" (p. 489). Cognitive challenges increase as instruction in reading and mathematics begins. Receptive and expressive language is increasingly used for abstract concepts and for comprehension of complex tasks. Typically, Piaget's concrete operations stage is achieved by 9–11 years of age and during this time children, for example, learn logic, reversibility, mathematical concepts, and conservation. Peer and social relationships gain importance, and interactions with other children become multifaceted. Most 6-year-old children have internalized societal rules (e.g., right and wrong), although they may not have complete understanding of causative factors. Values tend to be reflections of family values or those of the society or peer group mores (Fiegelman, 2007; Stein, 2006b).

From a physiologic standpoint, the rapid growth of earlier years begins to slow. The brain has reached about 90% of its adult size. By around age 7, myelinization of the central nervous system is achieved. However, the brain is not fully mature, as synapse and neuronal connections continue to form with concomitant progression of learning. Motor development increases. Improved coordination leads to recreational activity, such as bicycle riding, skate boarding, skiing, and/or snow boarding. Because these activities can present safety risks, the use of helmets and other protective equipment is important (Stein, 2006b).

Children with identified IDD usually require special education and related services that are focused on enhancing the child's educational capacity. For children who are at risk of IDD, such as those who were born prematurely, academic expectations often unmask disability in the form of intellectual disabilities, learning disabilities, and/or attention difficulties. ADHD is most often diagnosed during first or second grade, if not identified earlier in significantly affected children. Children with ADHD have a high rate of comorbidity with other conditions, such as depression, anxiety disorders, obsessive-compulsive disorder, and bipolar disorder. Autism spectrum disorders, fragile X syndrome, intellectual disabilities, and other neurodevelopmental conditions may also co-occur with ADHD. The impulsivity that often accompanies ADHD may make safety an issue (Wolraich, 2006).

Social interaction problems become most apparent during middle childhood because of the importance of peer groups and friends in the child's life. Children with IDD may often have difficulty making and keeping friends. Communication disorders, particularly nonverbal communication problems and difficulty with pragmatics or the social use of language, affect social skills. Learning about behavior and communication from past encounters is an important factor in development of social skills.

A significant problem for many children with IDD in grade school and middle school is bullying. Physical bullying is more common with boys, whereas verbal or social abuse is more frequent with girls (Horowitz et al., 2004). Children with IDD are often victims of bullies due to social communication problems, emotional problems, physical disabilities, and simply being different, particularly during this developmental period when conforming to the norm is so important. Bullying victims experience social isolation and suffer from poor self-esteem and depression, and thus may avoid school. While they are most often victims, children with IDD may also be bullies if they are more likely to deal with conflict by aggressive behavior. Bullying is a significant problem that always requires intervention for both the bully and the victim (Wells & Stein, 2006).

School Accommodations and Adaptation

In most cases, the IEP guides the provision of special education and related services for the child with IDD. Section 504 of the Rehabilitation Act of 1973 (PL 93-112) includes a wider definition of disability than IDEA and allows schools to offer special education to children and youth who do not qualify for IDEA. Children with IDD may receive special education services through both IDEA and Section 504 of the Rehabilitation Act. For more information on Section 504, see Table 4.4.

Table 4.4.   Facts about Section 504 of the Rehabilitation Act of 1973

Purpose is to ensure that children with disabilities have equal access to an education

Defines a person with a disability as someone with a physical or mental impairment that substantially limits one or more major life activity, has a record of such impairment, or is regarded as having such an impairment

Pertains to individuals with disabilities in federally funded programs such as preschools, schools, employment practices, or health and social welfare programs

Requires planning, but does not require an individualized education program or a written plan for the student

Does not require the presence of the student's parent during the planning process

Unlike IDEA, has fewer procedural safeguards than IDEA to protect the student and parent

Includes children with

        Communicable diseases (e.g., human immunodeficiency virus)

        Chronic illness (e.g., asthma, diabetes)

        Life-threatening disorder (e.g., severe peanut allergy)

        Substance abuse (e.g., alcohol, drugs)

        Temporary disabilities (e.g., fracture) for which short-term homebound services are required

        Attentional disorders without significant academic problems

        Tourette syndrome

Source: Clair, Church, and Batshaw (2006); Wrightslaw (2008).

Children who receive special education services often receive accommodations or modifications to their curriculum as specified in their IEP. Examples of accommodations include taping a lecture for a child who is unable to take notes, providing a separate room without distractions for a child to complete a test, and/or providing materials in Braille for a child who is blind. A modification is a change to an assignment that makes the assignment easier or more accessible to the student. For example, instead of providing a specific reading assignment, an alternative assignment would be offered, which covers the same material but at an easier reading level; or instead of requiring the student to read the entire chapter, a chapter summary can be provided (Families and Advocates Partnership for Education, 2001). Special education includes direct academic instruction, as well as training in functional and social skills. Teachers may provide information on getting along with others, making change and money management, and other life skills. Safety is an important topic, and many schools include curricula on prevention of abuse and victimization.

In addition to accommodations and modifications, many students with IDD receive related services, such as speech and language therapy, physical therapy, or occupational therapy. Therapy may be provided within the student's classroom and include the child with IDD in context within his class or in a pull-out model, in which the student receives the therapy in another room. Although related services per the student's IEP are provided for by IDEA, if the child is covered, many schools have begun billing Medicaid for therapy services to defray costs. Medicaid billing must first be negotiated within the state by legislation or changes in regulations.

Family Challenges and Adaptation

School is a major focus of the child and family during this period. Families often work closely with school, teachers, and therapists to ensure that their child receives the necessary education, and that gains in school are transferred to the home setting. While IDEA implementation for the child usually goes smoothly, differences of opinions between parents and the school or differing evaluations from professionals may occur. Challenging the school system is exhausting for families and may lead to an oppositional relationship between the parties. While procedural safeguards are ensured by IDEA with rights for parents and students who disagree with the school, consultation with experts in special education law may be necessary.

Families whose child develops a disability during the school years from injury, disease, or a genetic condition must cope with the loss of the typically developing child, and now include a "new" child into the family with his or her physical and behavioral changes (Trachtenberg, Batshaw, & Batshaw, 2006). Families may benefit from support from other families who have had similar experiences, as well as from nurses and other professionals.

Transition: Elementary to Middle School

Entry into middle school presents a different school environment than in the elementary grades. Students must change rooms for classes and cope with multiple teachers with different teaching styles. The pool of students is much larger and more diverse than in previous grades, and there may be fewer familiar faces. For children with IDD with mobility impairments, such as cerebral palsy, moving from room to room while carrying books may be very difficult. Negotiating lockers is also a challenge, particularly in the limited amount of time between classes. The environment itself may present challenges to the student with autism who has difficulty adjusting to schedule changes and sensory overload.

As in earlier shifts to new service systems, careful preparation in the form of a transition plan can benefit the student and the teachers. Opportunities to visit the school and classrooms and walk the route from room to room may be helpful. Social stories depicting key aspects of the new school may help students with autism. Staff and teachers at the middle school who are familiarized with the new student will be better able to provide assistance and ease the transition. Parents who are proactive and meet with teachers and school staff on a regular basis to solve problems can promote a collaborative relationship that can benefit the student (Vicker, 2003).

CONCLUSION

This chapter provided an overview of children with IDD from before birth through middle childhood. Age-related and developmentally based risk factors for IDD were presented, as well as common conditions and family concerns. The importance of family support and education was also emphasized.

REFERENCES

Adams-Chapman, I., & Stoll, B.J. (2007). The fetus and the neonatal infant: Nervous system disorders (Chapter 99). In R.M. Kleigman, R.E. Behrman, H.B. Jensen, & B.F. Stanton (Eds.), *Nelson textbook of pediatrics* (18th electronic ed.). Philadelphia: W.B. Saunders.

Americans with Disabilities Act (ADA) of 1990, PL 101-336, 42 U.S.C. §§ 12101 *et seq.*

Bashiri, A., Burstein, E., & Mazor, M. (2006). Cerebral palsy and fetal inflammatory response syndrome: A review. *Journal of Perinatal Medicine, 34,* 5–12.

Bhasin, T.K., Brocksen, S., Avchen, R.N., & Braun, K.V. (2006). Prevalence of four developmental disabilities among children aged 8 years—Metropolitan Atlanta Developmental Disabilities Surveillance Program, 1996 and 2000. *Morbidity and Mortality Weekly Report, 55,* 1–9.

Capper-Michel, B. (2004). Bronchopulmonary dysplasia. In P. Jackson Allen & J.A. Vessey (Eds.), *Primary care of the child with a chronic condition* (4th ed., pp. 282–298). St. Louis: Mosby Elsevier.

Chapman, R. (2008). *For some families there's no place like home: The IDEA and home schooling.* Retrieved February 7, 2009, from http://randychapman.wordpress.com/2008/10/09/for-some-families-theres-no-place-like-home-the-idea-and-home-schooling/.

Child Care Law Center. (2007). *Questions and answers about the Americans with Disabilities Act. A quick reference (information for childcare providers).* Retrieved February 1, 2009, from http://www.childcare law.org/docs/qanda-ada.pdf.

Clair, E.B., Church, R.B., & Batshaw, M.L. (2006). Special education services. In M.L. Batshaw, L. Pellegrino, & N.J. Roizen (Eds.), *Children with disabilities* (6th ed., pp. 523–538). Baltimore: Paul H. Brookes Publishing Co.

Cormier, E. (2008). Attention deficit/hyperactivity disorder: A review and update. *Journal of Pediatric Nursing, 23,* 345–357.

Davies, L. (2008). Influences on the health of the newborn, before and during pregnancy. In L. Davies & D. McDonald (Eds.), *Examination of the newborn and neonatal health: A multidimensional approach* (pp. 79–94). Edinburgh: Churchill Livingstone.

Davies, L., & Richards, J. (2008). Maternal and newborn transition: Adjustment to extrauterine life. In L. Davies & S. McDonald (Eds.), *Examination of the newborn and neonatal health: A multidimensional approach* (pp. 107–140). Edinburgh: Churchill Livingstone.

Dixon, D.P. (2008). Informed consent or institutionalized eugenics? How the medical profession encourages abortion of fetuses with Down syndrome. *Issues in Law & Medicine, 24,* 3–59.

Dixon, S.D. (2006a). Three to four months: Having fun with the picture book baby. In S.D. Dixon & M.T. Stein (Eds.), *Encounters with children: Pediatric behavior and development* (4th ed., pp. 252–267). Philadelphia: Mosby Elsevier.

Dixon, S.D. (2006b). Eight to nine months: Exploring and clinging. In S.D. Dixon & M.T. Stein (Eds.), *Encounters with children: Pediatric behavior and development* (4th ed., pp. 292–321). Philadelphia: Mosby Elsevier.

Dixon, S.D., & Hennessy, M.J. (2006a). Six months: Reaching out. In S.D. Dixon & M.T. Stein (Eds.), *Encounters with children: Pediatric behavior and development* (4th ed., pp. 268–291). Philadelphia: Mosby Elsevier.

Dixon, S.D., & Hennessy, M.J. (2006b). One year: One giant step forward. In S.D. Dixon & M.T. Stein (Eds.), *Encounters with children: Pediatric behavior and development* (4th ed., pp. 322–251). Philadelphia: Mosby Elsevier.

Dixon, S.D., & Vaucher, Y.E. (2006). The NICU: Special issues in the at-risk infant and family. In S.D. Dixon & M.T. Stein (Eds.), *Encounters with children: Pediatric behavior and development* (4th ed., pp. 170–199). Philadelphia: Mosby Elsevier.

Dykens, E.M. (2005). Happiness, well-being, and character strengths: Outcomes for families and siblings of persons with mental retardation. *Mental Retardation, 43,* 360–364.

Dykens, E.M., Hodapp, R.M., & Finucane, B.M. (2000). *Genetics and mental retarda-*

tion syndromes. A new look at behavior and interventions. Baltimore: Paul H. Brookes Publishing Co.

Education of the Handicapped Act Amendments of 1986, PL 99-457, 20 U.S.C. §§ 1400 *et seq.*

Families and Advocates Partnership for Education (2001). *FAPE-27. School accommodations and modifications.* Retrieved February 14, 2009, from http://www.fape.org/.

Fiegelman, S. (2007). Middle childhood (Chapter 11). In R.M. Kleigman, R.E. Behrman, J.B. Jensen, & B.F. Stanton (Eds.), *Nelson textbook of pediatrics* (18th electronic ed.). Philadelphia: W.B. Saunders.

Giallo, R., & Gavidia-Payne, S. (2006). Child, parent and family factors as predictors of adjustment for siblings of children with a disability. *Journal of Intellectual Disability Research, 50,* 937–948.

Gibbins, S., Hoath, S.B., Coughlin, M., Gibbins, M., & Franck, F. (2008). The universe of developmental care: A new conceptual model for application in the neonatal intensive care unit. *Advances in Neonatal Care, 8,* 141–147.

Gilbert, E.S. (2007). *Manual of high risk pregnancy and delivery* (4th ed.). St. Louis: Mosby Elsevier.

Greater Boston Physicians for Social Responsibility. (2000). *In harm's way: Toxic threats to child development.* Retrieved November 28, 2008, from http://www.psr.org/site/PageServer?pagename=boston_ihw-report.

Guralnick, M.J., & Conlon, C.J. (2007). Early intervention. In M.L. Batshaw, L. Pellegrino, & N.J. Roizen (Eds.), *Children with disabilities* (6th ed., pp. 511–521). Baltimore: Paul H. Brookes Publishing Co.

Hibbard, R.A., Desch, L.W., Committee on Child Abuse and Neglect, & Council on Children with Disabilities. (2007). Maltreatment of children with disabilities. *Pediatrics, 119,* 1018–1025.

Horowitz, J.A., Vessey, J.A., Carlson, K.L., Bradley, J.F., Montoya, C., McCullough, B. et al. (2004). Teasing and bullying experiences of middle school students. *Journal of the American Psychiatric Nurses Association, 10,* 165–172.

Howland, L.C. (2007). Preterm birth: Implications for family stress and coping. *Newborn and Infant Nursing Reviews, 7,* 14–19.

Hummel, P., & Cronin, J. (2004). Home care of the high-risk infant. *Advances in neonatal care, 4,* 354–364.

Individuals with Disabilities Education Improvement Act (IDEA) of 2004, PL 108-446, 20 U.S.C. §§ 1400 *et seq.*

Keogh, J.M., & Badawi, N. (2006). The origins of cerebral palsy. *Current Opinion in Neurology, 19,* 129–134.

Lavoie, P.M., Pham, C., & Jang, K.L. (2008). Heritability of bronchopulmonary dysplasia, defined according to the consensus statement of the National Institutes of Health. *Pediatrics, 122,* 479–485.

Levetown, M., & Committee on Bioethics. (2008). Communicating with children and families: From everyday interactions to skill in conveying distressing information. *Pediatrics, 121,* 1441–1460.

Lin, C.C., Wang, J.D., Hsieh, G.Y., Chang, Y.Y. & Chen, P.C. (2008). Increased risk of death with congenital anomalies in the offspring of male semiconductor workers. *International Journal of Occupational & Environmental Health, 14,* 112–116.

Lobato, D.J., Kao, B.T, & Plante, W. (2005). Latino sibling knowledge and adjustment to sibling chronic disability. *Journal of Family Psychology, 19,* 625–632.

Macdonald, H., & Callery, P. (2008). Parenting children requiring complex care: A journey through time. *Child: Care, Health, & Development, 34,* 207–213.

Maine Parent Federation. (2002). *Preschool to public school: Preparing for the transition.* Retrieved February 12, 2008, from http://www.mpf.org/faqs.htm.

McGrath, M.M., Sullivan, M., Devin, J., Fontes-Murphy, M., Barcelos, S., DePalma, J.L., et al. (2005). Early precursors of low attention and hyperactivity in a preterm sample at age four. *Issues in Comprehensive Pediatric Nursing, 28,* 1–15.

Milham, S., & Ossiander, E.M. (2007). Low proportion of male births and low birth weight of sons of flour mill worker fathers. *American Journal of Industrial Medicine, 51,* 157–158.

National Head Start Association. (2007). *About the National Head Start Association.*

Retrieved February 12, 2009, from http://www.nhsa.org/about_nhsa.

Odent, M. (2008). The neonatal period and beyond: Short- and long-term consequences of intrapartum events. In L. Davies & S. McDonald (Eds.), *Examination of the newborn and neonatal health: A multidimensional approach* (pp. 95–106). Edinburgh: Churchill Livingstone.

Olshansky, S. (1962). Chronic sorrow: A response to having a mentally defective child. *Social Casework, 51,* 190–193.

Rais-Bahrami, K., & Short, B.L. (2004). Premature and small-for-dates infants. In M.L. Batshaw, L. Pellegrino, & N.J. Roizen (Eds.), *Children with disabilities* (6th ed., pp. 107–122). Baltimore: Paul H. Brookes Publishing Co.

Ramirez, M., Peek-Asa, C., & Kraus, J.F. (2004). Disability and risk of school related injury. *Injury Prevention, 10,* 21–26.

Rehabilitation Act of 1973, PL 93-112, 29 U.S.C. §§ 701 *et seq.*

Rehm, R.S., & Bradley, J.S. (2005). Normalization in families raising a child who is medically fragile/technology dependent and developmentally delayed. *Qualitative Health Research, 15,* 807–820.

Stein, M.T. (2006a). 15 to 18 months: Declaring independence and pushing the limits. In S.D. Dixon & M.T. Stein (Eds.), *Encounters with children: Pediatric behavior and development* (4th ed., pp. 352–381). Philadelphia: Mosby Elsevier.

Stein, M.T. (2006b). Six to seven years: Reading, relationships and playing by the rules. In S.D. Dixon & M.T. Stein (Eds.), *Encounters with children: Pediatric behavior and development* (4th ed., pp. 477–501). Philadelphia: Mosby Elsevier.

Stoneman, Z. (2005). Siblings of children with disabilities: Research themes. *Mental Retardation, 43,* 339–350.

Taylor, H.G., Klein, N., Drotar, D., Schlucter, M., & Hack, M. (2006). Consequences and risks of <1000-g birth weight for neuropsychological skills, achievement, and adaptive functioning. *Developmental and Behavioral Pediatrics, 27,* 459–469.

Trachtenberg, S.W., Batshaw, K., & Batshaw, M. (2006). Caring and coping, helping the family of a child with a disability. In M.L. Batshaw, L. Pellegrino, & N.J. Roizen (Eds.), *Children with disabilities* (6th ed., pp. 601–612). Baltimore: Paul H. Brookes Publishing Co.

United States Government Accountability Office. (2005). *Education should provide additional guidance to help states smoothly transition children to preschool. GAO Highlights, GAO-06-26.* Retrieved February 8, 2009, from http://eric.ed.gov/ERICWebPortal/contentdelivery/servlet/ERICServlet?accno=ED489095.

Vicker, B. (2003). Transition to middle school. *The Reporter, 8,* 19–21. Retrieved February 12, 2009, from http://www.iidc.indiana.edu/irca/education/middleSchool.html.

Wells, R.D., & Stein, M.T. (2006). Seven to ten years: The world of middle childhood. In S.D. Dixon & M.T. Stein (Eds.), *Encounters with children: Pediatric behavior and development* (4th ed., pp. 504–533). Philadelphia: Mosby Elsevier.

Wolraich, M.L. (2006). Attention-deficit/hyperactivity disorder. In I.L. Rubin & A.C. Crocker (Eds.), *Medical care for children and adults with developmental disabilities* (2nd ed., pp. 470–483). Baltimore: Paul H. Brookes Publishing Co.

Wrightslaw. (2008). *Early intervention: Part C of IDEA.* Retrieved February 6, 2009, from http://www.wrightslaw.com/info/ei.index.htm.

Yang, Q., Wen, S.W., Leader, A., Chen, X.K., Lipson, J., & Walker, M. (2007). Paternal age and birth defects: How strong is the association? *Human Reproduction, 22,* 696–701.

CHAPTER 5

Developmental Transitions for Individuals with Intellectual and Developmental Disabilities

Adolescence and Beyond

Mary Theresa Urbano

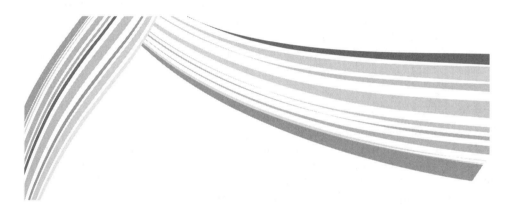

In 2000, the U.S. Department of Health and Human Services, Maternal and Child Health Bureau sponsored the National Survey of Children with Special Health Care Needs. This project was implemented by the Centers for Disease Control and Prevention in 2000–2002 and repeated in 2005–2006. The purpose of these surveys was to provide detailed information on the prevalence of children with special health care needs (CSHCN) at the national and state levels and to examine supports and access issues (U.S. Department of Health and Human Services [DHHS], 2006a). The 2006 survey, which represented great diversity among racial and ethnic groups, ages, family income levels, and functional abilities, found that 13.9% of U.S. children had CSHCN. The survey documented that CSHCN frequently required supports, such as medications, therapies, special educational provisions, or assistive technology (DHHS, 2006a).

These findings did not come as a surprise to health care professionals. Since the 1980s, improvements in health care, surgical procedures and technology have allowed individuals with intellectual and developmental disabilities (IDD) to live longer and more fulfilling lives. However, these individuals often have difficulty mastering functional skills. Support requirements also may change as people with IDD transition between developmental periods. Yet, educational, health, financial, and social systems are not always prepared to meet the special challenges that individuals with IDD experience as they move through life.

This chapter examines changes and challenges that require behavioral responses to adapt to changing environmental circumstances in the time period from middle school and beyond. Relevant nursing strategies for supporting individuals during these transitions are suggested.

ADOLESCENCE: MIDDLE SCHOOL TO HIGH SCHOOL

Historically, individuals with IDD have not reached the same life outcomes (i.e., employment and involvement in social activities) as their typically developing peers. The recognition of these discrepancies led to acknowledgement of the importance of appropriate planning and supports for transition (American Association on Intellectual and Developmental Disabilities, 2008). To begin transition planning, one must consider developmental tasks for particular age periods and the special needs experienced by individuals with IDD.

Students with special health care needs account for 16.8% of 12–17 year olds. Almost 75% of these youths take prescription medications; 39% require extra medical, mental health, or educational services; and 28% have a diagnosed emotional, behavioral, or developmental problem (DHHS, 2006a). These statistics indicate additional complexity in the lives of CSHCN during the period from middle school to high school.

Addressing Puberty

Attainment of developmental tasks during early adolescence is often more difficult because of unprecedented physical, cognitive, and social changes. Puberty generally occurs between 8.5 and 13 years of age in girls and between 9 and 14 years of age in boys (Murphy & Elias, 2006). Many children with IDD experience even earlier puberty (Siddiqi, Van Dyke, Donohoue, & McBrien, 1999). During this period of early adolescence, there is a focus on physical maturation, developing peer relationships, and sexuality. Erickson (1963) called the task of this period *group identification versus alienation.*

Physically, puberty is associated with rapid growth in height and weight. Changing hormones result in the development of secondary sexual characteristics, such as growth of pubic and underarm hair, growth of facial hair and penis in boys, and breast development and the beginning of menstrual periods (menarche) in girls. Psychosocial development is characterized by the need to become more independent, develop an individual identity, and become more comfortable with intimacy and sexuality. These rapidly occurring body changes can affect developing body image. Nurses can help by providing patient education about body changes, the typical development of secondary sex characteristics, gender differences, and sexuality.

Assessment of sexuality and reproductive concerns is important because youth vary in their readiness to explore these topics. While many youth benefit from a general discussion of these topics, others need more intensive and simplified explanations. Teaching and reinforcement of skills promotes development of socially appropriate behavior (Murphy & Elias, 2006). For example, nurses can teach boys about the proper terminology for intimate body parts and the appropriate use of such terms in public. Instruction should include appropriate behaviors, such as which personal activities are to take place in private and how to avoid unnecessary exposure of genitalia. While boys can easily become focused on normal physiological reactions, such as erections, they can also be taught to redirect to other activities. When instruction on socially correct actions is not provided, the innocent behavior of children may be inaccurately perceived by others as criminal acts or sexual deviancy.

Girls must also be taught how to manage changes, especially menstruation. Many girls need reminders of when to use and change sanitary napkins. They need to be reminded to use toilet paper wipes from front to back to avoid frequent urinary tract infections. Preadolescent girls can also benefit from frank discussions about appropriate dress, body positioning, and socially acceptable behaviors.

Intellectual and emotional development continues during this period. Brain development is demonstrated by evolution of advanced reasoning skills and abstract thinking for those without significant intellectual disability (Piaget, 1972, 1976, 1990). Hormone changes may contribute to fluctuating moods (Betz & Sowden, 2008).

Increasing Independence

For students in middle school to high school, a critical component of independence is self-care (e.g., getting up in the morning, bathing, hair care, dental hygiene, dressing). Youth with IDD may need physical assistance or verbal reminders to accomplish these tasks. Nurses and parents can promote gradual independence in daily personal care by breaking down complex activities into small steps, repeating the sequence in a ritual way, and providing consistent reinforcement and praise. Anticipatory guidance, explanations, and role playing can prepare a child for those activities that require greater independence.

Students with chronic health problems may need adult support for medicine administration and/or assistance with daily health-related procedures during the school day. Nurses can also assure that individualized education programs (IEPs) include plans for provision of necessary health care procedures, or guidance on the use of adaptive equipment such as communication devices to foster greater inclusion and classroom participation.

Orem (1995) presented the self-care deficit theory of nursing, which provides a useful framework for self-care activity by addressing universal, developmental, and health deviations. Although it originally addressed the adult population, the theory is also applicable for adolescents. Using Orem's model, Dashiff, McCaleb, and Cull (2006) found that early adolescence is an appropriate time for interventions related to self-care for adolescents with diabetes. A study of self-care in adolescents with cystic fibrosis found that those who were more highly satisfied with their family and those of higher socioeconomic status were more likely to have higher universal self-care scores (Baker & Denyes, 2008).

Health Promotion

Historically, professionals have focused on an individual with an IDD in terms of the disease or condition, not the person. That approach is now changing. There now are campaigns to educate the public about "people first" language, in which the focus is on the person, not the disability. For example, the appropriate language is *a person with autism*, not *an autistic person* (Snow, 2008).

Concurrent with these changing attitudes and terminology is the concept that an individual with an IDD has strengths as well as challenges and—even more revolutionary to some—that people are all more alike than different. There is growing recognition that the traditional medical model is limited. The implementation of concepts such as family-centered care and individual/family supports has altered service delivery. The resulting life span approach focuses on supporting people with lifelong health conditions in all facets of their lives, not just their health care.

In addition to this strengths-based approach to disability, it is being recognized that health promotion is beneficial to individuals with IDD. The *Surgeon General's Call to Action to Improve the Health and Wellness of Persons with Disabilities* introduced the concept of healthy living through health promotion and disease prevention for people of all ages and abilities (DHHS, 2005). Daily healthy choices are manifested by improved body function, mental function, mental health, and the avoidance of secondary adverse consequences of inactivity and obesity.

The prevalence of overweight was 17% for adolescents age 12–19 years during the period 2001–2004 (DHHS, 2006b). (Note that health care providers do not distinguish between overweight and obesity in children.) Because obesity and disability are often interrelated, nurses can make valuable contributions by initiating activities related to healthy food choices, exercise, and inclusion of individuals with IDD into recreation activities. Resources for nurses include the Bright Futures program, a national health initiative that focuses on health promotion and disease prevention (Hagan, Shaw, & Duncan, 2008).

The promotion of daily exercise, healthy food choices, and adequate sleep is not always easy. Sleep problems may begin to surface during this age period (e.g., sleep apnea; Myers & Challam, 2008). Middle school and high school students may not understand the long-term advantages of healthy choices. Similarly, they may lack resources (e.g., equipment, clothing, transportation) or inclusionary opportunities that would make exercise enjoyable. Nurses can contact agencies, such as the National Center on Physical Activity and Disability (2008), to obtain information on adapting exercise to meet special needs.

Health promotion extends to personal safety. Safety instruction includes learning how to avoid dangerous situations that could lead to accidents, physical or emotional injury, or abuse. Many strategies are easy and inexpensive, and parents can promote safety by adapting devices to special needs. Local fire departments often conduct school assemblies to orient students to safety measures and personal protection equipment. Every student can be taught how to call 911 for emergency assistance. Parents can place a card with the home address and phone number by each phone so that emergency information can be easily accessed. Parents also should notify local emergency officials that a person with special needs resides at that address in the event of an emergency (from fire to natural disaster) in which evacuation is needed. Cardiopulmonary resuscitation and first aid are important knowledge and skill sets for all, especially those who spend time with individuals with IDD.

Health Care

During the early adolescent years, all students should participate in routine screening to identify problems early. Routine health guidance and supervision (frequently conducted by school nurses) is recommended for all students. Attention should also be given to special needs. School nurses should participate on IEP teams. Planning for transition to adult health care services begins with a written health care transition plan included in the IEP by the time the student is 16 years of age. The nurse provides background information about a particular condition, therapy, or medication. The nurse also explains how a particular disability affects the acquisition of developmental milestones, as well as the ability to learn, live independently, work, and become a member of the community.

Transition to Adult Medical Care

Every year, 750,000 adolescents with IDD or special health care needs move into adulthood (Scal & Ireland, 2005). This is a critical transition because teens with IDD or special health care needs are particularly vulnerable when medical care becomes disrupted (Lotstein, McPherson, Strickland, & Newacheck, 2005). Healthy People 2010 called for services to assist all youth with special needs to receive supports in transition to health, work, and independent living (DHHS, 2000). The importance of a smooth transition from pediatric care to adult health care has been established by consensus of major professional health care organizations: the American Academy of Pediatrics (AAP), the American Academy of Family Physicians (AAFP), and the American College of Physicians [ACP]–American Society of Internal Medicine (2002).

While pediatric care is family-centered, adult health care focuses on the individual and concentrates on specialty care, rather than care coordination around a key health care provider. Adults benefit from receiving care from a provider familiar with adult medicine (AAP, 1996). A challenge arises when one considers that many adult health care providers are simply unfamiliar and uncomfortable with providing services to individuals with special health care needs (Smith, 2007).

Nurses can assist in coordinating the complexities of health care from many different providers in varying health care systems with diversity in eligibility and payment/reimbursement guidelines. The development of nursing roles as transition service coordinators demonstrates an advanced nursing practice model in service delivery and transition from pediatric to adult health care (Betz & Redcay, 2005).

Central to health care transition is the concept of a medical home. Key components include

1. A family-centered partnership
2. A family-centered, community-based network promoting development and well-being
3. High-quality, developmentally appropriate transitions
4. Appropriate financing (AAFP, AAP, ACP, and American Osteopathic Association, 2007)

In a medical home, a child receives health care from a consistent health care provider who works in collaboration with other clinical services and community agencies to promote access and coordinated health care (AAP, 2007). Specific guidelines exist for follow-up of particular medical conditions and associated co-morbidity, such as those developed for surveillance of individuals with Down syndrome (AAP, 2001). The National Center of Medical Home Initiatives for Children with

Special Needs has prepared a training packet entitled *Every Child Deserves a Medical Home* (AAP, 2008). Training materials contain sample slides, care plans, and tools.

Transition coordination is also important because insurance coverage changes in adulthood. Most children are covered under a parent's family health insurance plan or through government-supported health care initiatives. As one enters adulthood, insurance programs may shift to the individual based on one's employment. Insurance policies may preclude payment for a preexisting condition (see Chapter 3).

Large health care systems are moving from paper to electronic records to improve health care efficiency and safety (Hillestad et al., 2005). For individuals with IDD, these electronic approaches increase accessibility and provide critical information necessary for individualized health care.

Nurses support transition by providing community referrals within a framework that is family-centered and youth-centered, coordinated, and responsive to cultural diversity. The dimensions of caring, cultural sensitivity, cultural knowledge, and cultural skills provide for delivery of culturally competent community care. Thus, unique cultural characteristics (e.g., ethnic, racial, linguistic) that each person brings to the setting can be considered in all phases of nursing care at the individual, family, and community levels. This strategy will help to reduce racial and ethnic health disparities (Kim-Godwin, Clarke, & Barton, 2001).

The school system and organizations that provide information and referral services are invaluable. Some areas have a One-Stop employment center and housing-related agencies; consumer access is facilitated when the offices are located together. Localities may have a 211 telephone information line. Each state has a council on developmental disabilities, a disability law and advocacy center, and a university center for excellence in developmental disabilities. These organizations can provide additional information on resources and connections.

However, services are not always available. Of the 11.5% of children with disabilities who have poor psychosocial adjustment, only 41.8% of them receive services. The finding that children were more likely to receive mental health services when a health professional coordinated care emphasizes the role of the nurse in care coordination and advocacy (Witt, Kasper, & Riley, 2003).

Changing Social Roles

The period from middle school into the high school years is accompanied by changes in the child–parent relationship. Prior to this time, parents made the majority of decisions about almost all facets of the child's life. Increasing age brings a desire to make one's own decisions. Students with IDD (as all adolescents) will begin to discuss their dreams for the future.

Changing social relationships may be very difficult for parents. Skär (2003) found that relationships between youth with IDD and adults were often "simultaneously helpful and supportive" yet "overprotective and dominant" (p. 635). Whereas parents' lives have often focused on meeting their children's needs, they must now realize that parental and child roles are evolving. This realization often leaves a void and a sense of rejection. Parents and other family members benefit from encouragement to support their children's independence.

During the adolescent years, relationships with authority figures also change. A desire for independence, perhaps combined with a more limited understanding of the roles of those in authority, can lead to acting-out behavior or misunderstood comments. Sometimes, negative comments directed to police officers result in arrests. Prevention strategies, education, and role playing may help youth practice more socially acceptable responses.

Leisure and Recreation

The development of self-esteem in children with IDD is important (Murphy & Elias, 2006). People with IDD have both strengths and challenges. Leisure and recreational activities, such as youth leadership programs, community sports leagues, Special Olympics, and the YMCA, are ideal venues for the development of strengths, interests, self-esteem, and good health. Recreational programs, such as Best Buddies, promote friendships between those who have an IDD and those who do not, with resulting lifetime rewards for both (see http://www.bestbuddies.org).

Decision Making

Students benefit from the development of knowledge and skills of decision making. Guided experience with progressively more complex situations assists students in differentiating right from wrong, considering alternatives, determining priorities, and making appropriate decisions. Programs in self-advocacy may help students to value their positions and advocate for themselves appropriately (Powers et al., 1996).

The development of self-care skills and long-term disability management becomes especially important in the transition to adult health care providers (Betz & Ayres, 2007). Nurses can help adolescents to identify and communicate about medical conditions and needed accommodations (Geenen, Powers, & Sells, 2003). They can also assist the youth in determining the best personal action plan.

Healthy decision making means making the right choices about health behaviors. Specifically, this includes avoiding smoking, alcohol, and illicit drug use. Patient education can focus on adverse effects of such activities and self-advocacy to say "no" to uncomfortable situations. Self-advocacy includes attending one's own IEP meeting and discussions with health care providers and other professionals. Programs, such as Partners in Policymaking (2008), teach self-advocates and their families how to apply concepts such as self-determination, family support, community living, and assistive technology.

ADOLESCENCE AND EARLY ADULTHOOD: HIGH SCHOOL TO POSTSECONDARY EDUCATION

During young adulthood, students begin to face the developmental task of finding oneself. Erikson (1963) described the stage as *intimacy versus isolation*. At this time, individuals face the task of forming healthy friendships and intimate relationships with others. Failure to do so will result in isolation.

Havighurst (1953) detailed the developmental tasks that begin in this period and extend into adulthood:

1. Selecting a mate
2. Learning to live with a significant other, partner, or spouse
3. Beginning a family

4. Raising children

5. Maintaining a residence

6. Beginning to work in an occupation/profession

7. Becoming involved in community/civic activities

8. Creating a network of friends

Developing Healthy Friendships and Intimate Relationships

Individuals want to be loved and to love in return. Initially, reciprocal relationships center on respect, trust, and turn-taking. They may later evolve into complex roles with a significant other, in intimate relationships, with sexual experiences, and even in marriage. Related topics, such as sex education and protection from sexually transmitted diseases, become important. Sexuality includes issues related to beliefs, values, body image, and social relationships (Murphy & Elias, 2006).

One must be aware of the risk of dysfunctional or abusive relationships. It is well documented that children with IDD are at increased risk for abuse (Fisher, Hodapp, & Dykens, 2008). The National Center on Child Abuse and Neglect reported that children with disabilities are 2.2 times more likely to be abused than their typically developing peers (Cross, Kaye, & Tanofsky, 1993). A meta-analysis performed by Horner-Johnson and Drum (2006) revealed that maltreatment of individuals with IDD ranged between 11.5% and 28%, compared to a rate of 1.24% for children without IDD. This abuse may be physical, sexual, or emotional.

The ability for those with IDD to establish appropriate social boundaries may help to reduce the risk of abuse. Such boundary setting is difficult for most people, but it is further complicated when youth with disabilities—especially intellectual disabilities—perceive friendship differently than others in the relationship. Skär (2003) found that adolescents with IDD view themselves as a typical member of their peer group; however, their peers view them differently. In this study, the relationships between youth with IDD and their peers either did not exist or were "markedly defective" (p. 635). Youth, especially some with intellectual disabilities, may perceive that a helping or friendly person is their "best friend" or they may interpret a potentially sexually abusive situation as someone loving them. Thus, all adults who interface with a middle or high school student must promote safe and healthy relationships and realistic interpretations of the overtures from others.

Peer pressure and abuse involving the threat of violence, actual violence, sexual attack, or bullying are issues of particular concern. Students should be taught about appropriate behaviors and the recognition of inappropriate situations, including unwanted physical, verbal, or sexual advances. Students should be given a safe environment for honest and frank dialogue when they have questions about what is right or wrong.

Youth should also be cautioned about potentially high-risk behaviors and their consequences. This includes the use of alcohol and illicit drugs, as well as reckless, delinquent, and criminal behaviors. Frequently, individuals with disabilities—especially intellectual disabilities—are enticed into risky or illegal behaviors without understanding the full potential consequences. Participation in such risky behaviors could result in the development of physical and/or emotional problems or social problems, such as incarceration for criminal acts.

Self-Directed Choices

Self-advocacy becomes increasingly important as the adolescent moves closer to early adulthood. Earlier self-advocacy and self-determination efforts can be further supported through informal means in the family and at school. They can be further developed through person-centered training and formalized training sessions. At this time, self-advocacy can extend to decisions about postsecondary educational options, housing, and employment (Betz & Nehring, 2007).

Postsecondary Educational Options

The federal government has committed supports so students with disabilities can complete high school and be prepared for postsecondary education or employment (U.S. Department of Education, 2001). Postsecondary institutions receiving federal funding must comply with the Rehabilitation Act of 1973 (PL 93-112) and Titles II and/or III of the Americans with Disabilities Act (PL 101-336). The National Longitudinal Transition Study (NLTS) in 1987 and the NLTS-2 in 2003 examined the experiences of postsecondary students with IDD. A comparison of the two studies found significant increases in enrollment in postsecondary educational programs, employment, and participation in organized community groups (Wagner, Newman, Cameto, & Levine, 2005).

In 2003–2004, 11% of undergraduates reported a disability. Most commonly, students attending colleges and universities identified their disability as an orthopedic condition (25%), mental illness or depression (22%), or health impairment (17%) (U.S. Department of Education, 2006). Colleges and universities have formal offices, known by various titles such as Disabled Students Services, to support students with disabilities. These offices help students to receive the needed disability and health-related accommodations to be successful in the postsecondary setting. Additionally, the offices guide university faculty in making accommodations so that the student's educational experience can be successful and enjoyable.

In the last few years, there has been growing concern about the unmet educational needs of those with intellectual disabilities. Today, a growing number of community colleges and universities are offering pilot programs for those with intellectual disabilities. Programs fall into three categories: 1) substantially separate; 2) mixed; or 3) inclusive, individual support (Hart, Mele-McCarthy, Pasternack, Zimbrich, & Parker, 2004). Some programs combine self-help and functional training with specially developed content. Other programs provide inclusive options in which students with intellectual disabilities participate in general classroom activities, supported by a peer volunteer or paid support person. Students are encouraged to participate in social and group activities. Most programs culminate in a certificate rather than a college diploma. Graduates are generally prepared to enter the work force. For more information about postsecondary educational programs for students with intellectual disabilities, go to http://www.think college.net.

Life After Formal Education

Knowledge and experience from formal educational programs help a student prepare for life as an adult. Ultimately, educational programs can contribute to a life of increased independence, productivity, and integration into the community. Being a part of the community means assumption of responsibility to give back to society. Many people with disabilities say they also want to contribute, not just be the object of someone else's good deeds. An ideal way to get involved in the community, have rewarding interactions, make friends, and gain productive skills is through volunteerism. Programs such as AmeriCorps offer inclusive volunteer opportunities for youth and adults (Corporation for National and Community Service, 2009; see also Chapter 3). Volunteer experiences provide youth with opportunities to acquire job skills. Documentation of these skills is helpful when the individual seeks job training possibilities through programs such as those offered by state departments of vocational rehabilitation.

Housing

Decisions about housing are often determined by the individual's strengths and needs for support, family finances, individual financial supports, and available community options. Based on the NLTS-2, 75% of youth with disabilities live in the family home (Wagner et al., 2005).

Living at home or with siblings allows for individualized supports based on the individual's needs. This option is good for individuals who are not yet interested or able to live more independently. However, this arrangement tends to retain family/child social relationships and increase dependency roles.

Living with others with support is an evolution of the former group home experience. Most commonly, individuals with IDD, usually three or fewer, live together in a shared house or apartment, often with paid staff members providing intermittent or constant supports. This is a good option if the family is unable or unwilling to share living arrangements or if the individual wants to be more independent but still needs supports. Living in one's own home with supports provides options for someone with more developed independent living skills. Support personnel may be involved for a limited time each day or may assist with specific tasks such as cooking, bathing, or medical procedures that are done on a daily basis (Benjamin, 2001).

Preparation for Work

When students with all types of disabilities were surveyed in the NLTS-2, the number participating in employment was 44%. However, individuals with chronic health problems did not share improved high school completion or employment rates (Wagner et al., 2005). Nurses have an important role in encouraging students with health challenges to complete high school and assure employment-related goals on the IEP. The Healthy and Ready to Work web site provides information and toolkits in areas such as quality care, mental health, school-based services, and transition services (National Resource Center, 2008).

Completion of Transition to Adult Health Care

By age 18, transitional health care plans should have been completed. Students should have access to adult medical homes, have health insurance or government-supported health care, and participate in transportation and community services.

Work environments may be modified to meet health care needs. Principles of universal design can make access easier for all with temporary or long-term disabilities. Many times, the solutions require only creativity and perspective, not necessarily expensive modifications.

ADULTHOOD: ADULT TO AGING

In the 2000 Census, 33,153,211 individuals age 16–64 years (17.6% of the population) reported a disability (U.S. Department of Commerce [DOC], 2003). That group reported the following distribution of disabilities:

1. Employment disability (10.9%)
2. Physical disability (6.4%)
3. Difficulty going outside the home (6.4%)
4. Mental disability (3.7%)
5. Self-care difficulty (1.9%)
6. Sensory disability (1.9%)

As individuals with disabilities progress into middle adulthood, they experience the *generativity versus stagnation* stage described by Erickson (1963). Individuals in this stage want to help members of the younger generation to grow and develop their own productive lives. The converse can be reflected in personal dissatisfaction and frustration of things they did not accomplish. This stage may not be reached by all individuals with IDD depending on the severity of the intellectual disability.

Physical/Mental Health Challenges

Healthy People 2010 identified the 10 top issues affecting the health status of Americans: health care access, immunizations, overweight and obesity, physical activity, tobacco use, mental health, substance use, sexual behavior, injury, and environmental quality (DHHS, 2000). Data have shown that people with IDD are less likely to have health insurance and participate in physical activity than their typically developing peers. Individuals with IDD are also more likely to be obese and smoke (DHHS, 2006b).

For these reasons, health promotion is important for adults with IDD. Appropriate diet, regular exercise (cardiovascular, flexibility, and strength training), and sleep contribute to healthy lifestyles and the avoidance of chronic disease. However, performing health promotion activities may be a challenge. Ruffing-Rahal has developed a nursing health promotion model that focuses on self-care skills, emotional and spiritual integration, and social integration (Ruffing-Rahal, 2007). Unfortunately, there are limited health education materials adapted to meet the special needs of those with disabilities. Similarly, there are limitations in adaptive equipment or even accessible locations for exercise for adults with IDD. Resources and information about adaptive equipment for people with IDD can be obtained from the National Center on Physical Activity and Disability (2008).

Individuals with disabilities are prone to all the ailments associated with gradual aging in individuals with typical development. Diabetes, cancer, and cardiovascular disease are major sources of mortality. Indeed, individuals with IDD overall report a worse health status than their peers (Harris, Hendershot, & Stapleton, 2005).

Governmental and professional organizations provide guidelines to reduce morbidity and mortality. The American Cancer Society detailed guidelines for the early detection of breast, colon and rectal, cervical, endometrial, and prostate cancer (American Cancer Society, 2008). The National Institutes of Health provided guidelines for asthma, high blood cholesterol, high blood pressure, overweight and obesity, and sickle cell (DHHS, 2008). The American Heart Association detailed guidelines for blood pressure readings (American Heart Association, 2008). The Centers for Disease Control and Prevention provided recommendations for adult immunization schedules (DHHS, 2007).

In addition to the health concerns of all adults, individuals with IDD are often at risk for more specific co-occurring conditions as part of the normal course of the condition. For example, individuals with Down syndrome are at increased risk for disordered breathing, obesity, and hypothyroidism (Dykens, 2007). Individuals with Down syndrome are also more likely to develop neuropathological changes typical of Alzheimer disease by their fifth decade (Roizen & Patterson, 2003).

Health care for individuals with IDD includes both physical and mental components. In the past, health care providers attributed psychiatric symptoms in people with intellectual disabilities as part of the intellectual disability (Dykens & Hodapp, 2001). This tendency is known as *diagnostic overshadowing* (Reiss, Levitan, & Szyszko, 1982). Providers are beginning to realize that multiple conditions can be present in one individual at the same time. Adults with a disability are four times more likely to develop a mental illness (Rush, Bowman, Eidman, Toole, & Mortenson, 2004). In addition, there is the growing recognition that behavioral issues may be the result of boredom, or lack of meaningful work or activities, brought on by lack of services. Sometimes it is hard to separate the frustrations from the disability (see Chapter 14).

Finding appropriate services is a major challenge for many adults with IDD. Even when services are obtained, individuals with IDD may find it difficult to identify and/or articulate their concerns. They may have difficulty in becoming active participants in the intervention process due to cognitive or physical disabilities. They may also find it difficult to access necessary supplies and/or equipment for self-care or to locate consistent caregivers to provide long-term needs. Finding appropriate services is even more difficult if the adult is one of the many with limited financial resources or one whose care is limited by governmental benefits and related rules and regulations.

Access to appropriate community-based health care is critical when the individual has both an IDD and a psychiatric condition. Although discrimination is illegal, many individuals with IDD find facilities unwilling to admit someone with a co-occurring morbidity. Generally, reasons relate to the perceived inability of the facility to deal with special needs. More than likely, it is a lack of knowledge and preparation regarding how to make necessary accommodations (Betz & Nehring, 2007).

Health insurance is a related challenge. Many health care plans are geared to employment, which is a problem if one is not employed. Privately obtained insurance is often difficult to obtain when pre-existing conditions exist and may be prohibitively expensive. Nurses can become active in policy-making roles by sharing information with legislators and encouraging policy development that promotes access to needed specific screening, diagnosis, treatment, and rehabilitation services.

Societal Changes

Adults with IDD have experienced dramatic social changes. In the 1970s, many individuals with an IDD lived in an institution for their entire lives. Today, individuals are supported in increasingly inclusive community life. With the realization that adults have strengths, there is more emphasis on meaningful involvement. There is also increasing realization that individuals with IDD want and deserve to have a choice in decisions that affect their lives. Thus, new models of service delivery continue to evolve (Bradley, 1994).

Person-centered funding, goal setting and decision making by the individual, the development of self-advocacy skills, and the use of natural supports all contribute to increasing control over one's future. Person-centered planning acknowledges that the individual and significant others should drive the decisions made about one's life. It promotes services that are based on an individual's vision and desires. Person-centered planning becomes increasingly important as individuals with IDD age, since aging parents may not always be able to support their child. Many individuals with IDD have not developed concrete plans for care and services for the future (Heller & Caldwell, 2006). Nurses are frequently involved in conducting seminars about planning for the future, using tools such as Making Action Plans (Falvey, Forest, Pearpoint, & Rosenberg, 1997) and Planning Alternative Tomorrows with Hope (Pearpoint, O'Brien, & Forest, 1993).

Planning can include in-depth assessments of the individual's and family's needs across a variety of variables (e.g., living arrangements, future vocational and recreational desires, lifestyle choices, financial support, legal issues such as conservatorship and guardianship). This data is the basis for the identification of a nursing diagnosis and intervention plan. Family futures-planning intervention based on a model of peer support has proven to be very effective in reducing perceived caregiver burden and increasing person-centered decision making (Heller & Caldwell, 2006).

Social Relationships

Interpersonal relationships continue to have great importance in adulthood. However, for many, there are insufficient opportunities to meet and relate to others as one ages. Structured day programs and group living facilities, as well as community-sponsored recreation and social activities, provide some opportunities. But, for many, social relationships are limited to family and neighbors. Adults with intellectual disabilities receive much of their support from professionals (Lunsky & Benson, 2001).

Similarly, individuals with physical disabilities often face environmental barriers, such as transportation challenges, that limit social interaction. Nurses can promote opportunities for social gatherings, facilitation of agencies promoting friendships and social opportunities, and newer forms of social networking using the Internet. Participation in the arts or in a senior citizen center promotes positive self-concepts and opportunities for social interactions. Participation in community activities, such as a faith-based organization, a volunteer activity, or a more informal social group, helps consumers to gain acceptance and a sense of belonging (Harlan-Simmons, Holtz, Todd, & Mooney, 2001).

For those who are interested in having children, health care professionals can assess the individual situation and assist the person in determining the probability of a successful pregnancy. For some, physical and anatomical diversity may make conceiving and/or carrying a child more difficult. Nurses can also be helpful in modifying positioning for gynecological or obstetrical examinations (Simpson & Lankasky, 2001). Adults should also be knowledgeable about safe sex and methods of preventing disease.

Adults with disabilities are at risk for abuse, especially those with intellectual disabilities (Ammerman, Hersen, Van Hasselt, Lubetsky, & Sieck, 1994). This abuse may be sexual, emotional, physical, or financial. Education about setting limits, being comfortable with saying "no" in uncomfortable situations, and promoting self-advocacy are appropriate nursing interventions.

Jobs

Historically, most adults with an IDD have not had gainful employment. In the 2000 census, there were 18.6 million people age 16–64 years with all types of disabilities who were employed (DOC, 2003). However, many people with disabilities remain unemployed because they simply cannot find employment. Barriers to employment include the following (Loprest & Magg, 2001):

1.   No appropriate jobs available (52%)

2.   Family responsibilities (34%)

3.   Lack of transportation (29%)

4.   No appropriate information about jobs (23%)

5.   Inadequate training (21.6%)

6.   Fear of losing health insurance or Medicaid (20.1%)

7.   Discouraged from working by family and friends (14%)

Employers and publicly funded programs for individuals with IDD are beginning to recognize the social and financial advantages that work provides to those who are able. Postsecondary educational options, volunteerism, and supported employment are all slowly contributing to the changing employment scene. Increasingly, organizations are helping to focus on the development of job skills, dependability in job-related functions, and the social skills to be successful. The most common means for promoting employment are workplace accommodations, including accessible parking, elevators, adaptations to workstations, modified work hours or job responsibilities, physical accommodations such as handrails, and job coaches (Loprest & Magg, 2001).

Housing

Today, 60% of adults with disabilities live with their parents in a family setting (Hodapp & Urbano, 2007). However, many face increasing challenges as their own parents begin to age. Many aging individuals with disabilities do not receive governmental or community resources until their own parents need outside supports. Nurses can assist individuals and families in obtaining resources for personal care services, home health care, or assistive technology. Mobility devices and communication equipment, ramps, and safety bars and alerts can promote independence and allow individuals to live in their homes for a longer period of time. Nurses can assist individuals and family in determining appropriate housing by assessing personal and financial resources, community supports, transportation options to health care, needed physical accommodations, maintenance issues, and legal considerations.

Transportation

Even when one finds a suitable job or home, individuals with physical disabilities experience difficulty finding transportation to and from the job, health care, or recreational activities (Ho, Kroll, Kehn, Anderson, & Pearson, 2007). Public transportation is not available in all areas or at all times of the day and night. Not all transportation is accessible, and even accessible transportation can be unreliable. Adaptive driving equipment can meet these challenges for some.

Leisure and Recreation

Organized community activity programs are often filled with a variety of leisure activities such as arts and crafts sessions or exercise classes. Nurses can promote the inclusion of individuals with IDD in organizational programming. Nurses can also monitor the extent to which consumers are involved in community activities that reflect their needs, interests, preferences, and abilities. Nurses working in community settings that include exercise programs can ensure that activities are appropriate for one's physical abilities and assist agency personnel in making necessary modifications to promote optimal activity and enjoyment.

One resource for leisure and recreation is faith-based communities. While many faith-based organizations make accommodations for those who wear hearing aids, need sound amplification, or use wheelchairs, most do not go further. Simple approaches are helpful in promoting inclusion. Examples include having a support person provide transportation, providing peer support during services, and having individualized teaching sessions to assist an individual in preparing for rituals such as a wedding or a funeral.

Emergency Preparedness

Tragic events such as fires, flooding, and hurricanes take a disproportionate toll on individuals with IDD and those who are aging. The consequences are even more serious for individuals with IDD who are also aging, due to co-occurring morbidities or difficulty getting medicines after the disaster (Fordyce, Kenny, & Oettinger, 2006).

In 2006, after a series of natural disasters and their aftermaths, federal and state governmental officials realized that those with IDD needed to be included more fully in emergency preparation and response plans. Since that time, state governments have begun to include individuals with IDD on state planning committees and address the needs of individuals with IDD in training for first responders. Individuals with IDD, with the support of family members and support personnel, must also assume responsibility for emergency preparation and response plans that include accommodations for their individual needs. Specifically, this includes provision of supplies, medications, and backup for electrical equipment for a period of up to 2 weeks. Family members and/or support personnel should be prepared to meet any unusual situations with little or no assistance from governmental personnel.

Nurses can promote state and local planning that includes individuals with IDD. They can also facilitate communication among consumers, governmental officials, and emergency responders prior to a disaster. Such collaboration breaks down turf issues and communication barriers.

Coping with Loss

Loss is a part of the human experience. However, individuals with IDD experience more potential of loss, often with fewer coping strategies. Loss can result from a disability, an illness, or a surgery. It can also result from transitions in support staff, loss of a job, divorce, moving, or death of a pet, friend, coworker, or parent. The impact is especially intense when the loss is sudden. The death of a parent or family member is probably the most overwhelming loss.

Successful strategies for supporting the grieving individual include being honest about the death in terms that the individual can understand. Individuals benefit from the option of participating in the funeral or other religious or spiritual ritual. The individual can be encouraged to discuss the person who has died or participate in nonverbal activities, such as painting a picture of the deceased. Individual and/or group counseling can provide support during this process and has been found to improve symptoms of depression in individuals with IDD (Stoddart, Burke, & Temple, 2002).

AGING AND DYING

Developmentally, older individuals are in the final stage described by Erickson (1963), known as *integrity versus despair*. During this period, individuals evaluate life accomplishments. If they are content with their life, they are satisfied. If they feel they have not accomplished their goals, they experience dissatisfaction.

The estimated number of individuals with disabilities age 60 and older is 710,000 (Hodapp & Urbano, 2007). The 2000 U.S. Census reported disability in 43% of people age 65 and older (DOC, 2003). Individuals reported the following distribution of disabilities:

1. Physical disability (30.7%)
2. Difficulty going outside the home (23%)
3. Sensory disability (13.2%)
4. Self-care difficulty (11.4%)
5. Mental disability (11.4%)

Physical Concerns

Aging individuals with IDD experience age-related disorders in a similar pattern to their typically developing peers. Frequent disorders include cardiovascular disease, respiratory problems, and neoplastic disease (Janicki, Dalton, Henderson, & Davidson, 1999). The onset and severity of age-related physical difficulties and related secondary conditions can be positively affected by health promotion routines (Janicki et al., 1999).

While the incidence and prevalence of medical concerns increase with age, so do the complexities. Co-occurring morbidity means the potential treatment for one condition could influence the other condition. Assessments of functional capacity guide interventions related to health promotion, management of health concerns, and developmental issues (Service & Hahn, 2003).

Disorders related to aging often result in decreased functional ability. Those who are 60 years of age and older may find supports through the Older Americans Act of 1965 (PL 89-73). This legislation funds comprehensive support service, such as home meal delivery, homemaker services, nutritional support, and care coordination. Statewide programs in aging and disabilities and area agencies on aging can assist in identifying resources.

Mental and Emotional Health

Aging individuals are at risk for mental and emotional problems, especially loneliness, depression, and isolation. Memory problems increase. Certain disabilities are associated with particular sequelae. For example, individuals with Down syndrome are at risk for developing dementia (Seltzer, Heller, & Krauss, 2004). Thus, physical and mental/emotional assessment is critical in planning comprehensive heath care.

Individuals who are aging are particularly vulnerable to elder abuse and neglect and misappropriation of funds by others. Estimates are that between 1 and 2 million Americans are abused, neglected, or exploited by someone they thought would provide care or protection (National Research Center, 2003). Financial exploitation is believed to affect at least 5 million individuals yearly (Waski, 2000). These numbers are believed to be even higher in individuals with IDD.

Social and Recreational Activities

As people age, their circles of friends, social interactions, and leisure/recreational activities often decrease. Peers often face similar mobility and transportation problems, so interaction is difficult. Because many elders are not comfortable with or cannot afford computers, technology's role in reducing barriers is not as evident as with younger persons.

Coping with Loss

The potential for loss increases with age. Loss of friends and family is more likely to increase. New types of loss may arise: personal dignity, support personnel, and income potential. Losses have ripple effects on quality of life. Decreased independence may be reflected in an out-of-home placement or a move to a family setting, long-term care facility, or hospice.

Historically, professionals felt that individuals with an intellectual disability did not understand the finality of death nor experience grieving with a death (Botsford, 2000). However, a person does not have to be able to conceptualize death to feel its results (Dodd, Dowling, & Hollins, 2005). Adults with moderate to severe intellectual disabilities experience grief, sometimes lasting for a year or more, and understand that death is final (Harper & Wadsworth, 1993). Developmental stage and intellectual level influence the expression—not the feeling—of loss or grief (Botsford, 2000).

Approaching Dying

Fear of dying, or at least a concern about personal demise, is shared by most people. Nurses can play a valuable role in death education. Experiences in the life and death cycle of living things, as well as supported participation in rituals such as funerals, can help people prepare for death.

Futures planning, including wills, trusts, financial and funeral arrangements, and plans for distribution of assets, is important for individuals and families to consider. Just as person-centered decision making is important earlier in life, it is also important as one approaches dying (Kingsbury, 2005). Nurses can support those approaching dying by focusing on person-centered decision making, dignity, and physical/emotional comfort. Earlier roles related to assessment, problem identification, and empirically-based interventions are appropriate at this life transition, as is education of the individual, family, and collaborating personnel. At this stage, content may focus on promotion of comfort, signs of impending physical decline, and symptoms of imminent death. Nurses may also be involved in comfort to the family members following death, as well as custodial and legal concerns. Through it all, recognition of the value of the individual and the contribution that person made to life is important.

CONCLUSION

Life has changed dramatically for individuals with IDD since the 1970s. Today, individuals with an IDD have the potential for greater life expectancy and possible life experiences that could never have been conceived in an earlier time. Nurses are in a pivotal position to support these improvements in health and quality of life. Nurses have critical roles in assessment, diagnosis, nursing intervention, and individual and family supports throughout the life span. A nurse's appreciation for the strengths and challenges experienced by a person with IDD can contribute greatly to an enhanced sense of what is possible. Technical support in nursing assessment and procedures, family support and referral to community agencies, and coordination of care at the systems level all take advantage of the nurse's broad background and extensive knowledge and skills.

REFERENCES

American Academy of Pediatrics. (1996). Transition of care provided for adolescents with special health care needs. *Pediatrics, 98,* 1203–1206.

American Academy of Pediatrics. (2001). Health supervision for children with Down syndrome. *Pediatrics, 107,* 442–449.

American Academy of Pediatrics. (2007). Role of the medical home in family-centered early intervention services. *Pediatrics, 120,* 1153–1158.

American Academy of Pediatrics. (2008). *Every child deserves a medical home.* Retrieved November 24, 2008, from http://www.medicalhomeinfo.org/training/materials/April2004Curriculum/Transitions/Transitions%20Participant.doc.

American Academy of Pediatrics, American Academy of Family Physicians, & American College of Physicians–American Society of Internal Medicine. (2002). A consensus statement on health care transitions for young adults with special health care needs. *Pediatrics, 110,* 1304–1306.

American Academy of Family Physicians, American Academy of Pediatrics, American College of Physicians, & American Osteopathic Association. (2007). *Joint principles of the patient-centered medical home.* Retrieved November 3, 2008, from http://www.medicalhomeinfo.org/Joint%20Statement.pdf.

American Association on Intellectual and Developmental Disabilities. (2008). *Fact sheet on transition: What led to the realization of the need for transition?* Retrieved November 3, 2008, from http://www.aaidd.org/content_197.cfm?navID=12.

American Cancer Society. (2008). *American Cancer Society guidelines for the early detection of cancer.* Retrieved November 3, 2008, from http://www.cancer.org/docroot/PED/content/PED_2_3X_ACS_Cancer_Detection_Guidelines_36.asp?sitearea=PED.

American Heart Association. (2008). *Home monitoring of high blood pressure.* Retrieved November 25, 2008, from http://www.americanheart.org/presenter.jhtml?identifier=576.

Americans with Disabilities Act of 1990, PL 101-336, 42 U.S.C.A. §§ 12101 *et seq.*

Ammerman, R.T., Hersen, M., Van Hasselt, V.B., Lubetsky, M.J., & Sieck, W.R. (1994). Maltreatment in psychiatrically hospitalized children and adolescents with developmental disabilities: Prevalence and correlates. *Journal of the American Academy of Child and Adolescent Psychiatry, 33,* 567–576.

Baker, L.K., & Denyes, M.J. (2008). Predictors of self-care in adolescents with cystic fibrosis: A test of Orem's theories of self-care and self-care deficit. *Journal of Pediatric Nursing, 23,* 37–48.

Benjamin, A.E. (2001). Consumer-driven services at home: A new model for persons with disabilities. *Health Affairs, 20,* 80–95.

Betz, C.L., & Ayres, L. (2007). Promoting health care: Self care and long-term disability management. In C.L. Betz & W.M. Nehring (Eds.), *Promoting health care transitions for adolescents with special health care needs and disabilities* (p. 49–78). Baltimore: Paul H. Brookes Publishing Co.

Betz, C.L., & Nehring, W.M. (2007). *Promoting health care transition planning for adolescents with special health care needs and disabilities.* Baltimore: Paul H. Brookes Publishing Co.

Betz, C.L., & Redcay, G. (2005). Dimensions of the transition service coordinator role. *Journal for Specialists in Pediatric Nursing, 10,* 49–59.

Betz, C.L., & Sowden, L.A. (2008). *Mosby's pediatric nursing reference* (6th ed.). St. Louis: Mosby Elsevier.

Botsford, A.L. (2000). Integrating end of life care into services for people with an intellectual disability. *Social Work in Health Care, 31,* 35–48.

Bradley, V.J. (1994). Evolution of a new service paradigm. In V. Bradley, J. Ashbaugh, & B. Blaney, (Eds.), *Creating individual supports for people with developmental disabilities* (p. 11–32). Baltimore: Paul H. Brookes Publishing Co.

Corporation for National and Community Service. (2009). *Americorps.* Retrieved on January 21, 2009, from http://www.americorps.org/.

Cross, S., Kaye, E., & Tanofsky, A. (1993). *A report on the maltreatment of children with disabilities*. Washington, DC: National Center on Child Abuse and Neglect.

Dashiff, C., McCaleb, A., & Cull, V. (2006). Self care of young adolescents with Type 1 diabetes. *Journal of Pediatric Nursing, 21*, 222–232.

Dodd, P., Dowling, S., & Hollins, S. (2005). A review of the emotional, psychiatric and behavioural responses to bereavement in people with intellectual disabilities. *Journal of Intellectual Disability Research, 49*, 537–543.

Dykens, E.M. (2007). Psychiatric and behavioral disorders in persons with Down syndrome. *Mental Retardation and Developmental Disabilities Research Reviews, 13*, 272–278.

Dykens, E.M., & Hodapp, R.M. (2001). Research in mental retardation: Toward an etiologic approach. *Journal of Child Psychology and Psychiatry, 42*, 49–71.

Erickson, E.H. (1963). *Childhood and society*. New York: W.W. Norton.

Falvey, M., Forest, M., Pearpoint, J., & Rosenberg, R. (1997). *All my life's a circle: Using the tools: Circles, MAPS and PATHS*. Toronto: Inclusion Press International.

Fisher, M., Hodapp, R.M., & Dykens, E.M. (2008). Child abuse among children with disabilities: What we know and what we need to know. *Institutional Review of Research in Mental Retardation, 35*, 251–289.

Fordyce, C., Kenny, D., & Oettinger, E. (2006). *Just in case: Emergency readiness for older adults and caregivers*. Dayton, OH: Caresource Healthcare Communications.

Geenen, S.J., Powers, L.E., & Sells, W. (2003). Understanding the role of health care providers during the transition of adolescents with disabilities and special health care needs. *Journal of Adolescent Health, 32*, 225–233.

Hagan, J., Shaw, J., & Duncan, P. (2008). *Bright futures guidelines for health supervision of infants, children and adolescents* (3rd ed.). Elk Grove Village, IL: American Academy of Pediatrics.

Harlan-Simmons, J.E., Holtz, P., Todd, J., & Mooney, M.F. (2001). Building social relationships through valued roles: Three older adults and the community membership project. *Mental Retardation, 39*, 171–180.

Harper, D., & Wadsworth, J. (1993). Grief in adults with mental retardation: Preliminary findings. *Research in Developmental Disabilities, 14*, 313–330.

Harris, B.H., Hendershot, G., & Stapleton, D.C. (2005). *A guide to disability statistics from the National Health Interview Survey*. Ithaca, NY: Rehabilitation Research and Training Center on Disability Demographics and Statistics, Cornell University.

Hart, D., Mele-McCarthy, J., Pasternack, R., Zimbrich, K., & Parker, D.R. (2004). Community college: A pathway to success for youth with learning, cognitive, and intellectual disabilities in secondary settings. *Education and Training in Developmental Disabilities, 39*, 54–66.

Havighurst, R.J. (1953). *Human development and education*. New York: Longman, Green.

Heller, T., & Caldwell, J. (2006). Supporting aging caretakers and adults with developmental disabilities in future planning. *Mental Retardation, 44*, 189–202.

Hillestad, R., Bigelow, J., Bower, A., Girosi, F., Meili, R., Scoville, R., et al. (2005). Can electronic medical record systems transform health care? Potential health benefits, savings, and costs. *Health Affairs, 24*, 1103–1117.

Ho, P., Kroll, T., Kehn, M., Anderson, P., & Pearson, K. (2007). Health and housing among low-income adults with physical disabilities. *Journal of Health Care for the Poor and Underserved, 18*, 902–915.

Hodapp, R.M., & Urbano, R.C. (2007). Adult siblings of individuals with Down syndrome versus with autism: Findings from a large-scale US Survey. *Journal of Intellectual Disability Research, 51*, 1018–1029.

Horner-Johnson, W., & Drum, C.E. (2006). Prevalence of maltreatment of people with intellectual disabilities: A review of the recently published research. *Mental Retardation and Developmental Disabilities, 12*, 57–69.

Janicki, M.P., Dalton, A.J., Henderson, C.M., & Davidson, P.W. (1999). Mortality and morbidity among older adults with intellectual disability: Health services considerations. *Disability and Rehabilitation, 21,* 284–294.

Kim-Godwin, Y.S., Clarke, P.N., & Barton, L. (2001). A model for the delivery of culturally competent community care. *Journal of Advanced Nursing, 35,* 918–925.

Kingsbury, L.A. (2005). Person-centered planning and communication of end-of-life wishes with people who have developmental disabilities. *Journal of Religion, Disability & Health, 9,* 81–90.

Loprest, P., & Magg, E. (2001). *Barriers and supports for work among adults with disabilities: Results from the NHIS-D.* Washington, DC: The Urban Institute.

Lotstein, D.S., McPherson, M., Strickland, B., & Newacheck, P.W. (2005). Transition planning for youth with special health care needs: Results from the national survey of children with special health care needs. *Pediatrics, 115,* 1562–1568.

Lunsky, Y., & Benson, B.A. (2001). Association between perceived social support and strain, and positive and negative outcome for adults with mild intellectual disability. *Journal of Intellectual Disability Research, 45,* 106–114.

Murphy, N.A., & Elias, E.R. (2006). Sexuality of children and adolescents with developmental disabilities. *Pediatrics, 118,* 398–403.

Myers, S.M., & Challam, T.D. (2008). Psychopharmacology: An approach to management in autism and intellectual disabilities. In P.J. Accardo (Ed.), *Capute & Accardo's neurodevelopmental disabilities in infancy and childhood* (3rd ed., Vol. 2, pp. 577–613). Baltimore: Paul H. Brookes Publishing Co.

National Center on Physical Activity and Disability. (2008). *Exercise and fitness.* Retrieved November 3, 2008, from http://NCPAD.org/exercise.

National Research Center. (2003). *Exploitation in an aging America.* Washington, DC: Author.

National Resource Center. (2008). *Tools and checklists.* Retrieved May 7, 2008, from http://www.hrtw.org/tools/check.html.

Older Americans Act of 1965, PL 89-73, 42 U.S.C. §§ 3001 *et seq.*

Orem, D.E. (1995). *Nursing: Concepts of practice.* St. Louis: Mosby-Year Book.

Partners in Policy Making. (2008). *Partners in policymaking.* Retrieved November 3, 2008, from http://www.partnersinpolicymaking.com/.

Pearpoint, J., O'Brien, J., & Forest, M. (1993). *PATH: A workbook for planning positive possible futures.* Toronto: Inclusion Press International.

Piaget, J. (1972). *The psychology of the child.* New York: Basic Books.

Piaget, J. (1976). *The psychology of intelligence.* Towota, NJ: Littlefield, Adams.

Piaget, J. (1990). *The child's conception of the world.* New York: Littlefield, Adams.

Powers, L., Sowers, J., Turner, A., Nesbitt, M., Knowles, E., & Ellison, R. (1996). Take charge: A model for promoting self-determination among adolescents with challenges. In D. Sands & M. Wehmeyer (Eds.), *Self-determination across the life span: Independence and choice for people with disabilities* (pp. 291–322). Baltimore: Paul H. Brookes Publishing Co.

Rehabilitation Act of 1973, PL 93-112, 29 U.S.C.§§ 701 *et seq.*

Reiss, S., Levitan, G.W., & Szyszko, J. (1982). Emotional disturbance and mental retardation: Diagnostic overshadowing. *American Journal of Mental Deficiency, 86,* 567–574.

Roizen, N., & Patterson, D. (2003). Down's syndrome. *The Lancet, 361,* 1281–1289.

Ruffing-Rahal, M. (2007). Rationale and design for health promotion with older adults. *Public Health Nursing, 8,* 258–263.

Rush, K.S., Bowman, L.G., Eidman, S.L., Toole, L.M., & Mortenson, B.P. (2004). Assessing psychopathology in individuals with developmental disabilities. *Behavior Modification, 28,* 621–637.

Scal, P., & Ireland, M. (2005). Addressing transition to adult health care for adolescents with special health care needs. *Pediatrics, 115,* 1607–1612.

Seltzer, M.M., Heller, T., & Krauss, M.W. (2004). Introduction to the special issue on aging. *American Journal on Mental Retardation, 109,* 81–82.

Service, K.P., & Hahn, J.E. (2003). Issues in aging: The role of the nurse in the care of older people with intellectual and developmental disabilities. *Nursing Clinics North America, 38,* 291–312.

Siddiqi, S.U., Van Dyke, D.C., Donohoue, P., & McBrien, D.M. (1999). Premature sexual development in individuals with neurodevelopmental disabilities. *Developmental Medicine & Child Neurology, 41,* 392–395.

Simpson, K.M., & Lankasky, K. (2001). *Table manners and beyond: The gynecological exam for women with developmental disabilities and other functional limitations.* Retrieved November 3, 2008, from http://www.bhawd.org/sitefiles/TblMrs/cover.html.

Skär, L. (2003). Peer and adult relationships of adolescents with disabilities. *Journal of Adolescence, 26,* 635–649.

Smith, K. (2007). Care coordination. In C.L. Betz & W.M. Nehring (Eds.), *Promoting health care transitions for adolescents with special health care needs and disabilities* (pp. 255–267). Baltimore: Paul H. Brookes Publishing Co.

Snow, K. (2008). *People first language.* Retrieved November 24, 2008, from http://ftp.disabilityisnatural.com/documents/PFL8.pdf.

Stoddart, K.P., Burke, L., & Temple, V. (2002). Outcome evaluation of bereavement groups for adults with intellectual disabilities. *Journal of Applied Research in Intellectual Disabilities, 15,* 28–35.

U.S. Department of Commerce. (2003). *United States Census 2000: Disability status: 2000.* Retrieved November 3, 2008, from http://www.census.gov/prod/cen2000/doc/sf3.pdf.

U.S. Department of Education. (2001). *Government Performance and Report Act (GPRA) performance report FY 2000 and FY 2002 performance plan.* Washington, DC: Author.

U.S. Department of Education. (2006). *Profile of undergraduates in U.S. post secondary education institutions: 2003–2004.* Washington, DC: U.S. Government Printing Office.

U.S. Department of Health and Human Services. (2000). *Healthy people 2010: Understanding and improving health and objectives for improving health.* Washington, DC: U.S. Government Printing Office.

U.S. Department of Health and Human Services. (2005). *The Surgeon General's call to action to improve the health and wellness of persons with disabilities.* Washington, DC: U.S. Government Printing Office.

U.S. Department of Health and Human Services (2006a). *The national survey of children with special health care needs chartbook 2005–2006.* Rockville, MD: Author.

U.S. Department of Health and Human Services (2006b). *Disability and health: Leading health indicators data from Healthy People 2010.* Retrieved November 3, 2008, from http://www.cdc.gov/ncbddd/dh/hplhidata.htm.

U.S. Department of Health and Human Services. (2007). Recommended adult immunization schedule, United States, October 2007–September 2008. *Morbidity and Mortality Weekly Report, 56,* Q1–Q4.

U.S. Department of Health and Human Services (2008). *Current clinical practice guidelines and reports.* Retrieved November 3, 2008, from http://www.nhlbi.nih.gov/guidelines/current.htm.

Wagner, M., Newman, L., Cameto, R., & Levine, P. (2005). *Changes over time in the early post-school outcomes of youth with disabilities. National Longitudinal Transition Study (NLTS) and the National Longitudinal Transition Study-2 (NLTS2).* Menlo Park, CA: SRI International.

Waski, J. (March/April, 2000). The fleecing of America's elderly. *Consumers Digest, 38,* 77–81.

Witt, W.P., Kasper, J.D., & Riley, A.W. (2003). Mental health services use among school-aged children with disabilities: The role of sociodemographics, functional limitations, family burdens, and care coordination. *Health Services Research, 38,* 1441–1466.

CHAPTER 6

Continuum of Nursing Care

Dalice L. Hertzberg

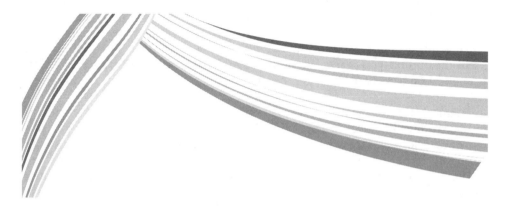

Nurses provide comprehensive services and supports for people with intellectual and developmental disabilities (IDD) and their families in a variety of roles. Hospitals, clinics, schools, and community and public health agencies are just a few of the settings where nurses are involved in promoting and maintaining the health of children, youth, and adults with IDD and their families. The professional registered nurse (RN) fills a unique role due to the depth and breadth of preparation in the biopsychosocial aspects of the human health and illness continuum. Of all the health professions involved with people with IDD, nurses have the capability to provide holistic care. In collaboration with families, other professionals, and individuals with IDD, nursing care seeks to maximize health and function in order to endorse full participation in society. In this chapter, the educational preparation of nurses is described, as well as the various roles and settings in which nurses may care for people with IDD.

EDUCATIONAL PREPARATION

Nurses enter into practice as an RN via either an associate's degree (about 2 years at a community college after high school), a diploma (a 2-year hospital-based nursing program after a year of community college obtaining prerequisites in arts and sciences), or a bachelor's degree (2 years of university education in liberal arts and sciences and 2–3 years of nursing). Associate's degree and diploma program graduates are prepared as technical nurses, whereas graduates of a Bachelor of Science in Nursing program are prepared as professional nurses and receive the educational foundation to obtain an advanced degree. Once the educational program is completed, the graduate must pass the National Council Licensure Examination for Registered Nurses, a national standardized examination, which confers the title RN. Licensure ensures that the entry-level RN has the necessary knowledge, skills, and independent decision-making abilities to safely provide care within the scope of practice. The board of nursing oversees licensure in each state (National Council of State Boards of Nursing, 2009).

Advanced practice nurses (APNs) have a master's degree and are prepared to work autonomously as clinical experts. APNs may be clinical nurse specialists, nurse practitioners, certified nurse midwives, or certified registered nurse anesthetists, and specialize in a specific area of care, such as a nurse practitioner in a primary health care clinic for children, families, and/or older adults. APNs must obtain national certification in a specialty (i.e., mental health) or subspecialty (i.e., palliative care) to practice, as well as undergo a credentialing process by the employer, which confirms the APN's education and certification. The state board of nursing grants the authority to practice as an APN within the specified state. Certification is renewed on a regular basis, and continuing education is mandatory to renew certification.

Clinical nurse specialists frequently practice in acute care settings, such as hospitals. They may specialize in any medical specialty area, such as gastroenterology, or may focus on an aspect of subspecialty care such as wound and ostomy care or organ transplantation. Nurse practitioners generally specialize in one of the following areas: newborn intensive care (neonatal nurse practitioner); pediatric primary care (pediatric nurse practitioner); adults and older adults (adult nurse practitioner); families, including children, childbearing and childrearing families, and elderly (family nurse practitioner); women's health (women's health nurse practitioner); mental health (psychiatry and mental health nurse practitioner); or eldercare (geriatric nurse practitioners). Subspecialty training and certification is also available in areas such as diabetes, spiritual care, or pain management. In addition, nurses may seek education and certification as certified nurse midwives or certified RN anesthetists.

Master's degree programs generally take between 2–5 years to complete for the RN with a bachelor's degree. The nurse with a master's degree who wishes further educational advancement may choose a clinical doctorate, the Doctor of Nursing Practice (DNP) degree; or a Doctor of Philosophy (PhD) degree, which prepares the nurse for roles in research, nursing education, and nursing theory development. A DNP may take 2–3 years to complete, while a doctorate generally takes 3–5 years. The DNP, which is a relatively new degree and role, focuses on developing advanced clinical and leadership skills for the increasingly complex health care environment. Nurses prepared as DNPs engage in evidence-based, outcome-focused care; in clinical nursing education; and outcome-based translational research. PhD-prepared nurses are more involved in theory development and original research (American Association of Colleges of Nursing, 2006). Academic nurses who teach in universities are usually prepared at the doctoral level.

Practicing RNs who do not have graduate education may prepare for and take national certification exams in various skill-based specialties. These certifications are offered by nursing organizations and are not specific to a graduate education. Some examples are rehabilitation nursing offered by the Association of Rehabilitation Nurses, pediatric nursing offered by the Society of Pediatric Nurses (2009) and the American Nurses Credentialing Center (2009), and IDD nursing offered by the Developmental Disabilities Nursing Association (DDNA, 2008). Certification is also available in specific aspects of care such as ostomy nursing (Wound, Ostomy, and Continence Nurses Society, 2007), or as a diabetes nurse educator (Pediatric Endocrinology Nursing Society, 2009).

Other care providers assist nurses in acute and community settings. Certified nursing assistants (CNAs) are unlicensed assistive personnel who provide very basic care and support services to people with IDD, under direct supervision from an RN. CNAs receive brief (several weeks) training and a state-level certificate to work in hospitals, home care, or congregate settings. Licensed practical nurses (LPNs) and licensed vocational nurses (LVNs) are trained at the community-college level for about 1 year; they are licensed by the state to work under the supervision of an RN, giving medications, providing basic health monitoring, and administering technical treatments.

Few educational programs exist at the college or university level to prepare nurses specifically to work with people with IDD. At least two graduate programs, at the University of Colorado Health Science Center and the University of Minnesota School of Nursing (funded by grants from the U.S. Maternal and Child Health Bureau), provide nursing education in leadership skills on behalf of children with special health care needs and their families, and include some content on children with IDD. However, no nursing programs address adults or aging adults with IDD. There are interdisciplinary doctoral programs across the United States in disability studies. Nurses may also obtain interdisciplinary fellowships at some universities across the country where University Centers for Excellence in Developmental Disabilities (UCEDDs) are located. Continuing education is available from professional associations at the national or state level and through HealthSoft, a private company that provides continuing education for nurses.

Nurses of all educational levels may care for people with IDD and their families. Direct nursing care is most often provided by RNs and LPN/LVNs. RNs often provide supervision, service coordination, and overall management of the health needs of people with IDD, and engage in providing education to direct care staff, individuals with IDD, and their families. APNs provide consultation, in areas such as wound and skin care, or function as a nurse practitioner to provide primary health care in community or specialized clinics. At the college or university level, academic nurses educate students in the care of the population, develop curricula in nursing addressing the health care needs of people with IDD, perform research in knowledge development regarding disabilities, and work with APNs in establishing standards and guidelines for nursing care.

One of the barriers to quality health care for people with IDD is negative or devaluing attitudes on the part of health care providers. Nurses are not immune to these negative attitudes, which may spring from a lack of experience with the population, as well as a lack of understanding of their behavior or causes of IDD (Smeltzer, 2007). Most nursing education programs lack any information at all about children or adults with IDD, as do most clinical experiences. Only those nursing students with placements in pediatric specialty clinics are likely to come into contact with children with IDD or their families. Nurses are in a unique position to move to eliminate the health disparities that people with IDD experience; however, before that happens, nurses will need to explore their attitudes toward people with IDD and other disabilities, and examine values that fail to support equal rights and opportunities for the population (U.S. Public Health Service, 2001).

CORE KNOWLEDGE BASE

To work with people with IDD, nurses need a core knowledge base. In addition to the basics of adult and pediatric nursing care, information tailored to the health

Table 6.1.   Knowledge base for nurses working with people with intellectual and developmental disabilities (IDD)

Categories of Care	Knowledge Foci
Physiologic	Causes of IDD
	Genetic conditions and syndromes
	Secondary conditions of specific diagnoses
	Common medications used
	Medication effects and side effects
	Influence of IDD on common chronic diseases (e.g., type II diabetes, cardiac disease)
Psychosocial	Co-occurring mental health diagnoses
	Challenging behavior and the importance of environment on behavior
	Communication disorders (e.g., nonverbal, speech processing problems)
	Social communication disorders (e.g., autism spectrum disorders)
	Level of social skills
	Developmental effects of growing up with an IDD
	Importance of self-advocacy
Family	Family-centered care and collaboration
	Family adaptation
	Response to stigma
	Effects on the family of initial diagnosis of child and how diagnosis was given to family
	Understanding that parents experience joy from their child with IDD as well as chronic sorrow
	Lifetime economic and health effects on caregivers
Community service system	Early intervention service system and the Individualized Family Service Plan
	Educational system planning
	Individualized education program and transition planning
	Health disparities and quality of health
	Preventative care
	Living situation (e.g., large institutionalized population versus group homes or other settings)
	IDD service system in state of practice
	Advocacy and support for self-advocacy for people with DD
	Funding issues
	Policy issues

This table was published in *Intellectual and developmental disabilities nursing: Scope and standards of practice*, Nehring, W.M., et al., p.1, Copyright American Nurses Association and Nursing Division of the American Association on Mental Retardation (2004). Reprinted by permission.

Reprinted with permission from American Nurses Association on Mental Retardation, *Intellectual and developmental disabilities nursing: Scope and standards of practice*, © 2004 Nursebooks.org.

care needs of the individuals with IDD being served is necessary. In Table 6.1, a summary of essential topic areas for nurses working with people with IDD is presented. Skills in behavioral management, skin and wound care, bowel and bladder management, and feeding and nutrition are also very useful. Specialization in a particular age group, such as elderly individuals or children, requires specific knowledge and skills targeted to the population.

There are a number of issues regarding IDD of which nurses should be aware, including (but not limited to) informed consent for people with IDD; state laws and regulations concerning long-term care facilities; surrogate decision making and guardianship; health care proxies; issues related to end-of-life care for people with IDD; do not resuscitate orders; and state board of nursing regulations regarding scope of practice, delegation, and supervision. Models of care and service for people with IDD and civil rights issues are also important topics. Nurses seeking education and training in these topics can contact their state IDD nurses association, the DDNA (2008), or the American Association of Intellectual/Developmental Disabilities. State IDD agencies and UCEDDs may also have courses or continuing education programs (Association of University Centers on Disabilities, 2009).

STANDARDS OF CARE

In an effort to define quality and excellence in nursing, standards of care have been developed. Research-based standards have been developed for nursing in general, as well as for specialty practice, by professional nursing organizations, government agencies, and other health care quality organizations. The American Nurses Association establishes standards of care for the profession of nursing and oversees the development of standards by specialty nursing organizations. The publication *Intellectual and Developmental Disabilities Nursing: Scope and Standards of Practice* (Nehring et al., 2004) established the standards of care for nurses working with individuals with IDD and their families. DDNA has also published a set of standards (Willis, 2008).

Health care standards that are interdisciplinary, or are not specific to a single discipline, are generally established by government agencies, such as the Joint Commission on Accreditation of Healthcare Organizations or the Agency for Healthcare Research and Quality. Standards exist for various aspects of health care (e.g., effectiveness of health care services) or for the care of people with specific conditions (e.g., diabetes). Nurses involved in the aforementioned health care services or patient care must consider these standards in their practice.

RESEARCH

Professional nurses take part in research concerning people with IDD and their families, as well as initiate it. Currently, nursing research concerning children and adults with IDD is limited. In 2004, DDNA launched the *International Journal of Nursing in Intellectual and Developmental Disabilities*, the first nursing journal focused entirely on IDD nursing. Prior to this publication, nursing research articles concerning IDD were published in a wide array of journals, including those focused on pediatric nursing, nurse practitioners, rehabilitation nursing, and others. Interdisciplinary professional journals such as *Intellectual and Developmental Disabilities* (previously *Mental Retardation*) have also published nursing research on IDD.

Evidence-based practice is the hallmark of quality nursing and medical practice, yet there is little evidence that may be applied directly to the health care of people with IDD (Nehring, 2005). Standard immunizations and preventative services for all people provide some guidance, but many situations exist where evidence for or against interventions simply is not available (Nehring et al., 2004; U.S. Public Health Service, 2001). Nurses have a responsibility to contribute to the body of knowledge and evidence for this population, both in independent and interdisciplinary practice and research.

Lack of funding, shortages of professional nurses in the field, and lack of recognition of the specialty, particularly in the United States, all contribute to the dearth of nursing research in the area (Smeltzer, 2007). International nursing research addresses topics of concern similar to those in the United States, such as efficacy of nursing interventions. The United Kingdom recognizes what they term *learning disabilities nursing* and offers the specialty in colleges and universities, supporting scholarly research (National Health Service, 2007). Interdisciplinary research addresses care, services, and outcomes for people with IDD, but even interdisciplinary or medical research is lacking, particularly when compared to research on other chronic conditions.

To improve care and promote the visibility of nursing in the lives of people with IDD and their families, nurses must participate in and initiate research on behalf of people with IDD. More information is necessary on condition-specific interventions, pharmacological treatments, and health promotion for children, men, and women, and their families. Nurses are uniquely situated to recognize and investigate the impact of systems of care across the life span, as well as the influence of caregiver burden on the health of mothers and other family members. These topics and many others provide fertile ground for future nursing research (Nehring, 2004).

INTERDISCIPLINARY FOCUS

The interdisciplinary team collaborates to provide services and supports using a problem-solving process that goes beyond discipline boundaries yet includes discipline-specific contributions (Lutz & Davis, 2008). Coordination of care is a primary goal of the team. The child or adult with IDD and/or their family are intrinsic members of the team. Team members may include (but are not limited to) RNs or APNs, physicians, psychologists, physical and/or occupational therapists, speech and language pathologists, audiologists, dentists, specialists in special education, and social workers.

While members of individual disciplines commit to working together on the team, at times discipline-specific loyalties may interfere with the work of the team and cause conflict between team members. Respect for the scope of knowledge of other team members and the ability to tolerate ambiguity in role boundaries are important characteristics in nurses working within interdisciplinary teams (Nehring et al., 2004). Leadership on the team may rotate among members, or be designated according to the service recipient's needs (e.g., a psychologist may be the team leader if the individual with IDD has autism). Table 6.2 presents the definition of interdisciplinary practice developed by the UCEDD, which is a federally funded program promoting research, education, and service on behalf of people with IDD and their families.

Although the interdisciplinary team remains the philosophical cornerstone of services and supports for people with IDD, economic constraints and health care reform have worked to erode its position. Many insurance companies—particularly Medicaid, which is the primary source of health care funding for people with IDD—are reluctant to pay for the comprehensive services provided by the interdisciplinary team; more frequently, they are opting for specific targeted services on a limited basis. For example, a full-team diagnostic evaluation (e.g., psychology, speech-language pathology, occupational therapy, special education, pediatrician) for a child suspected of having an autism spectrum disorder may be limited to an evaluation by a psychologist and speech-language pathologist. Consultations by other disciplines may then be obtained as needed or recommended. In the following sections, different settings where nurses care for persons with IDD will be discussed.

Table 6.2.   Definition of interdisciplinary practice according to the Association of University Centers on Developmental Disability (UCEDD)

Interdisciplinary practice is a team approach for providing services and supports to people with disabilities that

- Supports shared decision making by valuing and respecting the contributions of each individual, family, and professional discipline
- Demonstrates shared leadership, accountability, and responsibility for individualized planning of services and supports to improve the quality of life for everyone
- Is comprehensive, holistic, and inclusive across communities and which generates synergistic problem solving to meet the individual's needs

Interdisciplinary practice creates an integrated effort that exceeds the abilities and resources of any single professional discipline, provider agency, family, or individual.

Successful application of interdisciplinary practice in UCEDD Leadership Education in Neurodevelopmental Disability programs is grounded in the principles of inclusion with team collaboration among professionals, state and community partners, individuals, and their families for the delivery of health and human services, training, policy analysis, and research that addresses the complex life-span needs of people with disabilities.

From Council for Interdisciplinary Services, Association of University Centers on Disability (2007). Retrieved March 1, 2009, from http://www.aucd.org/docs/councils/cis/board_iddef_2007.pdf; reprinted by permission.

EARLY INTERVENTION

In this section, family-centered care, family support, child find, and child care consultation will be discussed.

Family-Centered Care and Family Support

The philosophy of family-centered care includes families as part of the care team and considers the family as intrinsic to the care and development of the child. Nurses are important proponents of family-centered care, as they are in the ideal position to advocate for families and to enable families to advocate for themselves and their children. At no other time during the life span is this more important than during infancy and early childhood, when the infant is completely dependent on the care of families. Family-centered nursing care begins very early, as nurses are often in the position to counsel families in the preconception stage. During pregnancy, teaching is focused on prevention of complications and maintenance of a healthy pregnancy, as well as preparing the parents for a significant lifestyle change. When prenatal diagnosis identifies a challenge to the family's expectations, the professional nurse can ensure that families have the information they need to make an informed decision about the pregnancy outcome.

Family support and education is a nursing role throughout the life span. Nurses are often the first professionals to refer families to parent support groups. While professional support and counseling is important, only other parents who have gone through the same things can relate to the day-to-day experience of caring for a premature infant or child with disabilities (Guralnick & Conlon, 2007; Howland, 2007). Family support organizations run the gamut between those formed solely for education (e.g., Parents Educating Parents) to those focusing on a specific condition, such as the Spina Bifida Association. Refer to Chapters 3 and 4 for additional information on early intervention programs.

Child Find

Nurses often serve on Child Find assessment teams, which determine if young children are eligible for early intervention programs, and if they are eligible, what services they might require (U.S. Office of Special Education Programs, n.d.). Care coordination or service coordination is a federally mandated component of the early intervention system and one for which nurses are well suited due to their knowledge of health needs and community resources. Early intervention centers that provide socialization, play, and therapeutic treatment for young children with IDD usually have an RN on staff (or available as a consultant) to meet the health and safety needs of the children. Home-based early intervention teams visit the child and family at home; teams often include an RN to assist with feeding problems, information on medication and medical concerns, and family teaching. Finally, nurses working in acute or community health settings, in clinics, or as APNs are in an ideal position to recognize developmental delays in young children and make referrals to the early intervention system and Child Find. Refer to Chapter 4 for additional information about early intervention.

Child Care Consultation

As more young children with IDD survive and thrive, child care centers are increasingly providing care for children with a variety of special health care needs and disabilities. Child care health consultants, who are usually RNs, provide information on child safety and different disabilities and health care concerns. For child care health consultants to be effective, they need not only the knowledge and skills related to child safety and health, but also familiarity with child care practices and state regulations (Alkon, Farraer, & Bernzweig, 2004). Health consultants formulate health care plans for children with potentially labile conditions, such as asthma or seizure disorders, which provide teachers with a step-by-step plan to follow in case the child's condition deteriorates.

For children who require medication during the hours they are in child care, nurse consultants instruct selected child care staff in medication administration; in most states, nurses delegate that task to the staff member to perform. Delegation of invasive procedures to unlicensed personnel (in this case, the child care provider), as outlined in the state Nurse Practice Act, is performed by RNs (not LPN/LVNs) and must be accompanied by specific procedures and documentation. The RN who delegates is responsible for supervising the unlicensed person; if the unlicensed person makes an error, both the person and the RN are held responsible. Invasive procedures that are commonly performed in child care centers include medication administration, gastrostomy tube feedings, and intermittent urinary catheterization (American Academy of Pediatrics [AAP] & American Public Health Association, 2002; Heschel, Crowley & Cohen, 2005; New Hanover County Health Department, 2009).

COMMUNITY CARE AND HABILITATION

This section will include discussions of public health nursing, home care, home visiting, group homes, and IDD services nursing.

Public Health Nursing

IDD nursing has a long history in public health, with early public health nurses often providing the only habilitative care to children with disabling conditions living in tenements with their families in the early 20th century (Wald, 1915). Public health nurses working in state and county health departments provide care coordination and consultation to children with special health care needs under programs funded by the U.S. Maternal and Child Health Bureau block grant to states, under Title V of the Social Security Act (U.S. Department of Health and Human Resources, n.d.). Title V nurses also administer and evaluate programs, as well as provide family and provider education.

State outreach and/or diagnostic clinics, provided by state Title V agencies at intervals throughout the year, offer services that might not have been available otherwise to rural populations; they are coordinated by public health nurses. Public health nurses, usually APNs, also provide preventative and wellness care, including immunizations, to low-income children and families in county health department clinics. In rural areas, these health department clinics may be the main source of pediatric care for families.

Home Care

Home care nursing for the medically fragile infant requires the knowledge and skills of a neonatal intensive care unit (NICU) nurse, combined with the ability to work in the much less controlled environment of the home and problem solve without the resources typically available in the hospital. Home care nurses are responsible for direct care of the infant or young child who is dependent on technology, physical and emotional assessment of the child and family, care coordination, ensuring that all medical supplies are available, development of an emergency plan, and family support and education.

When working in the home, nursing interventions are by necessity family-centered and include all family members, including siblings. The home environment is very beneficial for the infant and family. Medicaid waivers are available in most states, which allow children who are technology dependent to receive care in the home instead of an institutional setting (Hummel & Cronin, 2004).

Home Visiting

Nurse home visiting programs, similar to the practice of the early public health nurses, have experienced resurgence since the 1980s. Research has supported that home visits performed by RNs for child health monitoring, parenting instruction and support, and resources and referrals (when needed) provide high-risk children and families with improved health and well-being. Nurse home visiting has been shown to improve parenting skills and child health and development, prevent child abuse, improve pregnancy outcomes, prevent unwanted pregnancy, and improve mothers' job prospects (AAP, 2009; Olds et al., 2004). Funding sources that states may use for nurse home visiting include the U.S. Maternal and Child Health Bureau Title V block grant funds, Medicaid, state children's health insurance plans, and Temporary Assistance to Needy Families (Izzo et al., 2005; National Governors Association, 2002). Some private health insurance companies, such as Kaiser Permanente, also provide nurse home visiting programs.

Nurses with solid experience in pediatric health care, maternal and child health care, child and family assessment, child development, and family teaching and education are good candidates for positions in nurse home visiting programs. In addition, nurse home visitors must be knowledgeable about community resources (particularly those for children with developmental concerns), be comfortable providing interventions in the home, and have skills in culturally competent care.

Group Homes and IDD Services Nursing

With the push toward deinstitutionalization for people with IDD, community settings, such as group homes, host homes (adult foster care), and supported living programs are much more common. Agencies providing services and supports for people with IDD usually employ one or more professional RNs or nurse consultants to monitor the health status of residents, coordinate health services, and provide resources to direct care staff. Nurses instruct direct care providers in the health-related care of people with IDD, on such topics as medications and side effects, correct hygiene, skin care, and dental care. In the IDD systems of most states, direct care providers who have been trained in medication administration are able to administer medications in group homes or day programs under the supervision of an RN, who delegates the responsibility to them. Other responsibilities of the nurse include health promotion interventions and teaching. Nurses are usually responsible for infection control and hand washing in group homes and other community settings, as well as for monitoring outbreaks of infectious disease, which are more common in congregate settings (Lashley, 2005).

INSTITUTIONAL CARE

Approximately 30% of people with IDD reside in large congregate care settings, such as intermediate care facilities, nursing homes, and state-run institutions. About 21,000 people with IDD (6%) live in state-run institutions (Braddock, Hemp, & Rizzolo, 2008). Most state institutions are self-contained, providing residential, recreational, health, medical, rehabilitative, and dental care on campus for people with IDD with complex health or behavioral conditions. As a result, extensive nursing services with 24-hour coverage are necessary.

In a state-run institution, nursing responsibilities may range from staff education to direct nursing care to primary health care provided by an APN. Timely physical assessment, administration of injectable or intravenous medications, monitoring of minor acute or chronic illness, and participation as a member of the interdisciplinary care team are all nursing responsibilities. Other responsibilities include assessment and monitoring for side effects of psychoactive medications; and prevention of, and monitoring for, other complications of treatment, as well as secondary conditions that may arise from the individual's disability. In addition, the RNs on staff are responsible for supervision of LPN/LVNs and nursing assistants, as well as for delegation of invasive procedures to those ancillary nursing staff and unlicensed care givers who have undergone special training to administer medications or treatments. RNs and APNs are usually responsible for much of the direct care staff education, particularly in the areas of personal assistance for people with IDD, health issues, infection control, lifting, and positioning. In fact, nurses are generally responsible for infection control practice, policies, and procedures in long-term care facilities (Lockhart & Yamauchi, 2007).

HOSPITALS AND SPECIALTY CLINICS

Hospitals provide acute and surgical care for people with IDD, yet medical and nursing staff rarely have the expertise necessary to care for the population. Communication and behavioral issues, combined with complex medical needs, can make acute or postsurgical care very challenging, particularly if there are not any family members involved. Nurse specialists in rehabilitation, wound and ostomy care, geriatrics, and pediatrics may provide helpful information to hospital staff nurses, as can nurses consulting with group homes or developmental centers (Nehring et al., 2004).

Particularly during hospitalization, when individuals with IDD are away from their usual caregivers or family members, communication problems are often a source of great frustration for nurses and patients alike. Patients may be unable to get the nurse's attention or may be unable to explain their discomfort. Busy hospital nurses may feel that they do not have the time to interpret slow dysarthric speech, so questions may go unanswered. Medication errors may occur as can inappropriate care (e.g., a pressure ulcer resulting from the patient's difficulty in communicating discomfort). Communication devices may not be used because of real or perceived time constraints, limiting the ability of an individual with IDD to participate in care. Finally, people with communication disorders are often treated with condescension, or like they are children instead of adults (Balandin, Hemsley, Sigafoos, & Green, 2007).

Nurses working in pediatric hospitals or clinics generally have experience with children with IDD, who may be hospitalized at birth in the NICU, and throughout childhood for acute and chronic illness management as well as corrective surgeries, such as orthopedic surgery for club feet or hip dysplasia. Some units may specialize in caring for children with disabilities, such as rehabilitation, neurology and neurosurgery, orthopedics, or cardiology (Nehring, 2003). Coordination and discharge planning for children with IDD who have been hospitalized is generally the responsibility of RNs or APNs. Discharge planners may have on-the-job training or may have attended short courses in case management or funding issues. For example, when infants born prematurely or with congenital or genetic conditions are preparing for discharge to home from the NICU, nurses are usually the professionals responsible for orchestrating the complex discharge plan. Providing for parent education, evaluating the family's readiness and ability to take the infant home, obtaining equipment that will be needed in the home, setting up a home nursing agency, assisting the family with an emergency plan, and setting up the necessary follow-up visits is all part of discharge planning.

Prior to initiating discharge planning, the nurse must determine the type of health insurance the family has, and what will or will not be covered. Usually, it is necessary to obtain prior authorization for services and durable medical equipment, as well as establish medical necessity. When the family lives in a nearby urban area, the task of discharge planning is usually easier than determining the community resources in a faraway rural area, or even another state. Finally, the nurse works with the family on community agency referrals, such as to Child Find and the early intervention system. To formulate and carry out a successful discharge plan, the nurse must be knowledgeable not only about the infant's and family's needs while in the NICU, but what they will need in the future when they go home (Hummel & Cronin, 2004).

While any outpatient specialty clinic may see children with disabilities and their families, those clinics that provide care for children with complex conditions are more likely to have experience with them. Specialty clinics such as these are commonly found in regional pediatric centers or in large urban hospitals. Nurses are valuable team members in these clinics, providing care coordination, assessment and treatments, and collaborating with specialists. Coordination with other specialists and health care providers that the child sees is particularly important, as a child with IDD with a complex condition may receive services from as many as six or more medical specialists (e.g., neurology, orthopedics) and four or five ancillary service providers (e.g., physical therapists, home care nurses, speech language pathology). In addition, clinic nurses and nurse practitioners often take part in the child's individualized education program (IEP), which guides school-based services.

PRIMARY HEALTH CARE

Nurse practitioners are equipped to provide primary health care, including preventative and wellness care, management of minor acute illness, management of uncomplicated chronic conditions, and patient education. Many children and adults with IDD are basically well and very much in need of good preventative care and education tailored to their developmental level and understanding (Van Cleve, Cannon, & Cohen, 2006; Van Cleve & Cohen, 2006). However, nurse practitioners are capable of more complex condition management. In one study, at least 10% of pediatric nurse practitioners were found to practice in tertiary care settings, such as hospitals—particularly in specialty clinics, which serve a large number of children with IDD and their families (Brady & Neal, 2000). Nurse practitioners have strong collaborative skills and flexibility; they are well suited for innovative primary care practices, such as house calls and prehospital management, which seeks to prevent frequent hospitalizations in people with chronic illness (Landers et al., 2005).

SCHOOL AND BEYOND

As a recognized specialty in nursing by the American Nurses Association, school nurses provide a broad spectrum of services to school age children and youth and their families. While school nurses may provide intermittent first aid to children who are typically developing, availability of nursing services to children with disabilities and chronic illness is mandated by the Individuals with Disabilities Education Improvement Act of 2004 (PL 108-446) and Section 504 of the Rehabilitation Act of 1973 (PL 93-112) (National Association of School Nurses, 2006).

Students with IDD may be included in regular classrooms full or part time, may receive special education in segregated "resource rooms," or may even attend separate schools that are designed specifically for children with complex disabilities and significant behavioral or technology needs. For students who depend on technology, school nursing responsibilities may include direct care; establishment of policies and procedures to manage health, safety and legal issues; delegation to and supervision of staff, such as LPNs; planning for health services within the school via the IEP; coordinating care between the school, the family, other agencies involved with the child and family, and the child's specialty and primary health care providers (Rehm, 2002). School nurses must not only be knowledgeable about different conditions that may affect students, but also must be conversant with federal, state, and district regulations and laws that affect students, families, and the nurses' role and scope of practice (Selekman, 2006).

Transition to Adulthood

As a youth with IDD approaches graduation from high school, both the youth and family anticipate emancipation. However, an effort must be made by the family, health and school service providers, and the youth to prepare for this process if it is to occur. Some adolescents with IDD are not capable of self-care and independent decision making, so their families will need to plan for guardianship, long-term care in the community, health care decision making, supported employment, and providing for as much of the young person's hopes and dreams as possible. Other youth may be capable of self-care and decision making, but they must learn the appropriate skills and knowledge to do so. In addition, funding sources and service agencies change at age 18 years and/or 21 years, which may be confusing and concerning for families and youth who have come to depend on certain health and service providers. Pediatric health providers may wish to discharge the young adult from their care, but adult-oriented health providers may not be willing to take Medicaid or other public insurance, and often lack knowledge of IDD and service systems (Betz & Nehring, 2007).

The above conundrums present immense opportunities for nurses working with youth with IDD and their families. Pediatric nurses, pediatric nurse practitioners, nurse specialists, home care nurses, and public health nurses are all in ideal positions to bridge the gap between pediatric and adult health care and other service systems. Through care coordination; family and youth education and training in health, social skills, systems of care; resource brokering; and collaboration with other school and health providers, nurses can facilitate this challenging process for families and youth with IDD. Collaborating with families, service agencies (e.g., schools, IDD service providers, health insurance plans), pediatric health providers and adult health providers, independent living centers, and vocational rehabilitation centers, nurses can energize the process to develop a transition plan. The transition plan ideally addresses not only the school-to-work aspect of the youth's life, but also his or her living situation, degree and type of formal and informal support, and plan for moving from the pediatric health care system to the adult health care system (Betz, 2007).

Finding a primary care provider is only part of the problem; many youth with IDD receive a variety of specialty medical services, and providers for those services must be found. For example, a young man with Down syndrome who had heart surgery at birth will need lifelong follow-up on the heart valve which was repaired. A cardiologist with an understanding of congenital heart disease, as well as the potential cardiac problems that develop with age, is necessary. Such specialists are not always found in all communities, particularly in rural areas, and travel may be necessary to meet the young person's health care needs.

Not only pediatric nurses are involved with transition; nurse practitioners in family practice are uniquely situated to provide family-centered care—whatever the age of the individual. Family nurse practitioners receive preparation in life-span health and illness issues, and they frequently work in settings where special or vulnerable populations seek care. Government-funded, low-income, or community health centers generally take public insurance like Medicaid, and have more resources available to assist individuals and families with chronic conditions and disadvantaged social situations.

Adulthood

As the life expectancy of individuals with IDD increases due to improvements in health care, technological and scientific advances nurses will continue to provide care in a myriad of settings and in a variety of roles to the adult and aging population of individuals with IDD. The organization and philosophical orientation of the adult health care system are distinctly different from the pediatric system of care and will bring challenges for individuals with IDD, their families, and their circles of social and service supports. Adult health care is person-centered rather than family-centered. The adult health care provider may be unaccustomed to including a family member or direct care staff member from the residential facility or group home during the clinic visit. Issues pertaining to conservatorship for health care decision making need to be clarified in advance of providing clinical care. Referrals to other specialists made by the primary care provider are more complicated. Unlike the integrated pediatric specialty care teams, there is no comparable model of care in the adult system of care. Accessing the care of adult specialists will require traveling to different locations and making multiple appointments. Coordinating care is inherently more difficult because the infrastructure for facilitating interdisciplinary care is lacking. Nurses are well positioned to facilitate care coordination based on the comprehensive framework of nursing practice, whether in an institutional or community setting as described previously.

Models of adult care have been developed to address the growing need for more proactive responsive models of health care for those with chronic conditions (Commonwealth Fund, 2004; Wagner, 1998). The chronic care model (CCM) is a comprehensive model of care developed to facilitate the care of adults who require chronic care management (Improving Chronic Illness Care, 2009; Wagner, 1998). The CCM comprehensive approach to addressing the individual's ongoing needs for services is similar to the concepts of the pediatric medical home.

A joint statement by the American Academy of Family Physicians, AAP, American College of Physicians, and American Osteopathic Association (2007) was issued presenting the principles of the patient-centered medical home (PCMH), similar to the pediatric medical home developed by the AAP. The principles of the PCMH are

1. Every patient has a personal physician.
2. Care is directed by the physician.
3. Care is oriented to the whole person.
4. Care is coordinated.
5. Quality and safety of care are foremost.
6. Enhanced access to services is available.
7. Medical home services are reimbursed.

Implementation of models of care such as the CCM and PCMH may provide a comprehensive and integrated approach similar to the pediatric model once they are applied by more primary care providers.

Nursing care and collaboration extend to new partners to meet the ongoing needs of adults with IDD. These partners include job developers, employers, rehabilitation specialists, and public agency representatives. Nursing collaboration involves working with employees with IDD in partnership with job developers and employers to institute the health-related accommodations needed in the workplace. Nurses serve as advocates to effect changes in the community such as improved paratransit services, more affordable housing, and infrastructure repairs (e.g., sidewalk repairs) to promote safety and more appropriately respond to the needs of individuals with IDD. These roles reflect the array of opportunities, besides those previously mentioned, available for nurses who work in community and institutional settings with adults with IDD. For additional information on adult issues, refer to Chapters 3, 5, 8, and 9.

CONCLUSION

This chapter provided an overview of the many roles and service settings where nurses may work with children, youth, and adults with IDD and their families. The scope of practice, knowledge, and values in which professional RNs need to provide holistic care for the population was discussed. Knowledgeable, evidence-based, and compassionate care that realizes the rights, value, and diversity of all individuals and supports self-determination is an important contribution of nursing to the many systems of care that serve people with IDD and their families.

REFERENCES

Alkon, A., Farraer, J., & Bernzweig, J. (2004). Child care health consultant's roles and responsibilities: Focus group findings. *Pediatric Nursing, 30,* 315–321.

American Academy of Family Physicians, American Academy of Pediatrics, American College of Physicians, & American Osteopathic Association. (2007). *Joint principles of the patient-centered medical home.* Retrieved on March 15, 2009, from http://www.pcpcc.net/content/joint-principles-patient-centered-medical-home.

American Academy of Pediatrics. (2009). The role of preschool home-visiting programs in improving children's developmental and health outcomes. *Pediatrics, 123,* 598–603.

American Academy of Pediatrics & American Public Health Association. (2002). *Caring for our children. National health and safety performance standards: Guidelines for out-of-home child care programs* (2nd ed.). Arlington, VA: National Center for Education in Maternal and Child Health.

American Association of Colleges of Nursing. (2006). *The essentials of doctoral education for advanced nursing practice.* Retrieved June 4, 2009, from http://www.aacn.nche.edu/DNP/pdf/Essentials.pdf.

American Nurses Credentialing Center. (2009). *Board credentialing of nurses makes a difference.* Retrieved on March 10, 2009, from http://www.nursecredentialing.org/default.aspx.

Association of University Centers on Disabilities (2009). *UCEDD directory.* Retrieved on March 10, 2009, from http://www.aucd.org/directory/directory.cfm?program=UCEDD.

Balandin, S., Hemsley, B., Sigafoos, J., & Green, V. (2007). Communicating with nurses: The experiences of 10 adults with cerebral palsy and complex communication needs. *Applied Nursing Research, 20,* 56–62.

Betz, C.L. (2007). Facilitating the transition of adolescents with developmental disabilities: Nursing practice issues and care. *Journal of Pediatric Nursing, 22,* 103–115.

Betz, C.L., & Nehring, W.M. (2007). *Promoting health care transition planning for adolescents with special health care needs and disabilities.* Baltimore: Paul H. Brookes Publishing Co.

Braddock, D., Hemp, R., & Rizzolo, M.C. (2008). *State of the states in developmental disabilities.* Retrieved March 8, 2009, from https://www.cu.edu/ColemanInstitute/stateofthestates/UnitedStates.pdf.

Brady, M.A., & Neal, J.A. (2000). Role delineation study of pediatric nurse practitioners: A national study of practice responsibilities and trends in role functions. *Journal of Pediatric Health Care, 14,* 149–159.

Commonwealth Fund. (2004). *Patient-centered primary care initiative.* Retrieved on March 15, 2009, from http://www.commonwealthfund.org/Content/Program-Areas/High-Performance-Health-System/Patient-Centered-Primary-Care-Initiative.aspx.

Council for Interdisciplinary Services, Association of University Centers on Disability. (2007). *Interdisciplinary practice.* Retrieved March 7, 2009, from http://www.aucd.org/docs/councils/cis/board_iddef_2007.pdf.

Developmental Disabilities Nurses Association. (2008). *An overview of certification.* Retrieved on March 10, 2009, from http://www.ddna.org/pages/certification.

Guralnick, M.J., & Conlon, C.J. (2007). Early intervention. In Batshaw, M.L., Pellegrino, L., & Roizen, N.J. (Eds.), *Children with disabilities* (6th ed., pp. 511–521). Baltimore: Paul H. Brookes Publishing Co.

Heschel, R.T., Crowley, A.A., & Cohen, S.S. (2005). State policies regarding nursing delegation and medication administration in child care settings: A case study. *Policy, Politics, & Nursing Practice, 68,* 86–98.

Howland, L.C. (2007). Preterm birth: Implications for family stress and coping. *Newborn and Infant Nursing Reviews, 7,* 14–19.

Hummel, P., & Cronin, J. (2004). Home care of the high-risk infant. *Advances in Neonatal Care, 4,* 354–364.

Improving Chronic Illness Care. (2009). *Chronic illness care model.* Retrieved on March 15, 2009, from http://www.improvingchroniccare.org/index.php?p=The_Chronic_Care_Model&s=2.

Individuals with Disabilities Education Improvement Act (IDEA) of 2004, PL 108-446, 20 U.S.C. §§ 1400 *et seq.*

Izzo, C.V., Eckenrode, J.J., Smith, E.G., Henderson, C.R., Cole, R., Kitzman, H., et al. (2005). Reducing the impact of uncontrollable stressful life events through a program of nurse home visitation for new parents. *Prevention Science, 6,* 269–274.

Landers, S.H., Gunn, P.W., Flocke, S.A., Graham, A.V., Kikano, G.E., Moore, S.M., et al. (2005). Trends in house calls to medicare beneficiaries. *JAMA, 294,* 2435–2436.

Lashley, F.R. (2005). Infection, infectious disease, and infection control. In W.M. Nehring (Ed.), *Core curriculum for specializing in intellectual and developmental disability.* Boston: Jones & Bartlett.

Lockhart, J., & Yamauchi, T. (2007). Influenza vaccination in a "special needs" extended care facility. *American Journal of Infection Control, 35,* E208–E209.

Lutz, B.L., & Davis, S.M. (2008). Theory and practice models in rehabilitation nursing. In S.P. Hoeman (Ed.), *Rehabilitation nursing: Prevention, intervention, & outcomes* (4th ed., pp. 14–29). St. Louis: Mosby Elsevier.

National Association of School Nurses. (2006). *Position statement: School nursing management of students with chronic health conditions.* Retrieved March 10, 2009, from http://www.nasn.org/Default.aspx?tabid=351.

National Council of State Boards of Nursing. (2009). *Practice.* Retrieved March 7, 2009 from https://www.ncsbn.org/1427.htm.

National Governors Association. (2002). *The benefits and financing of home visiting programs.* Retrieved March 8, 2009 from http://www.nga.org/Files/pdf/BENEFITS FINANCINGHOME.pdf.

National Health Service (2007). *Good practice in learning disability nursing.* Retrieved on March 11, 2009 from http://www.dh.gov.uk/en/Publicationsandstatistics/Publications/PublicationsPolicyAndGuidance/DH_081328.

Nehring, W.M. (2003). History of the roles of nurses caring for persons with mental retardation. *Nursing Clinics of North America, 38,* 351–372.

Nehring, W.M. (2004). Directions for the future of intellectual and developmental disabilities as a nursing specialty. *International Journal of Nursing in Intellectual and Developmental Disabilities, 1,* 2.

Nehring, W.M. (2005). *Health promotion for persons with intellectual and developmental disabilities: The state of scientific evidence.* Washington, DC: American Association on Mental Retardation.

Nehring, W.M., Roth, S.P., Natvig, D., Betz, C.L., Savage, T., & Krajicek, M. (2004). *Intellectual and developmental disabilities nursing: Scope and standards of practice.* Silver Spring, MD: American Nurses Association and Nursing Division of the American Association on Mental Retardation.

New Hanover County Health Department. (2009). *Smart start child care nursing program.* Retrieved on March 11, 2009 from http://www.nhcgov.com/AgnAndDpt/HLTH/PHS/Documents/ChildCareNewsletterMarch2009.pdf.

Olds, D.L., Robinson, J., Pettitt, L., Luckey, D.W., Holmberg, J., Ng, R.K., et al. (2004). Effects of home visits by paraprofessionals and by nurses: Age 4 follow-up results of a randomized trial. *Pediatrics, 114,* 1560–1568.

Pediatric Endocrinology Nursing Society. (2009). *Pediatric Endocrinology Nursing Society.* Retrieved on March 10, 2009, from https://www.pens.org/.

Rehabilitation Act of 1973, PL 93-112, 29 U.S.C. §§ 701 *et seq.*

Rehm, R.S. (2002). Creating a context of safety and achievement at school for children who are medically fragile/technology dependent. *Advances in Nursing Science, 24,* 71–84.

Selekman, J. (2006). *School nursing: A comprehensive text.* Philadelphia: F.A. Davis.

Smeltzer, S.C. (2007). Improving the health and wellness of persons with disabilities: A call to action too important for nursing to ignore. *Nursing Outlook, 55,* 189–195.

Society of Pediatric Nurses. (2009). *Certification.* Retrieved on March 10, 2009, from https://www.pedsnurses.org/certification.html.

U.S. Department of Health and Human Services. Health Resources and Services Administration, Maternal Child Health Bureau. (n.d). *Understanding Title V of the Social Security Act.* Retrieved on September 17, 2009, from ftp://ftp.hrsa.gov/mchb/titlevtoday/UnderstandingTitleV.pdf.

U.S. Department of Health and Human Services. Health Resources and Services Administration, Maternal Child Health Bureau. (n.d). *Title V block grants to state.* Retrieved March 8, 2009, from http://mchb.hrsa.gov/programs/default.htm.

U.S. Office of Special Education Programs. (n.d.). *About Child Find.* Retrieved on March 11, 2009, from http://www.childfindidea.org/overview.htm.

U.S. Public Health Service. (2001). *Closing the gap: A national blueprint for improving the health of individuals with mental retardation. Report of the Surgeon General's conference on health disparities and mental retardation.* Rockville, MD: U.S. Department of Health and Human Services.

Van Cleve, S.N., Cannon, S., & Cohen, W.I. (2006). Part II: clinical practice guidelines for adolescents and young adults with Down syndrome: 12 to 21 years. *Journal of Pediatric Health Care, 20,* 198–205.

Van Cleve, S.N., & Cohen, W.I. (2006). Part I: Clinical practice guidelines for children with Down syndrome from birth to 12 years. *Journal of Pediatric Health Care, 20,* 47–54.

Wagner, E.H. (1998). Chronic disease management: What will it take to improve care for chronic illness? *Effective Clinical Practice, 1,* 2–3.

Wald, L. D. (1915). *The house on henry street.* New York, NY: Henry Holt.

Willis, M.A. (2008). *Aspirational standards of developmental disabilities nursing practice.* Orlando, FL: Developmental Disabilities Nursing Association.

Wound, Ostomy, and Continence Nurses Society. (2007). *Education.* Retrieved on March 10, 2009, from http://www.wocn.org/Education/.

CHAPTER 7

Psychosocial Issues

J. Carolyn Graff

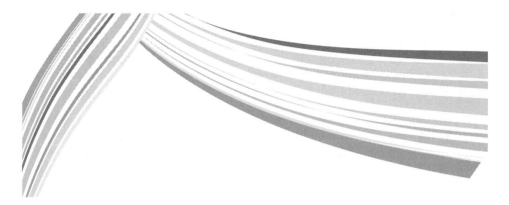

This chapter focuses on the psychosocial issues of individuals with intellectual and developmental disabilities (IDD) and the implications of these issues for individuals, families, nurses, and health professionals. Although dynamic approaches to social development, such as developmental science (Magnusson & Cairns, 1996) and life-course theory (Elder, 1996) have gained prominence over stage-based approaches, individuals' psychosocial development are considered from the perspective of psychosocial developmental theory in this chapter (Erikson, 1959). Erikson's stages of psychosocial development provide a solid foundation for thinking about psychological and social issues of individuals with IDD. In this context, the contributions of an individual's characteristics, behavior, and experience to psychosocial development are discussed. Relevant literature and research studies guide the consideration of nursing care to promote psychosocial development and well-being.

PSYCHOSOCIAL DEVELOPMENT: ERIKSON'S PSYCHOSOCIAL STAGES

The stages of psychosocial development are attributed to the work of Erik H. Erikson, a psychologist who expanded on Sigmund Freud's stages of psychosexual development (2000) by integrating society and culture into his theory. Erikson's orientation toward society and culture was largely due to the influence of anthropologists, such as Kurt Lewin, Margaret Mead, and Gregory Bateson, and his own observations of children of various cultural groups. His theory involves an eight-stage process of socialization from infancy to adulthood. It concentrates on the healthy personality rather than on neurotic behavior, which was the focus of Freud's theory. Erikson asserted that each individual achieves ego identity by solving identity crises at each stage of growth (Thomas, 2005). Erikson's stages serve as the background for considering psychosocial issues of individuals with disabilities. Individuals learn these tasks through complex social interactions with their family, school, and others. Each psychosocial crisis contains two dichotomous tasks; Erikson expected that individuals would learn both tasks to some degree.

For example, infants ideally learn trust but must know something about mistrust to avoid being deceived or taken advantage of in the future.

Erikson's theory provides a helpful context for regarding the psychosocial development and issues of individuals with IDD. Although this theory proposes distinct stages of development, dynamic approaches to social development, such as developmental science (Magnusson & Cairns, 1996) and life-course theory (Elder, 1996), can help nurses understand psychosocial variability within and among individuals with IDD. The following section provides an overview and discussion of Erikson's stages of psychosocial development. In subsequent sections of this chapter, Erikson's theory is applied to illustrate its usefulness to nurses working with individuals with IDD and their families.

Infancy

The first psychosocial crisis, *trust versus mistrust*, involves infants acquiring a sense of trust and overcoming a sense of mistrust (Erikson, 1959). Infants trust that their feeding, comfort, stimulation, and needs will be addressed. The quality of the relationship between infants and their parents (or caregivers) is important in achieving this developmental task. Providing food, warmth, and shelter alone will not lead to infants having a strong sense of self. Infants and parents learn to meet each other's needs for mutual regulation of frustration. When this mutual regulation does not develop, mistrust is the outcome. Infants' frustration increases when parents do not understand their behaviors and cues and when parents' responses to their behaviors and cues are prolonged and delayed. Infants become frustrated and eventually mistrustful when their needs are not met. From a different perspective, parents who always meet their infant's needs before the infant signals readiness are depriving the infant of the opportunity to test their ability to control their environment.

During the first 3–4 months of life, food intake is the most important social activity for infants. Infants have limited tolerance for frustration or delayed gratification. After initially being totally concerned for themselves, infants begin grasping and reaching out toward their parents. Grasping, initially a reflex, sends a powerful message to parents. When infants reach toward their parents and parents respond by holding or touching their infants' hands, mutual satisfaction for infants and parents results. The total quality of this parent–infant relationship, not single aspects of it, influences infants' gradual development of trust. Gaining a sense of trust and overcoming mistrust provide infants with the foundation for subsequent stages of psychosocial development.

Toddlerhood

The second psychosocial crisis, *autonomy versus shame and doubt*, spans the second and third year of life (Erikson, 1959). Once an infant's need for basic trust has been satisfied, a new sense of power provides the basis for the toddler to develop a sense of autonomy or ability to do some things without parents. Toddlers' differentiation of themselves from their parents can lead to excessive independence and negative responses from their parents. A balance between parental firmness and flexibility is needed as toddlers learn to tolerate separation from their parents, withstand delayed gratification, control their bowel and bladder functions, and communicate verbally with others. Parental firmness prevents toddlers from exceeding their safe limits, and parental flexibility allows toddlers to gain a sense of control.

Toddlers gain the skills of holding on and letting go as seen in their play and their behavior. They throw objects, take objects out of containers, and hold on tight when someone says "no" or tries to remove a toy from their hand. Although toddlers' negativism and strong emotions can be challenging to parents, they are evidence of the psychosocial function of holding on and letting go. From a different perspective, toddlers find comfort in sameness and ritualism. When they know that familiar routines, places, and persons continue to exist, they take advantage of opportunities to venture out and increase independence and autonomy. With an increased understanding of the differences between themselves and others, toddlers increase their sense of trust in themselves. This awareness of ability to achieve contributes to an awareness of ability to fail. Toddlers' awareness of their potential to fail can lead to doubt and shame.

Preschool

Initiative versus guilt, the third psychosocial crisis, refers to the preschool period when the children are gaining a sense of initiative (Erikson, 1959). Preschoolers' gains in language skills, ability to handle things, and ability to move about more freely contribute to their sense of accomplishment as they use these new skills in play and interacting with others. Conflict occurs when preschoolers exceed the limits of their abilities and when they experience a sense of guilt for not behaving according to their parents' expectations. Preschoolers may feel anxious, fearful, and guilty about having thoughts that differ from those expected by their parents. Development of the conscience is a task for preschoolers who are beginning to learn right from wrong and good from bad. They likely do not understand why something is acceptable or unacceptable. Preschoolers are beginning to make comparisons and develop curiosity about differences in sizes and gender as they learn about categories of things, objects, and people.

School Age

Industry versus inferiority is the psychosocial crisis that refers to latency or the period between toddlerhood and adolescence. The goal of this stage is to achieve a sense of personal and interpersonal competence by completing tasks that are worthwhile and by receiving attention and recognition for these accomplishments (Erikson, 1959). School-age children want to learn new skills, engage in meaningful and useful work, and complete tasks. They experience feelings of inferiority when they do not have a sense of accomplishing such tasks. Intrinsic and extrinsic motivation is associated with increased competence in mastering new skills and assuming new responsibilities. Intrinsic motivators include the satisfaction gained as children explore and manipulate aspects of their environment and interact with their peers. Extrinsic motivators include peer approval, grades, recognition, privileges, and concrete rewards that are clearly related to their accomplishments.

School-age children may experience feelings of inferiority that originate from themselves or from people in their environment. Children who are not well prepared for school life can experience feelings of inadequacy. A child whose ambition is greater than his or her ability will likely experience failure, whereas a child whose ambition is less than his or her ability will likely experience success. Feelings of inferiority may occur when children are compared to others who are similar in age or ability. Feelings of inferiority may occur when children's teachers, peers, or parents view something that children have learned to do as insignificant.

Adolescence

The psychosocial crisis of *identity and repudiation versus identity diffusion* occurs during adolescence, or between 12 and 18 or 20 years (Erikson, 1959). With the onset of puberty, adolescents experience rapid growth in their body and physical changes that signal sexual development is taking place. These changes influence body image and sexual behavior. Achievement of identity is strongly influenced by adolescents' interactions with others. These interactions teach them what behaviors they should and should not assume.

Society plays a role in determining the range of available opportunities open to the adolescent. At best, adolescents have opportunities to explore a range of possible options in forming an identity. In identity diffusion, adolescents do not recognize who they are to themselves or to others. Overidentification with others, such as peer groups, celebrities, or heroes, can lead adolescents to lose their sense of self. Adolescents give and receive help from other adolescents by forming cliques and being intolerant of those outside of their clique. This search for themselves can result in conflict with parents, siblings, and others. Adolescents who gain a sense of identity have a strong sense of individuality and recognition of acceptability to society. Adolescents who fail to work through their identity crisis continue demonstrating immature behaviors such as "intolerance, clannishness, cruel treatment of people who are 'different,' blind identification or loyalty to heroes and idols" (Thomas, 2005, p. 94).

Early Adulthood

The early adulthood psychosocial crisis that occurs among individuals in their 20s involves *intimacy and solidarity versus isolation*. Individuals who have moved from adolescence with a relatively sound and secure sense of identity are prepared to "establish a nonexploitative intimacy, sexually and intellectually, with a companion of the opposite sex" (Thomas, 2005, p. 94). Individuals with a secure identity are capable of defending their personal rights and individuality. The counterpart of intimacy is distancing or "the readiness to repudiate, to isolate, and, if necessary, to destroy those forces and people whose essence seems dangerous to one's own" (Erikson, 1959, pp. 95–96). This rejection in a more mature form is considered to be the result of prejudices that developed during the struggle for identity and the differentiation between the familiar and the less familiar.

Middle Adulthood

The middle adulthood psychosocial crisis is labeled *generativity versus self-absorption* and extends from the late 20s to the 50s. Individuals in partnership with another produce and care for their offspring. Individuals who do not produce offspring may focus their attention on "other forms of altruistic concern and of creativity, which may absorb their kind of parental responsibility" (Erikson, 1959, p. 97). According to Erikson, individuals who do not develop generativity through producing offspring or altruistic concern and creativity may become self-absorbed and develop a sense of "stagnation and interpersonal impoverishment" (Erikson, 1959, p. 97). Erikson pointed out that having children does not result in generativity since there are parents who remain self-absorbed and do not develop a sense of responsibility toward their children.

Later Adulthood

The final adult stage occurs in the later years, 50s and beyond, and involves the psychosocial crisis of *integrity versus despair and disgust*. Integrity involves accepting one's own life cycle, the people who are significant in it, and responsibility for one's own life. Integrity of the ego "implies an emotional integration which permits participation by followership as well as acceptance of the responsibility of leadership" (Erikson, 1959, p. 99). The responsibility of being a follower and leader is learned and practiced. The absence of integrity is despair, which may be hidden by disgust. Individuals in despair feel as if life is too short to start again and to strive for integrity.

PSYCHOSOCIAL DEVELOPMENT OF INDIVIDUALS WITH IDD

Cognitive, communication, and motor development and adaptive functioning are related to and interrelated with psychosocial development. Respecting and understanding these relationships and interrelationships are particularly important for nurses working to advance the development and well-being of individuals with IDD and their families. Psychosocial development is influenced by individuals' unique characteristics, their behaviors, and their experiences with parents, family, friends, and the community. The characteristics, behaviors, and experiences of individuals with IDD often result from and are related to the disability. This section begins with a discussion of characteristics and behaviors of individuals with IDD that influence psychosocial development.

Characteristics and Behavior

Psychosocial development can be seen and most easily understood through an individual's characteristics and behavior. Characteristics are the distinctive features and behavior is the visible evidence of the development and growth that are taking place within an individual. Psychosocial development of the individual with IDD is discussed from the perspectives of the individual's characteristics and behavior.

Difficulty communicating with and responding to others can impact the psychosocial development of individuals with IDD. The impact of a hearing loss in infants and young children on their psychosocial development is described by Rall (2007). Infants with a hearing loss may not be able to benefit from auditory cues (e.g., a parent's verbal attempt to soothe and offer affection, a ringing telephone that distracts a parent's attention away from them). These experiences can influence the infant's learning *trust versus mistrust*. Parents may focus their attention on adjusting to their infant's hearing loss and be less available to respond consistently to their infant's needs. For example, parents may overprotect toddlers with a hearing loss and not encourage them to try new activities or increase their independence. Overprotection can hinder toddlers' movement toward developing independence and learning to resolve the psychosocial crisis of *autonomy versus shame and doubt*. Overprotection of children with IDD can have undesirable consequences over the long term (Sanders, 2006). For example, 3- to 6-year-old children with hearing loss may find that access to aspects of their environment is limited, which can result in a lack of meaningful and consistent communication with their peers, teachers, and family members. These limitations can interfere with children's efforts to acquire a sense of accomplishment and learn *initiative versus guilt*.

Children with severe IDD may respond less frequently and differently from children with milder IDD or children without IDD. The diminished or lack of responsiveness observed in children with severe IDD may result in parents' reduced awareness of their children's cues (Woolfson & Grant, 2006). Parents may engage in an authoritative style of parenting to counter society's low expectations of children with disabilities and their children's future in society (Woolfson, 2004). As children with IDD grow older, parents' style of parenting becomes less authoritative (Woolfson & Grant, 2006). This change may reflect adaptive coping responses on the part of parents along with an increase in the child's ability and willingness to respond. Changes in children and adults with IDD influence and are influenced by the responses from parents, family members, and others.

The influence of behavior and characteristics of individuals with IDD on their psychosocial development is considered from the perspective of Prader-Willi syndrome (PWS). During their first 2 years, children with PWS tend to have noticeably low muscle tone and poor feeding skills, which can lead to failure to thrive. Feeding problems during infancy may affect infants' learning of *trust verus mistrust*. Parents of infants with PWS may view themselves as inadequate when they cannot respond successfully to their infant's cues and when their infant's cues are subtle or nonexistent. Similarly, infants with PWS may experience frustration when their parents do not respond to their cues or when their attempts at responding to their parents are unsuccessful. Low muscle tone may prevent infants from reaching toward and grasping their mother's finger or an object. This can affect parent–infant interactions; the mutual and reciprocal interactions that allow parents' and infants' needs to be met and that help establish a trusting relationship may be limited or absent.

Between ages 2 and 3 years, children with PWS surprise parents as they transition from being underweight to having an insatiable appetite and gaining weight. Initially, parents are pleased that their toddler is eating and eating often. In addition to having an insatiable appetite, these toddlers may have behavior problems, such as constant foraging for food, stubbornness, refusal, inflexibility, and tantrums. Marked obesity will occur if steps are not taken to restrict access to food items. Toddlers with PWS not only overeat and forage for food, but they may also eat nonfood items, such as garbage and dog food. Parents may then begin to restrict their toddlers with PWS from certain areas to prevent overeating and unsafe situations. They must closely monitor their children and prevent easy access to food in all settings. Because of these necessary restrictions and close monitoring, children with PWS may face challenges with learning *autonomy versus shame and doubt, initiative versus guilt,* and *industry versus inferiority* (Erikson, 1959). Parents may be challenged to find creative ways to guide their children toward learning these tasks. Intensive behavior management programs for individuals with PWS may start during the early childhood years and continue into adulthood to address behavior problems such as obsessive-compulsive disorder (Alexander, 2006a).

Experiences

Individuals with IDD participate in a variety of activities to expand their knowledge and skills. Full participation varies for each individual with IDD. Although opportunities for full participation depend on society's policies, attitudes, and commitment to quality of life, the role of families in making sure individuals have opportunities for full participation is crucial. This section focuses on the important role of families in promoting the psychosocial development of individuals with IDD.

All families are interestingly diverse; they develop, change, and live with change. However, the experiences of families of individuals with IDD may vastly differ from families that do not include individuals with IDD. Family members may provide direct care and assistance to the individual with IDD. They may engage in activities to assure that the individual with IDD is included in school, neighborhood, and community activities.

Research studies have focused on the stress, coping, and adaptation of parents of children with IDDs (Glidden, Billings, & Jobe, 2006; Plant & Sanders, 2007; Webster, Majnemer, Platt, & Shevell, 2008). The assumption has been that family members who provide care and assistance to individuals with an IDD experience increased stress and often have health problems related to their stress. Research studies have also focused on the experience of having a child with or being a relative of an individual with an IDD (Eddy & Engel, 2008; Paczkowski & Baker, 2007; Trute, Hiebert-Murphy, & Levine, 2007). It is thought that by understanding the experience of family members of individuals with IDDs, appropriate interventions can be developed to support the family. In turn, it is thought that family members who understand the unique behavior, temperament, and functional limitations of the individual with an IDD will respond appropriately to the individual's needs. This appropriate responding to the individual's needs is expected to then decrease the negative impact of the IDD on the individual and the family (Raina et al., 2005). Therefore, interventions and preventive strategies have focused on helping family caregivers remain healthy so they will be available to respond appropriately to the individual (Birdsong & Parish, 2008; Ha, Hong, Seltzer, & Greenberg, 2008; Magana & Smith, 2008; McCallion & Nickle, 2008).

When family members are healthy and available to individuals with IDD during stressful times, they promote greater trust and sense of security in individuals with IDD compared to families whose members are not available. In a study exploring their hospitalization experience, preschool and school-age children with IDD were found to be comforted by their parents, siblings, hospital staff, and toys or personal items (Angstrom-Brannstrom, Norberg, & Jansson, 2008). Contact with family members and knowledgeable and skilled hospital staff helped the children to trust, feel safe, and cope with stressful situations during their hospital stay. Parents were the most comforting to the children.

Parenting children with IDDs can be more stressful and problematic than parenting typically developing children (Woolfson & Grant, 2006). Parents' stress may be related to their involvement in addressing daily care needs of their children (Roberts & Lawton, 2000). Raina et al. (2005) described the challenging nature of this added stress in a study of adult caregivers of children with cerebral palsy. Child behavior, caregiving demands, and family functioning were the most important predictors of caregiver well-being. Caregivers had better physical and psychological health when they had fewer caregiving demands, children who had fewer behavior problems, and higher family functioning. In addition, caregivers who had a higher self-esteem, had sense of mastery over their caregiving situation, and used more stress management strategies had better psychological health. Social support provided by the immediate family had greater impact on caregiver health than social support provided by the extended family, friends, and neighbors. The day-to-day needs of the child with cerebral palsy and the support from immediate family members, not parents' sense of self or social supports, mediated the impact of the child's level of disability on parent health.

Parents' expectations and perceptions of both their child and their child's disability contributed to their own adjustment to the disability and the degree of their stress. In a study of relationships between toileting concerns, behavior problems, and parenting stress in children with neural tube defects, developmental-behavioral disabilities, and history of intraventricular hemorrhage, Macias, Roberts, Saylor, and Fussell (2006) found that parents whose children had toileting concerns that were expected due to the nature of their disability (i.e., neural tube defect) experienced less stress than parents whose children had toileting concerns that were not an expected part of their disability (i.e., attention-deficit/hyperactivity disorder [ADHD], learning disabilities). The education about their child's disability influenced parents' perceptions and expectations of their child. Parents who were educated about the likelihood of toileting concerns among their children with a neural tube defect were prepared to expect these concerns. Parents of children with ADHD and learning disabilities were most likely not educated about toileting concerns because these concerns typically do not co-occur with these two diagnoses. The experience of being educated about their children's IDD and future expectations of their children helped decrease parents' stress.

Mothers of children with Down syndrome found real differences between their own and others' expectations about having a child with Down syndrome (Lalvani, 2008). The predominantly negative societal expectations for families of children with Down syndrome were not experienced by these mothers. These mothers focused their attention not only on their child's diagnosis of Down syndrome but also on issues of social inclusion, acceptance, and rejection of their child. Expressions of sympathy from health professionals were viewed as counterproductive, as was the pressure from health professionals to terminate their pregnancy following prenatal testing. Limited opportunities to know individuals with Down syndrome and their families and a lack of accurate information about Down syndrome were sources of stress. These mothers viewed Down syndrome in the context of their children, their social environments, and their political environments.

Individuals with IDD who grow up in an environment in which their parents and family members promote inclusion and acceptance have very different experiences from children who grow up in an environment in which parents isolate themselves and their children from their family, friends, or the community (Sanders, 2006). Inclusion and full participation in chosen activities that occur within the context of family and friends provide individuals with opportunities for psychosocial development. An individual's choices, preferences, abilities, and opportunities help determine experiences; however, it is family members, friends, educators, nurses, and other health professionals who determine the breadth and diversity of these experiences.

NURSING CARE THAT PROMOTES PSYCHOSOCIAL DEVELOPMENT

The following section will present information on the nursing care to promote psychosocial development in individuals with IDD across the life span. Clinical approaches to screening, assessment and intervention and treatment plans are discussed.

Screening and Assessment

Screening for psychosocial concerns should be conducted at routine health visits and when concerns are expressed by individuals with IDD, their families, and other familiar persons. Individuals with IDD and their families should be expected to participate as fully as possible in screening and assessment and in developing and implementing intervention and treatment plans.

The prevalence of psychosocial concerns is evident from the data on the prevalence of emotional, behavioral, and developmental problems. In a report from the National Survey of Children's Health, parents reported on having a child with a chronic emotional, developmental, or behavioral problem that was expected to last 12 months or longer (Blanchard, Gurka, & Blackman, 2006). Slightly more than 5% of children between birth and 17 years (approximately 1.5 million children) were reported to have persistent emotional, developmental, and behavioral problems. The rates of parent concerns about their children's emotional, developmental, and behavioral problems were much higher. Parents of 6- to 17-year-old children expressed concerns about their children having learning difficulties, depression/anxiety, eating disorders, and substance use at rates of 41%, 36%, 25%, and 22%, respectively.

The prevalence of mental illness among individuals with an IDD is thought to be between 20% and 35% (Poindexter, 2002, 2003). However, the rates for psychosocial and mental health problems in individuals with IDD are thought to be unreliable because symptoms of mental health problems may be attributed to a IDD and remain undiagnosed. Individuals with IDD who also have psychosocial concerns may not receive a proper diagnosis and the services they need until behavior problems and disruptions occur.

This lack of diagnosing psychosocial and mental health problems due to the presence of IDD is referred to as *diagnostic overshadowing* (Reiss, 2001). In other words, psychosocial and mental health problems are attributed to the disability. Equally concerning is the attributing of physical disorders to a disability. Some physical problems may closely resemble or complicate mental health disorders in individuals with IDD (Ailey, 2005). For example, symptoms of a sleep disorder can include appetite changes, behavior changes, depression, and mood swings that may be mistakenly attributed to an IDD. Nurses and other health professionals focus their attention on an individual's IDD and may unconsciously deemphasize the individual's psychosocial well-being. Identification of psychosocial and mental health problems in individuals with IDD demands careful communication between nurses, individuals with IDD, their families, and other professionals. Individuals with IDD may not receive a proper mental health diagnosis because the symptoms and signs are attributed to the disability or other disorders and go unrecognized (Benson, 2005). An in-depth discussion of mental health issues can be found in Chapter 14.

Support for the screening and early detection of mental health problems in children is found in a report generated from the 2001 National Survey of Children with Special Health Care Needs (CSHCN) data. CSHCN who had chronic emotional, behavioral, and developmental problems were more likely to have diminished health and quality of life and have problems accessing and receiving needed care compared to CSHCN without emotional, behavioral, and developmental problems (Centers for Disease Control and Prevention, 2005). The prevalence of emotional, behavioral, and developmental problems was greatest among CSHCN who were living in poverty, adolescents, and boys. These findings from this report reinforced prior recommendations for expansion of screening and early detection of emotional, behavioral, and developmental problems and improved access, coordination, and quality of services for children with these problems.

Individuals with disabilities may be at increased risk for abuse by their parents or caregivers, assault, exploitation, incest, and rape (American Academy of Pediatrics, 2001). Although children with IDD have been reported to be at increased risk for abuse, the definitions of child abuse and IDD vary across studies (Alexander, 2006b). A study of risk for maltreatment by Jaudes and Mackey-Bilaver (2008) revealed that children who were younger than 6 years, who were from families with low incomes, and who had behavior/mental health problems were at highest risk for abuse or neglect. Disabilities did not appear to increase the children's risk for maltreatment. Friedlaender et al. (2005) found that children who were victims of serious abuse and neglect changed their primary care providers more often than nonabused children when the socioeconomic status, race, and health status of the children were controlled. They found that children who had been abused or neglected were seven times more likely to have changed health providers in the past year compared to children who had not been abused or neglected.

Although incorporating routine screening for psychosocial problems into clinical practice can result in increased identification of these problems, challenges related to screening and assessing individuals with IDD exist. In addition to the previously mentioned diagnostic overshadowing (Reiss, 2001), the following factors contribute to underidentification of psychosocial problems (Centers for Disease Control and Prevention, 2005):

1. Delay between the onset of signs and symptoms and diagnosis of psychosocial problems

2. Parent's lack of recognition of signs and symptoms as indicative of an emotional or behavioral disorder

3. Parent's belief that problems are not serious enough to warrant treatment or counseling

4. Lack of available resources and supports

5. Parent's lack of awareness of available resources and supports for their children

Advanced training in psychosocial issues for clinic staff and pediatricians has been recommended to improve the identification and management of children with psychosocial problems (Leaf et al., 2004).

Eliciting family members' and caregivers' concerns about psychosocial problems in individuals with disabilities can be challenging. Horwitz, Leaf, and Leventhal (1998) described issues encountered when eliciting parents' concerns about their child's psychosocial development. Parents were least likely to discuss their child's social/peer relationships with a pediatric health professional and most likely to discuss their child's annoying habits, learning difficulties, behavior problems, disciplinary issues, and family difficulties. Parents believed it was appropriate to discuss their child's psychosocial problems with a pediatrician, yet only 41% actually brought up these problems for discussion.

Although nurses face similar challenges when they screen and assess for psychosocial problems in individuals with IDD, nurses have options to consider. Benson (2005) proposed that health professionals who screen and assess individuals with IDD can

1. Use an instrument that was developed for the general population

2. Modify an instrument for use with individuals with IDD

3. Develop new instruments that are designed specifically for use with individuals with IDD

Benson exemplified this by pointing out that assessment of depression in individuals with a disability can be accomplished by administering the Beck Depression Inventory (Beck, Ward, Mendelson, Mock, & Erbaugh, 1961) which is used with the general population; the Children's Depression Inventory (Kovacs, 1981), which can be read to individuals with IDD; and the Reynolds Depression Scale (Reynolds & Baker, 1988), which was developed for individuals with IDD. Various instruments can be used to screen and assess psychosocial development (see Tables 7.1 and 7.2).

Communication between individuals with disabilities, their parents, their family members, their caregivers, nurses, and other health professionals provides opportunities for all to gain new information and insights and to clarify their understanding of previously acquired information. The use of medical jargon when communicating about IDD can hinder understanding if not properly used and explained. Farrell, Deuster, Donovan, and Christopher (2008) examined pediatric residents' use of medical jargon during their discussions with standardized patients about a child being a carrier for a genetic disorder. Residents commonly used medical jargon when they communicated with parents and seldom explained the meaning of the jargon. When they explained the meaning of the jargon, the explanation occurred far after the use of the word. Based on their results, these authors questioned whether parents were able to understand health professionals' explanations. They noted that parents who felt uncomfortable asking questions about the medical jargon may develop psychosocial issues of their own, have difficulty making informed decisions, and be unprepared to follow a recommended treatment plan. In short, the communication between health professionals and parents can be more harmful than beneficial if parents leave the discussion uninformed, anxious, and alienated. Pediatric residents seemed to be aware of the potential for parents to misunderstand medical jargon, as evidenced by 86% of the residents explaining one or more jargon words.

In summary, screening for psychosocial and mental health problems in individuals is necessary and should be integrated into routine health visits. Psychosocial issues should be considered by nurses during all contact with individuals with

Table 7.1. Psychosocial screening instruments

Instrument	Source	Age range	Time to administer
Ages & Stages Questionnaires® (ASQ-3), Third Edition[a]	Squires, J., & Bricker, D. (with Twombly, E., Nickel, R., Clifford, J., Murphy, K., Hoselton, R., Potter, L., et al.) (2009). *Ages & stages questionnaires® (ASQ-3): A parent completed, child monitoring system* (3rd ed.). Baltimore: Paul H. Brookes Publishing Co. http://www.brookespublishing.com	2–66 months	15–20 minutes
Battelle Developmental Inventory[a]	Newborg, J. (2004). *Battelle developmental inventory (BDI-2)* (2nd ed.). Itasca, IL: Riverside. http://www.riverpub.com	0–8 years	15–20 minutes
Denver II Developmental Screening Test[a]	Frankenburg, W.K., Dodds, J.B., Archer, P., Bresnick, B., Maschka, P., Edelman, N., & Shapiro, H. (1992). *Denver II* (2nd ed.). Denver, CO: Denver Developmental Materials. http://www.denverii.com	0–6 years	10–20 minutes
Developmental Observation Checklist System[a]	Hresko, W.P., Miguel, S.A., Sherbenou, R.J., & Burton, S.D. (1993). *Developmental observation checklist system (DOCS)*. Austin, TX: PRO-ED. http://www.proedinc.com	0–7 years	30 minutes
Eyberg Child Behavior Inventory; Sutter-Eyberg Behavior Inventory-Revised	Eyberg, S. (1999). *Eyberg child behavior inventory (ECBI) & Sutter-Eyberg student behavior inventory-revised (SESBI-R) (ECBI SESBI-R)*. Lutz, FL: Psychological Assessment Resources. http://www.parinc.com	2–16 years	10–15 minutes
Family Needs Scale[b]	Dunst, C.J., Trivette, C.M., & Jenkins, V. (1986). *Family needs scale*. Brookline, MA: Brookline Books. http://www.brooklinebooks.com	Families of young children	10 minutes
Family Resource Scale[b]	Dunst, C.J., & Leet, H.E. (1986). *Family resource scale*. Brookline, MA: Brookline Books. http://www.brooklinebooks.com	Families of children	10 minutes
Family Support Scale[b]	Dunst, C.J., Trivette, C.M., & Jenkins, V. (1986). *Family support scale*. Brookline, MA: Brookline Books. http://www.brooklinebooks.com	Families of young children	10 minutes
Home Observation for Measurement of the Environment[c]	Caldwell, B., & Bradley, R. (1984). *Home observation for measurement of the environment (HOME) inventory*. Little Rock, AR: University of Arkansas at Little Rock. http://ualr.edu/case/index.php/home/home-inventory	0–15 years	>60 minutes

Instrument	Citation	Age range	Administration time
Parenting Stress Index[b]	Abidin, R.R. (1995). *Parenting stress index (PSI)* (3rd ed.). Lutz, FL: Psychological Assessment Resources. http://www.parinc.com	1–12 years	20–30 minutes
Parents' Evaluation of Developmental Status[a]	Glascoe, F.P. (2007). *Parents' evaluation of developmental status (PEDS)*. Nolensville, TN: Ellsworth & Vandemeer Press. http://www.pedstest.com	0–8 years	2–10 minutes
Pediatric Symptom Checklist	Jellinek, M. (1999). *The pediatric symptom checklist*. Boston, MA: Massachusetts General Hospital. http://psc.partners.org/psc_contact.htm	4–16 years	10–15 minutes
Preschool and Kindergarten Behavioral Scales–Second Edition	Merrell, K. (2003). *Preschool and kindergarten behavior scales* (2nd ed.). Austin, TX: PRO-ED. http://www.proedinc.com	3–6 years	15–20 minutes
Strengths and Difficulties Questionnaire	Goodman, R. (1997). The strengths and difficulties questionnaire: A research note. *Journal of Child Psychology and Psychiatry, 38,* 581–586. http://www.sdqinfo.com	3–16 years	10 minutes

[a]Instrument measures multiple domains of development to include psychosocial development.
[b]Instrument used to screen family and family resources.
[c]Instrument used for screening and assessment.

Table 7.2. Psychosocial assessment instruments

Instrument	Source	Age range	Time to administer
Child Behavior Checklist	Achenbach, T., & Rescorla, L. (2000). *Child behavior checklist for ages 1½–5.* Burlington, VT: Achenbach System of Empirically Based Assessment. http://www.aseba.org	18–60 months	20–30 minutes
Assessment, Evaluation, and Programming System[a]	Bricker, D. (Series ed.). (2002). *Assessment, evaluation, and programming system (AEPS®) for infants and children* (2nd ed.). Baltimore: Paul H. Brookes Publishing Co. http://www.brookespublishing.com	0–6 years	>60 minutes
Bayley Scales of Infant Development[a]	Bayley, N. (2005). *Bayley scales of infant and toddler development (Bayley-III)* (3rd ed.). San Antonio, TX: Pearson. http://pearsonassess.com/	1–42 months	60 minutes
Behavior Assessment System for Children, Second Edition	Reynolds, C.R., & Kamphaus, R.W. (2004). *Behavior assessment system for children (BASC-2)* (2nd ed.). Circle Pines, MN: American Guidance Service Publishing. http://www.agsnet.com	2–21 years	20–30 minutes
Brief Infant Toddler Social Emotional Assessment	Briggs-Gowan, M., & Carter, A. (2005). *Brief infant toddler social emotional assessment (BITSEA).* San Antonio, TX: Pearson. http://pearsonassess.com/	12–36 months	7–15 minutes
Devereux Early Childhood Assessment Program	LeBuffe, P.A., Naglieri, J.A., & Foundation, D. (1999). *Devereux early childhood assessment.* Lewisville, NC: Kaplan Press. http://www.kaplanco.com	2–5 years	10 minutes
Early Learning Accomplishment Profile[a]	Glover, M.E., Preminger, J.L., & Sanford, A.R. (1988). *Early learning accomplishment profile for young children: Birth to 36 months.* Lewisville, NC: Kaplan Early Learning Company. http://kaplanco.com	0–36 months	>60 minutes
Functional Emotional Assessment Scale	Greenspan, S.I., DeGangi, G., & Wieder, S. (2001). *The functional emotional assessment scale (FEAS).* San Antonio, TX: Pearson. http://harcourtassessment.com/HAIWEB/Cultures/en-us/Productdetail.htm?Pid=015-8005-333	7–48 months	20 minutes
Infant-Toddler Developmental Assessment[a]	Provence, S., Erikson, J, Vater, S., & Palmeri, S. (1995). *Infant toddler developmental assessment (IDA).* Rolling Meadows, IL: Riverside Publishing. http://www.riverpub.com	0–42 months	>60 minutes
Infant Toddler Social Emotional Assessment	Carter, A., & Briggs-Gowan, M. (2005). *Infant toddler social emotional assessment (ITSEA).* San Antonio, TX: Pearson. http://pearsonassess.com/	12–36 months	30–45 minutes
Social Skills Rating System	Gresham, F.M., & Elliott, S.N. (1990). *Social skills improvement system rating scales.* Circle Pines, MN: American Guidance Service. http://www.agsnet.com	3–18 years	15–25 minutes
Vineland II: Vineland Adaptive Behavior Scales, Second Edition[a]	Sparrow, S.S., Cicchetti, D.V., & Balla, D.A. (2005). *Vineland adaptive behavior scales.* San Antonio, TX: Pearson. http://www.agsnet.com	0–90 years	20–60 minutes

[a]Instrument measures multiple domains of development to include psychosocial development.

IDD whether conducting screening, assessment, or intervention. Screening and assessment places nurses in a position of providing families with anticipatory guidance, information about the IDD and its current and future impact on the individual and family, and options for intervention and referral for developmental and psychosocial problems.

Interventions

Interventions for psychosocial concerns and problems typically focus on prevention and treatment, separately or in combination. Nurses' knowledge of the disability, communication skills, acceptance of and respect for individuals with IDD and their families, ability to form and sustain trusting relationships, and willingness to provide ongoing support are crucial to recognizing psychosocial concerns and preventing and treating psychosocial problems.

To be effective when trying to prevent psychosocial problems in individuals with IDD, nurses must have accurate and up-to-date knowledge of the disability and potential comorbid conditions. Nurses should educate parents, family members, and individuals with IDD about possible comorbid conditions. Education before or when early signs appear can lead to early treatment. Education can help prevent a psychosocial problem, lessen the psychosocial problem, and minimize the stress experienced by individuals with IDD and family members when a problem does occur.

Anticipatory guidance requires clear and careful communication between nurses, other health professionals, individuals with a disability, and family members. In addition to being accurate and up-to-date, the information being shared must be appropriate and timely. The content must be developmentally and emotionally appropriate for individuals with IDD and their family members. Deciding to extend anticipatory guidance to individuals with IDD depends on the views and abilities of individuals with IDD and on the views of parents or care providers. For example, many parents of children with PWS believed that informing their children about future prognoses would decrease their children's well-being (Wigren & Hanson, 2003) and place an unnecessary burden on the child (Van den Borne et al., 1999). Nurses should encourage education of individuals with IDD and involve them in the planning and implementation of their care.

Rall (2007) suggested that support of the family promotes the psychosocial development of infants with hearing loss. Health professionals who openly demonstrated acceptance of infants with a hearing loss and supported and encouraged their parents were preparing parents to be emotionally available to meet their infant's needs. Rall noted that health professionals should educate parents that their child with hearing loss may perceive situations very differently from children without hearing loss. Nurses' support of other professionals' efforts provides additional support to the individual and family. For example, nurses should support the audiologist's efforts to make certain that infants with a hearing loss have visual and auditory access to their parents' communication. This may require use of amplification, teaching parents about the characteristics of good listening environments, and advising parents to encourage developmentally appropriate activities. Parents can promote psychosocial development by encouraging their children to participate in developmentally appropriate tasks, such as hearing aid checks. Parents may contribute to their children's psychosocial development when they allow their children to experience failure and offer reassurance when mistakes are made (Rall, 2007).

In addition to acceptance of individuals with disabilities, nurses should avoid making assumptions that families of individuals with disabilities will have negative experiences and negative outcomes because of a family member's disability. Lalvani (2008) suggested that health professionals should ask parents of children with Down syndrome to share their experiences and the context of their family's experiences instead of assuming that their family will have negative experiences and negative outcomes.

Findings from a study of adult caregivers of children with cerebral palsy supported a biopsychosocial framework that was family-centered rather than a framework that focused mainly on the child and short-term rehabilitation (Raina et al., 2005). Strategies for maximizing caregiver physical and psychological health should include supports for behavioral management and daily functional activities, along with stress management and self-efficacy techniques. Focusing preventive strategies and interventions on caregivers of children with cerebral palsy can help caregivers understand their child's unique behaviors, temperament, and functional limitations and be more responsive to their child's needs. This can serve to decrease the impact of the disability on the child and family. By using cognitive and behavioral strategies to manage their child's behaviors, parents may not only improve their child's behaviors but experience positive changes in their own health.

Support for the importance of educating parents about their child's condition and normalizing aspects of their child's disability as a means of helping parents adjust their expectations and improve their coping was provided in the previously discussed study by Macias et al. (2006). They stressed the importance of attending to parents' reported and existing concerns, even when a primary disability requires much attention. In the absence of education and services, normalization of concerns in children with a disability could help parents adjust their expectations and improve their coping. Health professionals should provide parents with needed information about their concerns, help them design a plan to address their concerns, provide an ongoing evaluation of the treatment, modify the plan as needed, and offer psychological support to the family.

Individuals with IDD and their family members look to nurses and other health professionals for assistance with their spoken and unspoken concerns about psychosocial issues. Psychosocial interventions may consist of assessment and modification of the individual's environment, behavior management, intensive behavior program, parent training, play and cognitive therapy, psychotherapy, and therapeutic communication. Depending on a nurse's education, training, and experience, the nurse may initiate, fully implement, partially implement, or support these interventions. The intervention for psychosocial problems is dependent on the individual's IDD and its related symptoms and on the psychosocial problem and its related symptoms. The intervention must be developmentally appropriate for the individual with a disability and the family. Nurses must genuinely accept individuals with a disability and their families and reveal this acceptance.

Support is provided in numerous ways, such as when family members and individuals with a disability are educated about the disability and are given opportunities to educate nurses about their experiences. Nurses should ask parents regularly about their understanding of information being provided and avoid using jargon when communicating with individuals with IDD and their families whenever possible. Although more research about use of medical jargon with parents and family members is needed, Farrell et al. (2008) have provided some evidence that a jargon word should be followed by an explanation of the word to minimize confusion and misunderstanding.

END-OF-LIFE CARE

Twenty-first century advances in education, medicine, public health, science, and technology have contributed to an increased life expectancy of individuals with IDD, especially in developed countries, where most adults with disabilities reach their 30th birthday and many live into old age (World Health Organization, 2000). As individuals with IDD live longer, they begin experiencing chronic health problems and increase their risk for chronic health conditions that require palliative care (Beange, 2002). This increasing population of individuals with IDD (Boulet, Boyle, & Schieve, 2009; McCallion & Nickle, 2008) demands that nurses examine ways to provide support and address quality of life over the life course.

This section focuses on issues related to dying and death, assessment, and intervention strategies that are unique to individuals with IDD. Strategies for assessing and intervening with individuals without IDD should be used whenever possible; they can be adjusted or modified to meet each individual's and family's needs.

Terminology

The National Institutes of Health State of the Science Conference on improving end-of-life care identified two components of end of life. First, a chronic disease or diseases, symptoms, or functional impairments are present, persistent, and may vary in severity. Second, symptoms or impairments that result from an underlying irreversible disease are present and require formal or informal care and can lead to death (National Institutes of Health, 2004). End-of-life care is provided to persons in their final stages of life. Hospice care is provided in an individual's home or a facility for individuals who are dying (Pace, Burke, & Glass, 2006). Palliative care is provided to reduce pain and other symptoms with the aim of treating rather than curing (Stevens, Lynm, & Glass, 2006).

End-of-life care for individuals with disabilities may involve a palliative care approach, a curative care approach, or a combined or integrated palliative and curative care approach, depending on the circumstances and the desires of the individual and family. In many instances, a palliative care approach is preferred. In other instances, a palliative and curative care approach is preferred. An integrated palliative and curative care approach may be preferred for children with a neurodevelopmental disability to assure the ongoing treatment of the disability (i.e., curative care), while a palliative care approach is directed toward the superimposed life-threatening disease (Graham & Robinson, 2005).

Communication

Communication, cognitive, and motor abilities, as well as comorbid conditions, influence an individual's ability to comprehend and respond to the end-of-life experience. For example, an adult with Down syndrome may have cognitive and communication difficulties that are related to the genetic disorder and also experience dementia and depression as he or she ages. The individual's increased difficulty articulating and sharing thoughts and feelings can create additional challenges for family members and caregivers as they communicate with and attempt to support the individual with Down syndrome.

Decision Making

Communication and cognitive abilities of individuals with IDD influence their capacity to engage in decision making about their own health and future. If the capacity of individuals with IDD is difficult to assess, a competency evaluation or testing should be considered. Parents have the authority to make health-related decisions about their children, and surrogate decision makers may be needed for adults with IDD who cannot make informed decisions about their own health (American Association on Intellectual and Developmental Disabilities [AAIDD] Board of Directors, 2005).

The decision to accept or refuse health care and treatment requires an informed consent from individuals with IDD or their surrogate decision maker. This means that individuals with IDD have the legal capacity to give consent, have received adequate information to understand the benefits and risks of the treatment, have been offered the opportunity to ask questions and receive answers that they can understand, and have not been forced to accept a particular treatment (The Arc, Congress of Delegates, & AAIDD Board of Directors, 2002).

Two policies related to the principles for end-of-life care focus on permissible treatment options and physician behavior. End-of-life treatment options for individuals with an intellectual or developmental disability should be the same as for all individuals. Physicians should follow existing codes of medical ethics, state laws, federal laws, and their conscience (AAIDD Board of Directors, 2005). These two policies are directed toward physicians; however, they are relevant for nurses and other health professionals.

Assessment

Meaningful, clear, and productive communication is crucial to assessing and identifying the emotional, physical, psychosocial, and spiritual needs of individuals with an IDD. Communication can become problematic when individuals with IDD become frightened and anxious, when they experience pain, or when they must receive care in an unfamiliar environment. Nurses' interpretations of verbal and nonverbal signs of pain and distress become even more important when individuals have limited communication.

Nurses may effectively assess pain and distress in individuals with IDD using tools that were developed for individuals without a disability. The effective use of a tool depends on the individual's cognitive and communication abilities and the nurse's knowledge of the individual's abilities, knowledge of the tool, and ability to properly administer it. Special tools such as the Abbey Pain Scale (Abbey et al., 2004) and the Disability Distress Assessment Tool (Mencap, 2008; Regnard et al., 2007) have been recommended to assess individuals with communication problems (Read & Thompson-Hill, 2008). Brown, Burns, and Flynn (2005) developed a checklist to document the responses and experiences of the individual and staff members when the individual has an IDD and is terminally ill. This checklist also helps staff evaluate interventions that are geared toward managing pain and distress and guides them toward sensitively involving family members.

Intervention

End-of-life care requires collaboration among individuals with IDD, their family members, caregivers, nurses, and other professionals. Options for treatment at the end of life should be the same for individuals with and without IDD. Likewise, options for nursing interventions should be the same. Nursing interventions should be carefully adapted to the individual with IDD and the individual's own situation. Strategies that can be helpful to nurses in their work with individuals with IDD and their families are being identified and new strategies are being developed (Read & Thompson-Hill, 2008; Willis, 2007). Tools that can be useful to health professionals who are providing end-of-life care include the Gold Standards Framework (Gold Standards Framework, 2005), Liverpool Care Pathway, and the Preferred Priorities of Care (Read & Thompson-Hill, 2008).

Family members and caregivers helping individuals with IDD deal with loss and death of others can be the beginning step toward discussing issues related to end of life and end-of-life care. Hollins (n.d.) provided suggestions for assisting individuals with IDD deal with loss and death. Routine bereavement counseling should be offered to individuals with IDD rather than offering counseling when maladaptive behavior occurs. Death education should be provided to professionals working with individuals with IDD and parents and integrated into school and adult education curricula for individuals with IDD.

Meeting individual and family needs requires sensitive and caring nurses who are knowledgeable and informed about end-of-life care and IDD. Application of existing evidence on end-of-life care and generation of new evidence are needed to improve the end-of-life care received by individuals with IDD and their families.

CONCLUSION

Early detection of psychosocial concerns is crucial to promoting psychosocial development, identifying concerns when interventions can be most effective, and preventing further problems for individuals with IDD and their families. Psychosocial interventions that benefit individuals without IDD should be evaluated and interventions that address psychosocial development across the life span should be developed. Nurses should be able to distinguish psychosocial concerns from characteristics related to IDD by having accurate, up-to-date information about the disability. Communication among individuals with IDD, family members, caregivers, nurses, and other professionals should be meaningful and clear to assure that psychosocial problems are recognized and identified and interventions are properly evaluated. Nurses and professionals should assure that end-of-life care is adapted and suitable to meet the unique needs of each individual with IDD and the individual's family members.

REFERENCES

Abbey, J., Piller, N., DeBellis, A., Esterman, A., Parker, D., Giles, L., et al. (2004). The Abbey Pain Scale: A 1-minute numerical indicator for people with end-stage dementia. *International Journal of Palliative Nursing, 10,* 6–13.

Ailey, S.H. (2005). Behavior management and mental health. In W.M. Nehring (Ed.), *Core curriculum for specializing in intellectual and developmental disability: A resource for nurses and other health care professionals* (pp. 291–304). Boston: Jones & Bartlett.

Alexander, R. (2006a). Prader-Willi syndrome. In I.L. Rubin & A.C. Crocker (Eds.), *Medical care for children and adults with developmental disabilities* (2nd ed., pp. 188–194). Baltimore: Paul H. Brookes Publishing Co.

Alexander, R. (2006b). Abuse and neglect. In I.L. Rubin & A.C. Crocker (Eds.), *Medical care for children and adults with developmental disabilities* (2nd ed., pp. 663–671). Baltimore: Paul H. Brookes Publishing Co.

American Association on Intellectual and Developmental Disabilities Board of Directors. (2005). *Caring at the end of life position statement.* Retrieved January 31, 2009, from http://www.aamr.org/content_170.cfm?navID=31.

American Academy of Pediatrics. (2001). Assessment of maltreatment of children with disabilities. *Pediatrics, 108,* 508–512.

Angstrom-Brannstrom, C., Norberg, A., & Jansson, L. (2008). Narratives of children with chronic illness about being comforted. *Journal of Pediatric Nursing, 23,* 310–316.

Beange, H. (2002). Epidemiological issues. In V. Prasher & M. Janicki (Eds.), *Physical health of adults with intellectual disabilities* (pp. 1–20). Oxford, UK: Wiley-Blackwell.

Beck, A.T., Ward, C.H., Mendelson, M., Mock, J., & Erbaugh, J. (1961). An inventory for measuring depression. *Archives of General Psychiatry, 4,* 561–571.

Benson, B.A. (2005). Mental health. In W.M. Nehring (Ed.), *Health promotion for persons with intellectual and developmental disabilities: The state of scientific evidence* (pp. 73–86). Washington, DC: American Association on Mental Retardation.

Birdsong, S., & Parish, S.L. (2008). The Healthy Families Act: Vital support for families of people with developmental disabilities. *Intellectual and Developmental Disabilities, 46,* 319–321.

Blanchard, L.T., Gurka, M.J., & Blackman, J.A. (2006). Emotional, developmental, and behavioral health of American children and their families: A report from the 2003 National Survey of Children's Health. *Pediatrics, 117,* e1202–e1212.

Boulet, S.L., Boyle, C.A., & Schieve, L.A. (2009). Health care use and health and functional impact of developmental disabilities among US children, 1997–2005. *Archives of Pediatric and Adolescent Medicine, 163,* 20-26.

Brown, H., Burns, S., & Flynn, M. (2005). *Dying matters: A workbook on caring for people with learning disabilities who are terminally ill.* London, UK: The Mental Health Foundation.

Centers for Disease Control and Prevention. (2005). Mental health in the United States: Health care and well-being in children with chronic emotional, behavioral, or developmental problems—United States, 2001. *Morbidity and Mortality Weekly Review, 54,* 985–989.

Eddy, L., & Engel, J.M. (2008). The impact of child disability type on the family. *Rehabilitation Nursing: The Official Journal of the Association of Rehabilitation Nurses, 33,* 98–103.

Elder, G.H., Jr. (1996). Human lives in changing societies: Life course and developmental insights. In R.B. Cairns, G.H. Elder, Jr., E.J. Costello (Eds.), *Developmental science* (pp. 31–62). New York: Cambridge University Press.

Erikson, E.H. (1959). Identity and the life cycle [Monograph]. *Psychosocial Issues, 1,* 1–171.

Farrell, M., Deuster, L., Donovan, J., & Christopher, S. (2008). Pediatric residents' use of jargon during counseling about newborn genetic screening results. *Pediatrics, 122,* 243–249.

Freud, Sigmund (2000). *Three essays on the Theory of Sexuality,* trans. James Strachey. New York: Basic Books.

Friedlaender, E.Y., Rubin, D.M., Alpern, E.R., Mandell, D.S., Christian, C.W., Alessandrini, E.A. (2005). Patterns of health care use that may identify young children who are at risk for maltreatment. *Pediatrics, 116,* 1303–1308.

Glidden, L.M., Billings, F.J., & Jobe, B.M. (2006). Personality, coping style and well-being of parents rearing children with developmental disabilities. *Journal of Intellectual Disability Research, 50,* 949–962.

Gold Standards Framework (2005). *The Gold standards framework: A programme for community palliative care.* Retrieved January 31, 2009, from http://www.goldstandardsframework.nhs.uk.

Graham, R.J., & Robinson, W.M. (2005). Integrating palliative care into chronic care for children with severe neurodevelopmental disabilities. *Developmental and Behavioral Pediatrics, 26,* 361–365.

Ha, J., Hong, J., Seltzer, M.M., & Greenberg, J.S. (2008). Age and gender differences in the well-being of midlife and aging parents with children with mental health or developmental problems: Report of a national study. *Journal of Health and Social Behavior, 49,* 301–316.

Hollins, S. (n.d.). *Managing grief better: People with intellectual disabilities.* Retrieved January 31, 2009, from http://www.intellectualdisability.info/mental_phys_health/P_grief_sh.html.

Horwitz, S.M., Leaf, P.J., & Leventhal, J.M. (1998). Identification of psychosocial problems in pediatric primary care. *Archives of Pediatric and Adolescent Medicine, 152,* 367–371.

Jaudes, P.K., & Mackey-Bilaver, L. (2008). Do chronic conditions increase young children's risk of being maltreated? *Child Abuse and Neglect, 32,* 671–681.

Kovacs, M. (1981). Rating scales to assess depression in school-aged children. *Acta Paedopsychiatarica, 46,* 305–315.

Lalvani, P. (2008). Mothers of children with Down syndrome: Constructing the sociocultural meaning of disability. *Intellectual and Developmental Disabilities, 46,* 436–445.

Leaf, P.J., Owens, P.L., Leventhal, J.M., Forsyth, B.W.C., Vaden-Kiernan, M., Epstein, L.D., et al. (2004). Pediatricians' training and identification and management of psychosocial problems. *Clinical Pediatrics, 43,* 355–365.

Macias, M.M., Roberts, K.M., Saylor, C.F., Fussell, J.J. (2006). Toileting concerns, parenting stress, and behavior problems in children with special health care needs. *Clinical Pediatrics, 45,* 415–422.

Magana, S., & Smith, M.J. (2008). Health behaviors, service utilization, and access to care among older mothers of color who have children with developmental disabilities. *Intellectual and Developmental Disabilities, 46,* 267–280.

Magnusson, D., & Cairns, R.B. (1996). Developmental science: Toward a unified framework. In R.B. Cairns, G.H. Elder, Jr., E.J. Costello (Eds.), *Developmental science* (pp. 7–30). New York: Cambridge University Press.

McCallion, P., & Nickle, T. (2008). Individuals with developmental disabilities and their caregivers. *Journal of Gerontological Social Work, 50,* 245–266.

Mencap. (2008). *The Disability Distress Assessment Tool.* Retrieved June 26, 2009, from www.mencap.co.uk/displaypagedoc.asp?id=1477.

National Institutes of Health. (2004). *National Institutes of Health State-of-the-Science Conference statement on improving end-of-life care.* Retrieved January 31, 2009, from http://consensus.nih.gov/2004/2004EndOfLifeCareSOS024html.htm.

Pace, B., Burke, A.E., & Glass, R.M. (2006). Hospice care. *Journal of the American Medical Association, 295,* 712.

Paczkowski, E., & Baker, B.L. (2007). Parenting children with and without developmental delay: The role of self-mastery. *Journal of Intellectual Disability Research, 51,* 435–446.

Plant, K.M., & Sanders, M.R. (2007). Predictors of care-giver stress in families of preschool-aged children with developmental disabilities. *Journal of Intellectual Disability Research, 51,* 109–124.

Poindexter, A.R. (2002). *Cooperation between mental health and mental retardation/developmental disability systems.* Retrieved June 26, 2009, from http://www.nasmhpd.org/general_files/publications/MIDD%20report102704FINAL.pdf.

Poindexter, A.R. (2003). *Cooperation between mental health and mental retardation/devel-*

opmental disability systems—continuation of a dialogue. Retrieved June 26, 2009, from http://www.thenadd.org/pages/membership/bulletins/bullv6.shtml.

Raina, P., O'Donnell, M., Rosenbaum, P., Brehaut, J., Walter, S.D., Russell, D., et al. (2005). The health and well-being of caregivers of children with cerebral palsy. *Pediatrics, 115,* e626–e636.

Rall, E. (2007). Validating outcomes and supporting our youngest patients' development. *Perspectives on Hearing and Hearing Disorders in Childhood, 17,* 8–11.

Read, S., & Thompson-Hill, J. (2008). Palliative care nursing in relation to people with intellectual disabilities. *British Journal of Nursing, 17,* 506–510.

Regnard, C., Reynolds, J., Watson, B., Matthews, D., Gibson, L., & Clarke, C. (2007). Understanding distress in people with severe communication difficulties: Developing and assessing the Disability Distress Assessment Tool (DisDAT). *Journal of Intellectual Disability Research, 51,* 277–292.

Reiss, S. (2001). People with a dual diagnosis: America's powerless population. In A.J. Tymchuk, K.C. Lakin, R. Luckasson (Eds.), *The forgotten generation: The status and challenges of adults with mild cognitive limitations* (pp. 275–298). Baltimore: Paul H. Brookes Publishing Co.

Reynolds, W.M., & Baker, J.A. (1988). Assessment of depression in persons with mental retardation. *American Journal on Mental Retardation, 93,* 93–103.

Roberts, K., & Lawton, D. (2000). Acknowledging the extra care parents give their disabled children. *Child: Care, Health and Development, 27,* 307–319.

Sanders, K.Y. (2006). Overprotection and lowered expectations of persons with disabilities: The unforeseen consequences. *Work, 27,* 181–188.

Stevens, L.M., Lynm, C., & Glass, R.M. (2006). Palliative care. *Journal of the American Medical Association, 296,* 1428.

The Arc, Congress of Delegates, and the American Association on Intellectual and Developmental Disabilities Board of Directors. (2002). *Health care.* Retrieved January 31, 2009, from http://www.aamr.org/content_151.cfm?navID=31.

Thomas, R.M. (2005). *Comparing theories of child development* (6th ed.). Belmont, CA; Thomson Wadsworth.

Trute, B., Hiebert-Murphy, D., & Levine, K. (2007). Parental appraisal of the family impact of childhood developmental disability: Times of sadness and times of joy. *Journal of Intellectual and Developmental Disability, 32,* 1–9.

van den Borne, H.W., van Hooren, R.H., van Gestel, M., Rienmeijer, P., Fryns, J.P., & Curfs, L.M.G. (1999). Psychosocial problems, coping strategies, and the need for information of parents of children with Prader-Willi syndrome and Angelman syndrome. *Patient Education and Counseling, 38,* 205–216.

Webster, R.I., Majnemer, A., Platt, R.W., & Shevell, M.I. (2008). Child health and parental stress in school-age children with a preschool diagnosis of developmental delay. *Journal of Child Neurology, 23,* 32–38.

Wigren, M., & Hansen, S. (2003). Prader-Willi syndrome: Clinical picture, psychosocial support and current management. *Child: Care, Health & Development, 29,* 449–456.

Willis, E. (2007). Symptom care flowcharts: A case study. *Paediatric Nursing, 19,* 14–17.

Woolfson, L. (2004). Family wellbeing and disabled children: A psychosocial model of disability-related child behaviour problems. *British Journal of Health Psychology, 9,* 1–13.

Woolfson, L., & Grant, E. (2006). Authoritative parenting and parental stress in parents of pre-school and older children with developmental disabilities. *Child: Care, Health & Development, 32,* 177–184.

World Health Organization (2000). *Ageing and intellectual disabilities—improving longevity and promoting healthy ageing: Summative report.* Geneva: World Health Organization.

CHAPTER 8

Physical Care of Individuals with Intellectual and Developmental Disabilities

Lee Barks

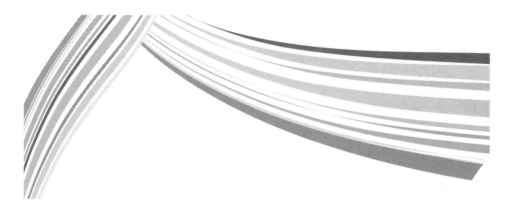

Nurses, by virtue of their professional training, are responsible for physical care when individuals or their families are unable to do so and are in a professional agreement for services. Although the nurse may do this directly, unlicensed staff (i.e., direct support professionals) or family members also may provide supports for physical care. For the latter, the nurse works as a consultant to direct support staff or family; in both situations, the nurse must provide assessment and rationale for payment to justify nursing care (i.e., health supports). In either case, the nurse may be challenged to state what seems obvious to nurses, but not to others.

This chapter describes topics that may need nursing assessment and planning in the physical care of people with intellectual and developmental disabilities (IDD). This chapter also discusses how these supports must be specialized for nursing care to be person-centered and developmentally appropriate. These health supports must be specialized and added to the fundamentals of nursing. The care of individuals with IDD differs from standard long-term care, rehabilitative care, or care in a nursing home setting because it is concerned with achieving new function and independence in addition to regaining, preserving, and maintaining function that has been present. The term *function* here refers to both daily living skills and physiologic function.

It is impossible to specify the physical care required for every possible IDD within this chapter; identifiable syndromes alone number in the thousands. In-

—Special thanks go to Terry Terrell Maas, RN, and Katherine Dula, LPN, of Quest, Inc., Tampa, Florida; and Kim Ramos, RN, Hillsborough County Developmental Center, Tampa, Florida, for their technical assistance with this chapter.

stead, an approach is offered that can be applied to the physical care of any person with IDD. As for all nursing care, a standard fundamentals of nursing textbook (e.g., Potter & Perry, 2009) and the evidence base for current clinical practice guidelines will provide support for how to perform the procedure and the rationale behind the process. Although nursing assessments abound, important assessment areas for IDD are included in this chapter.

Unless otherwise noted, the evidence base for physical nursing care specific for individuals with IDD is extremely limited, typically Level V (i.e., low level and from reviews of descriptive studies only, no experimental research designs) (Ackley, Ladwig, Swan, & Tucker, 2008). Enlarging the evidence base should be a high priority for developmental nurses.

HEALTH HISTORY AND PHYSICAL ASSESSMENT

A nursing physical assessment includes use of observation, auscultation, palpation, and percussion of individuals with IDD. When assessing nonambulatory individuals, nurses need to provide an increased level of observation and intervention. Ambulatory individuals tend to follow the usual nursing physical assessment components, except for syndrome- and diagnosis-specific features. See Table 8.1 for nursing assessment components, cues, and interventions to include in developmental nursing assessments.

MORBIDITY AND MORTALITY

The most common causes of disability-specific morbidity and mortality in people with IDD are respiratory causes (e.g., pneumonia, aspiration pneumonia), seizures, accidents, and gastrointestinal causes (e.g., perforated ulcer, intestinal obstruction; Eyman, Grossman, Chang, & Call, 1990). Physical nursing care addresses these risks as highest priority. Four issues predominate in nursing management: dysphagia (difficulty in swallowing) and prevention of aspiration, management of joint contractures and immobility, management of tracheostomies and enteral feeding, and prevention of seizures and accidents. Nurses initiate health supports and collaborate with the interdisciplinary team (IDT) to manage these threats to health and function, which are detailed in the following sections.

Dysphagia and Prevention of Aspiration

The nurse is responsible for oral medication administration, oral feeding, and assessing all data about the gastrointestinal (GI) tract, including bowel flow, intake monitoring, evidence of gastroesophageal reflux disease (GERD) and characteristics of reflux and elimination, including blood in the stool. There is a very high prevalence of dysphagia among people with IDD. Dysphagia may result in aspiration into the airway, which may lead to respiratory compromise, morbidity, and/or mortality. It also may confer nutritional risk and result in malnutrition. A nurse should look for the least restrictive treatment when addressing dysphagia. The opportunity for the person to continue to eat orally should be valued over staff convenience, and nursing interventions should center on making oral intake safe. For a detailed discussion of dysphagia, see Barks and Sheppard (2005).

Table 8.1. Nursing assessment components, cues, and interventions

Nursing assessment component	What to look for	Nursing intervention
Vital signs and anthropometric data	• Disability-specific anthropometric charts for assessing growth and nutrition	• Collaborate with registered dietitian (RD) to evaluate • Measurement of height may need to be segmental for nonambulatory individuals who cannot stand • Wheelchair scales may be needed for weights
Skin, hair, and nails	• Severe curtailment of positioning options by joint contractures if nonambulatory, and evidence of poor healing related to poor hydration or nutrition, related to dysfunctional, or primitive oral motor patterns (difficulties associated with oral intake related to cerebral palsy, resulting in dehydration or malnutrition) • Skin breakdown related to self-injurious behavior, related to sensory deprivation and altered ability to predict approach by others	• Monitor skin integrity meticulously using Braden or other scale • Provide physical management (frequent therapeutic positioning according to a 24-hour plan and avoidance of factors such as pressure, shearing or surface moisture that lead to breakdown) and use of oral motor therapy by the speech or occupational therapist, with use of specialized oral intake procedures for adequate nutrition/hydration • Provide frequent pleasant sensory input in a socially-appropriate context and provide advance notice of approach through intact sensory channels, such as speaking to the person before touching if the person can hear
Head, eyes, ears, nose, mouth, and throat	• Nutrition/hydration disturbance related to oral hypersensitivity or periodontal disease, which initially may present as avoidance/refusal of oral examination or food or fluid intake, along with white, purulent-appearing gum borders and red gums, or overgrown, or bleeding gums related to phenytoin (Dilantin) use • Abnormal swallow related to primitive or abnormal oral motor patterns such as tongue thrust, tonic biting, lip purse-stringing, and others • Iatrogenic influences, such as anticholinergic drugs, which can interfere with neural transmission and strength/coordination of muscle groups during the swallow	• Ensure frequent, thorough oral hygiene at home and dental prophylaxis and treatment by a qualified dentist • Oral hygiene may need to be adapted, using suction, if the person is prone to aspiration; the nurse should recommend referral to an oral motor specialist, especially with periodontal disease and hypersensitivity • Nursing interventions also include planning with the dentist and behaviorist for dental office visits, including compiling a dental history from health records, a medication history, and planning for sedation, if needed • Collaborate with an oral motor specialist (OMS) for all oral intake • Consider replacement of medication with nonmedical interventions where possible (e.g., therapeutic positioning and specialized handling techniques which result in decreased spasticity and more normal swallow, and specialized presentation of food and fluids)

(continued)

Table 8.1. *Continued*

Nursing assessment component	What to look for	Nursing intervention
Head, eyes, ears, nose, mouth, and throat (*continued*)		• Collaborate with physical and oral motor therapists if needed • Try oral motor therapy for saliva control • If the client has epileptic seizures, assist in classification of seizures and reevaluation of appropriateness of antiepileptic drug (AED) according to seizure classification, to avoid unnecessarily high dosages of inappropriate AEDs that interfere with alertness and oral intake
Neck	• Skeletal deformities such as neck hyperextension that may lead to aspiration	• Collaborate with therapists on positioning options
Chest and respiratory system	• In nonambulatory individuals look for unbalanced thoracic and abdominal respiratory movement; restriction of diaphragmatic movement by pelvis on either side of abdomen (may occur in scoliosis); restriction of thoracic movement by shoulder girdle and upper extremities • Upper airway obstruction related to abnormal muscle tone, prolonged immobility/supine positioning, and posterior placement of tongue and soft tissue over airway. • In all individuals, look for moist rales and/or fever indicating possible aspiration into upper or lower airway, or rhonchi (wheezing) indicating aspiration or reflux following oral intake, or at any time • Respiratory insufficiency evidenced by periodic sweats, anxiety, and agitation, scarring of lungs on X-ray, periodic wheezing following oral intake	• Collaborate with physical therapist to provide therapeutic positioning using gravity and firm support surfaces to elongate trunk, derotate spine, support upper extremities, and remove restriction of respiratory movement by shoulder girdle (e.g., wheelchair positioning or supported sidelying on apex of scoliotic curve) • Protect skin from pressure while positioned • Therapeutic positioning using gravity and firm support surfaces to allow soft tissue to move forward, out of airway space, such as supported prone positioning • Requires careful monitoring to prevent apnea due to the head falling downward • Collaborate with interdisciplinary team (IDT) to determine cause of aspiration: GERD or dysphagia. For dysphagia, collaborate with oral motor specialist to specify positioning and specialized procedures for all oral intake. For GERD, collaborate with physician and therapists for medical treatment and positioning options. • Collaborate with IDT physician for medical treatment options and OMS for effective oral motor intervention. These include altering oral intake texture and consistency which results in aspiration (example: liquids only, pureed food only, etc.) and oral motor therapy. • Therapeutic positioning with alignment and incline against gravity at mealtime, to provide postural stability which can influence the swallow

Problem	Indicators	Interventions
Disturbance in cardiovascular function related to immobility, prolonged supine positioning		• Often, a customized 24-hour therapeutic positioning system is indicated, if the person's contractures have limited positioning options. Consult PT and therapeutic equipment specialist. • Collaborate with physician to refer to pulmonologist
	Postural hypotension, anxiety, apprehension, behavior alterations upon repositioning into upright position	• Gradual therapeutic positioning with alignment and incline against gravity, to provide postural stability • Often, a customized therapeutic positioning system is indicated, if the person's deformities have limited positioning options. Consult PT and therapeutic equipment specialist.
Disturbance in peripheral vascular system function related to • Immobility, prolonged dependent positioning of lower extremities • Disturbance in nutrition/hydration (e.g., low serum protein, edema)	• Dependent edema • Low serum protein, edema	• Therapeutic positioning to support venous return of fluid from lower extremities, such as supported prone, left sidelying, avoiding GERD • Increase active movement where possible • Consult RD and physician to improve nutritional status
Alteration/disturbance of intestinal flow related to immobility or positioning	• Regurgitation, formula odor on breath, oral movements, and observation of re-swallowing of refluxate	• Therapeutic positioning, with alignment and about 30 degrees incline against gravity for a significant portion of the 24-hour day • For slow emptying and gastroesophageal reflux, inclined right or left sidelying (on the apex of the main scoliotic curve) for usually 1.5–2 hours following each meal, or for a representative gastric emptying time, obtained through upper GI series and gastric emptying test • Refer to a gastroenterologist
Disturbance of GI flow related to insufficient fluid/fiber/texture in diet	• History of constipation and inadequate fiber intake	• Collaborate with IDT to increase fiber and fluid in diet • Work with RD and OMS to implement oral motor interventions to increase fluid, fiber, and texture in oral diet

(continued)

135

Table 8.1. *Continued*

Nursing assessment component	What to look for	Nursing intervention
Disturbance of GI flow related to medications	• Slow gastric emptying, reflux, or constipation	• Collaborate with physician and pharmacist to find medications influencing GI flow and advocate for medication changes where possible • Where possible, substitute less invasive, nonmedical interventions (e.g., increase dietary fluid, soluble fiber)
Decreased level of consciousness, related to • Medications • Decreased oxygenation related to oral intake difficulty • Difficulty in maintaining airway patency, related to hydrocephaly and lack of head control • Insufficient hydration • Seizures	• Use of central nervous system depressing medications, such as phenobarbital • Low peripheral O_2 saturation values • Decreased alertness related to low fluid intake and associated decreased urination, high urine specific gravity, usual signs of dehydration. • Low level of alertness • Direct observation or eyewitness data	• Re-evaluate medications for possible substitution of less invasive, nonmedical interventions; collaborate with IDT • Collaborate with OMS and others for oral motor therapy and specialized oral intake protocols • Therapeutic positioning to increase airway patency and chest expansion • Therapeutic positioning to increase airway patency and chest expansion • Collaborate with RD and OMS to increase fluid intake • Collaborate with IDT for improvement in seizure control to improve alertness and fluid intake • Assist IDT to classify seizures and decrease seizure frequency through accurate data collection, use of drug of choice for classification, and control of influencing factors for seizures
Tardive dyskinesia	• Extrapyramidal signs: slowly increasing hand tremors, gait disturbances, and oral and facial movements, as revealed on Abnormal Involuntary Movement Scale, Dyskinesia Identification Scale/Coldwater, or other screening tool for dyskinesia related to medication side effects	• Refer to IDT, including prescriber of dyskinesia-producing medications; reconsider medication regimen • Consider behavioral programs where possible, to reduce or replace medication use
Decreased ability to communicate health needs and control environment, with associated greater health risk, related to difficulties with cognitive function	• Lack of (or limited) verbal ability	• With other IDT members, develop the use of augmentative communication means, including items relating to physical status and pain • Elicit use in all interaction
Alteration of bone density, related to • Immobility • Medications	• Radiologist's comments on osteoporosis/osteopenia • History of osteopenia-inducing medications such as phenobarbital or phenytoin, or on pharmacist's report	• Refer to physician, IDT for possible medical treatment and graduated program of increased weight bearing • Refer to physician, pharmacist, IDT; consider substitution, discontinuation of medications when possible

Positioning, Repositioning, and Contractures

The nurse is responsible for addressing contractures in people with IDD who are immobile. Contractures prevent positioning in functional and safe positions for oral intake and daily activities. Contractures can also predispose the individual to injury due to protrusion from wheelchairs during careless transportation or during transfers. Management for nonambulatory individuals entails development of a 24-hour positioning plan with frequency of repositioning determined by management of pressure on bony prominences, daily activities, and oral intake and digestion. The evidence base for patient positioning in nursing care is primarily Level III or below (moderately strong evidence) and includes some randomized control trials (Gavin-Dreschnack & Barks, 2008a).

Wheelchair seating is the most prevalent form of seated positioning in long-term care. Scientific evidence has shown that institutionalized older adults benefit from individually prescribed wheelchair seating. The use of towels, linens, or bandages to tie a person into a wheelchair constitutes restraint and also poses risk of entrapment (Gavin-Dreschnack & Barks, 2008b). The evidence base for patient positioning in wheelchairs is primarily Level III or above (medium to high-quality evidence), but research is needed with individuals with IDD (Gavin-Dreschnack & Barks, 2008b). For people with IDD, particularly those with spasticity, wheelchair seat belts provide pelvic stability and safety and do not constitute restraint. A recent clinical guideline showed that the evidence base supports wheelchair positioning using the following steps (Gavin-Dreschnack & Barks, 2008b):

1. Position a person in a wheelchair to prevent deformity by positioning the hips and trunk first (proximally) and then position the extremities (distally), with the centers of the head and trunk over the ischial tuberosities and buttocks touching the chair back.

2. Position the person with a comfortable symmetrical midline posture: the head in midline, trunk erect, hips flexed to 105 degrees, knees flexed at 90–100 degrees, feet neutral, spine stable, pelvis level, neck at 11–27 degrees of (slight) flexion, eyes looking straight ahead, and arms supported.

If this is impossible to achieve, the person should be referred for a wheelchair evaluation (see Figure 8.1).

Positioning for oral intake is more than just elevation of the head and neck into a sitting position. Alignment and symmetry are critically important in individuals without trunk control. All structures of the mouth, pharynx, and the neck are necessary for a normal swallow and the pelvis should form a firm base of support for a straight trunk; positioning equipment is often required (see Figure 8.2). The nurse should collaborate on the 24-hour positioning plan with the therapeutic equipment specialist, physical therapist, and other IDT members, as well as assist in positioning and repositioning.

Enteral Feeding

Enteral feeding requires the same positioning measures as oral intake. Food and fluids move superiorly to inferiorly in the GI tract, and from left to right in the stomach. Food must get down into the pylorus because peristalsis is not initiated in the fundus of the stomach, so lying in a supine position does not aid gastric outflow.

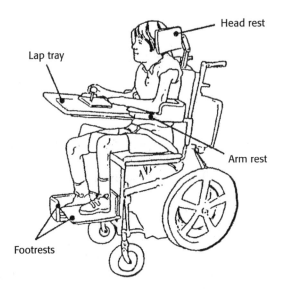

Head rest

Lap tray

Arm rest

Footrests

Alignment Checklist

- ☐ Is the pelvis at a slight anterior tilt and as level and derotated as possible?
- ☐ Is the seat belt snug over the pelvis?
- ☐ Is the trunk straight?
- ☐ Are the nose, navel, knees, and toes pointing in the same direction?
- ☐ Are the shoulders level?
- ☐ Is there weight bearing through the arms and shoulders?

Base of Support Checklist

- ☐ Is there adequate support to stabilize the pelvis in a slight anterior tilt?
- ☐ Do the seat and back provide firm cushioned support?
- ☐ Does the trunk need support on either side to keep it aligned?
- ☐ Is the person's head supported?
- ☐ Are the forearms supported (e.g. arm rest, lap tray)?
- ☐ Is additional support needed on either side of the knees?
- ☐ Do the shoulders need additional support (e.g. pads, shoulder harness)?
- ☐ Is there foot support to keep the base of support evenly distributed across the person's thighs and feet?

Figure 8.1.   Wheelchair positioning. (*Source:* Gerber, McAllister, and Tencza [1992]).

The same positioning is required for continuous enteral infusions. Bolus feeding is preferred, if possible. It should approach normal flow and peristalsis in the tract, with alternate filling and emptying, and a "sump" action in the tract. Continuous infusion feedings increase the risk of reflux and aspiration when either postural drainage or horizontal positioning is employed. Management of GERD is similar to usual medical treatment. The use of fundoplications (surgical treatment to tighten the cardiac sphincter) is not always effective and may result in lack of ability to belch, gastric distention, and pain due to unexpelled intestinal gas.

Tracheostomies

Tracheostomies require the same management as individuals without IDD. The nurse should place a high priority on affording more opportunities to vocalize using equipment (e.g., Passy-Muir valves) to facilitate speech in individuals with IDD.

Position the person in the order indicated. Use a firm, slow touch. The face and mouth are sensitive areas. Alignment for each person is individualized for his/her needs and may look different from person to person. The mealtime instructions include specific directions for positioning, alignment and handling.

Note: These techniques should only be used with the guidance of a therapist.

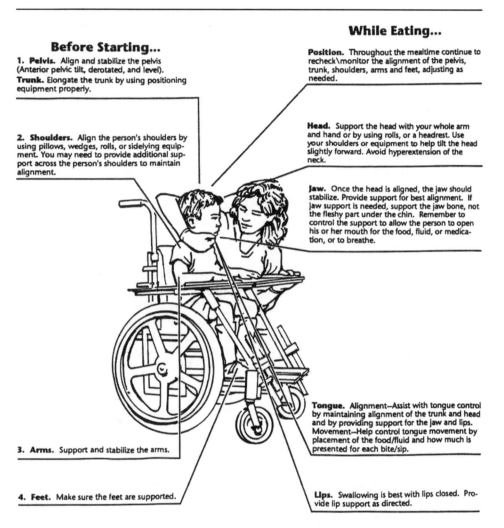

Before Starting...

1. Pelvis. Align and stabilize the pelvis (Anterior pelvic tilt, derotated, and level).
Trunk. Elongate the trunk by using positioning equipment properly.

2. Shoulders. Align the person's shoulders by using pillows, wedges, rolls, or sidelying equipment. You may need to provide additional support across the person's shoulders to maintain alignment.

3. Arms. Support and stabilize the arms.

4. Feet. Make sure the feet are supported.

While Eating...

Position. Throughout the mealtime continue to recheck\monitor the alignment of the pelvis, trunk, shoulders, arms and feet, adjusting as needed.

Head. Support the head with your whole arm and hand or by using rolls, or a headrest. Use your shoulders or equipment to help tilt the head slightly forward. Avoid hyperextension of the neck.

Jaw. Once the head is aligned, the jaw should stabilize. Provide support for best alignment. If jaw support is needed, support the jaw bone, not the fleshy part under the chin. Remember to control the support to allow the person to open his or her mouth for the food, fluid, or medication, or to breathe.

Tongue. Alignment—Assist with tongue control by maintaining alignment of the trunk and head and by providing support for the jaw and lips. Movement—Help control tongue movement by placement of the food/fluid and how much is presented for each bite/sip.

Lips. Swallowing is best with lips closed. Provide lip support as directed.

Figure 8.2. Positioning for oral intake. (From Beckman, D., Roberts, L., & Tencza, C. [1992]. *Mealtime challenges: eating assistance for individuals with severe oral motor challenges.* Winter Park, FL: Oklahoma Department of Human Services by Therapeutic Concepts.)

Seizures

People with epilepsy are at increased risk of nocturnal death while sleeping because of the occurrence of major motor seizures. Recent evidence indicates that heart arrhythmias during a seizure—not suffocation—may be the cause of death (Ryvlin, Montavant, & Kahane, 2006). Prevention should include good seizure management and control using classification and the drug of choice, while also avoiding polypharmacy if possible. Seizure management is generally the same for people with and without disabilities, but collection of seizure management data through other caregivers increases nursing responsibility. Ongoing training of caregivers in seizure observation, medication administration, and side effects is necessary.

Accidents

People with disabilities rely on others to assist with accident prevention. Accidents generally occur due to cognitive challenges associated with a developmental disability (e.g., overstuffing the mouth and choking on a large piece of food, drowning in a swimming pool); maladaptive behavior, such as pica (e.g., eating cigarette butts or other objects and choking); or severe immobility, such as an unattended person in a wheelchair rolling into a street or falling. Because it is not possible to predict all accidents, safety depends on a caregiver's ability to see the environment from the person's point of view and recognize unusual behavior. While providing the person privacy at some times, the nurse should also ensure that sufficient observation is provided for safety, which will be discussed later in the chapter.

Gastrointestinal Disorders

Helicobacter pylori is endemic in long-term care settings. The bacteria can result in peptic ulcers and GI bleeding, which necessitate increased patient monitoring and staff training on hand hygiene. Other GI disorders include dysphagia and intestinal obstruction resulting from constipation or pica. Meticulous monitoring of GI data is warranted, particularly in people who are nonverbal. Monitoring should include oral intake data; elimination frequency; care of ileal conduits, colostomies and surrounding skin; and evaluation of outcomes.

Skin Care, Wound Treatment, Bathing, and Skin Assessment

In the care of patients with disabilities, this nursing function relies more on assessment when patients have communication difficulties or are immobile. When a person with IDD is severely immobile, future skin breakdown is probable; therefore, skin care should be more proactive than usual. The Braden Scale for Predicting Pressure Sore Risk is most often used to identify and monitor individuals at high risk (Bergstrom, Braden, Laguzza, & Holman, 1987; Comfort, 2008; Potter & Perry, 2009). A low score of 6–23 on the scale indicates a high risk of developing pressure sores.

Skin care may be complicated by the individual picking at lesions or engaging in other behavior predisposing to secondary infection. Generally, restraints should not be used, so positive behavioral supports may be needed to assist the individual to allow healing to occur. The nurse should monitor for dryness, excessive skin moisture, common fungal infections (e.g., ringworm), candidiasis (i.e., yeast) in skinfolds, athlete's foot, fungal infections of the groin, scabies, and pediculosis. Nurses should also monitor pressure areas to prevent decubiti; administer treatment for minor illnesses (e.g., fungal or bacterial infections); perform routine nail and foot care, particularly for individuals with diabetes mellitus; and refer for more serious illnesses.

SUPPORTING PHYSIOLOGIC FUNCTION

Normal physiologic function is the foundation for learning and adaptive behavior. To support the patient in this area, the nurse should monitor seizures, psychotropic drugs, drug side effects, serum glucose, hemoglobin A1C, diabetes mellitus manifestations, foot care, and all other body systems. The nurse should ensure that individuals with IDD get to activities on time with proper shoes, properly fitting clothing, foot protection, glasses, hearing aids, dentures, and adaptive equipment (e.g., wheelchairs, communication devices). The nurse should also perform pain assessment in nonverbal individuals, as well as physical assessment for abdominal distention and urinary retention.

Dental Health

Periodontal disease may cause oral infections, pain, and cardiovascular disease. Therefore, caregivers should provide daily oral hygiene (Seirawan, Schneiderman, Greene, & Mulligan, 2008). The nurse often monitors daily oral hygiene and oral health in residential settings to ensure continued adequate oral intake and nutrition. Loss of upper incisors removes the barrier to tongue tip elevation that begins a normal swallow; therefore, natural teeth should be preserved if possible. The nurse usually ensures that the individual visits a dental practitioner at least once per year, has appropriate sedation for the visit as needed, and has anesthesia for scaling as needed. Fillings, crowns, and extractions should be addressed at this visit as well as monitoring for infections, abscesses, or needed hospitalization. The nurse should be prepared to recommend a dental practitioner who can treat people with disabilities.

Safety for the Individual and Caregiver

The nurse ensures safety of the individual with disabilities through use of bed rails, safe wheelchair positioning to avoid falls, and training for safe lifting. Because of the injuries that may occur if patients climb over bed rails, their use in hospitals has often been abandoned in favor of low beds and other safety measures. For nonambulatory individuals, however, more danger may result from falling out of bed, particularly during seizures. Assessment and planning are necessary.

Manual lifting may cause injury to both caregivers and patients; therefore, it is rarely used. Lifting of equipment in the care environment should adhere to National Institute for Occupational Safety and Health (1997) standards for vertical lifts and carrying. These standards vary for different tasks; manual lifting of anything should generally be avoided because of increased intervertebral disc pressure. Mechanical lifts are now indicated for patient lifting. Nurses should encourage employers and staff to make these lifts available, and should use them exclusively (Nelson & Baptiste, 2004). An incident report must be completed whenever an unusual incident occurs, both for documentation of appropriate staff actions and to collect safety data for future prevention of accidents.

Prevention of Secondary Conditions

Secondary conditions may occur in patients with IDD throughout the life span. These conditions are directly related to the disability, but sometimes they may be prevented or their effects may be mitigated. The nurse's role in this endeavor is to observe, advocate, and bring issues to medical attention, as well as to provide daily health supports that prevent development of secondary conditions. Secondary conditions may be screened as part of routine health care. Examples are scoliosis and repetitive stress (overuse) joint injuries in individuals with cerebral palsy, leukemia and Alzheimer's disease in some individuals with Down syndrome, and epilepsy in many individuals with undifferentiated developmental disabilities. Handmaker (2005, p. 52) stated

> Prevalence is correlated to the severity of the [developmental disability]. Greater than half of the children with severe [intellectual disabilities] have sensory impairments (55%), followed by mental health and behavioral problems (50%) and seizure disorders (21%). Children with mild [developmental disabilities] have secondary conditions less often, but when they do, they are most likely mental health and behavioral problems (25%) and sensory impairments (24%).

Nursing care should center on the surveillance for, mitigation of, and prevention of secondary conditions when possible, depending on the particular disability. An important part of physical nursing care for individuals with IDD is annual person-centered planning (habilitation planning), when the IDT addresses prevention or mitigation of expected secondary conditions for the coming year. IDD nurses should familiarize themselves with a person's disability, comorbidities, and potential secondary conditions for this process. For more information on specific secondary conditions, see Batshaw, Pellegrino, and Roizen (2007) and Rubin and Crocker (2006).

Other Responsibilities in Physical Care

The IDD nurse should monitor discomfort and wellness through ongoing physical assessment, including breast and testicular monthly checks. The nurse should coordinate physician and imaging appointments and laboratory work orders; interface with physicians; monitor vital signs and body temperature in minor illnesses; track abrasions, bruises, self-injurious behavior; manage sleep disturbances, interventions, and data collection; interface with behaviorists regarding behavior programs; and coordinate all of this in other environments, such as supported employment settings.

Infection Control

The nurse generally consults on infection control practices in home, school, employment, and recreational environments. Concerns for people with IDD include providing and teaching good hygiene practices for both caregivers and people with disabilities, including hand, oral, and personal hygiene, as well as care of personal articles such as combs, toothbrushes, and shavers. Showers should be routinely disinfected to prevent fungal and other infections. Immunizations are also routinely tracked by the nurse and usually include influenza vaccines and periodic immunizations; however, immunization tracking forms are often proprietary and not shared among providers. Hepatitis B virus (HBV), which can result in hepatic failure and liver cancer, has been endemic in institutional environments for many years due to drooling, personal contact, and other behaviors that predispose to transmission of HBV through body fluids. Consequently, extra vigilance is warranted in the care of individuals with IDD. HBV immunizations are now given, but when HBV titers need to be drawn to determine immunity levels, they are generally not covered by insurance and must be paid by the individual or residential provider. Isolating individuals with methicillin-resistant *Staphylococcus aureus* and other antibiotic-resistant infections from others is extremely difficult, often due to behavioral and cognitive challenges. Management of infection control is situational, according to the residence and staff solutions and policies; therefore, good staff disinfection practices are critical and periodic training is essential.

Transportation

Transportation of nonambulatory individuals is often arranged by the nurse through professional providers. Providing for the safety of riders includes planning for individuals with behavioral issues who could harm other riders or exit the vehicle in unsafe places, such as in traffic. The nurse should ensure that wheelchairs are ready to be tied down, that all necessary equipment accompanies the individual, that a staff member is available to accompany the client, and that adequate time has been provided for safe transit.

Movement to an Acute Care Setting

Because hospital admission must sometimes take place rapidly, annual person-centered planning should include plans for emergencies, an advocate to attend to the person during the stay, and continuing therapeutic positioning. All necessary communication, feeding, and mobility equipment should accompany the person to the hospital and return intact to the residential environment. Hospital staff who are unfamiliar with the person with IDD may draw incorrect conclusions about capabilities, so the person may be discharged with unnecessary treatments (e.g., enteral feeding tubes) when less restrictive means are feasible.

Universal Design

Use of universal design is a practice intended to create an environment accessible to and usable by all individuals, regardless of whether they need a wide doorway to accommodate a wheelchair or sign language during a performance. This practice has been legislated for public structures, but it includes all aspects of participation and access—visual, auditory, physical, and language—so that all citizens may participate actively in community life (Iwarsson & Stahl, 2003; Story, 1998). The nurse's role in universal design is to understand it as a support for people with IDD and to advocate for it when needed. Some nurses may consult on architectural design for the specialized needs of people with IDD.

Assistive Technology

Assistive technology is defined in the Assistive Technology Act of 1998 [PL 105-394] as

> Technology designed to be utilized in an assistive technology device or assistive technology service. An "assistive technology device" means any item, piece of equipment, or product system, whether acquired commercially, modified, or customized, that is

used to increase, maintain, or improve functional capabilities of individuals with dis- abilities. "Assistive technology service" means any service that directly assists an in- dividual with a disability in the selection, acquisition, or use of an assistive technol- ogy device. (p. 6)

Assistive technology for individuals with IDD usually refers to assisted mobility, such as wheelchairs, canes, or walkers and augmentative communication boards like computers, but may include a wide variety of other technologies, such as en- vironmental control switches, head wands, mouth switches, sensors, and telecom- munication devices for the deaf (ABLEDATA, n.d.). The individual with IDD and the IDT typically collaborate on selection of and training in device use, and the nurse reinforces use of the device with the individual.

CONCLUSION

IDD nursing includes the care of both ambulatory and nonambulatory people. Physical care by nurses must be specialized in order to be person-centered and de- velopmentally appropriate, but the evidence base for this care is very limited. IDD nurses should add specialized approaches to fundamental nursing methods and procedures. Physical nursing care focuses primarily on prevention of morbidity and mortality in this population, specifically in the areas of dysphagia and aspira- tion, enteral feeding, accidents, epilepsy, GI disorders, skin and wound care, oral and dental care, and secondary conditions. Other physical care nursing responsi- bilities are to monitor discomfort/pain and wellness through physical assessment, to coordinate medical tests and follow-up, and to coordinate health supports in all environments (e.g., residential, school, employment, recreational). The nurse often coordinates infection control, transportation, and movement to an acute care setting, and may consult on architectural design and assistive technology. Nursing approaches for physical assessment are specialized for the care of individ- uals with IDD. Enlarging the evidence base for this care should be a high priority for IDD nurses.

REFERENCES

ABLEDATA. (n.d.). *Your source for assistive technology information*. Retrieved December 5, 2008, from http://www.abledata .com.

Ackley, B., Ladwig, G., Swan, B., & Tucker, S. (2008). *Evidence-based nursing care guidelines: Medical-surgical interventions*. St. Louis: Mosby.

Assistive Technology Act of 1998, PL 105-394, 29 U.S.C. §§ 3001 *et seq.*

Barks, L., & Sheppard, J. (2005). Eating and swallowing disorders (dysphagia) in adults and children. In W. Nehring (Ed.), *Core curriculum for specializing in intellectual and developmental disability: A resource for nurses and other health care professionals* (pp. 271–292). Sudbury, MA: Jones & Bartlett.

Batshaw, M., Pellegrino, L., & Roizen, N. (Eds.). (2007). *Children with disabilities* (6th ed.). Baltimore: Paul H. Brookes Publishing Co.

Beckman, D., Roberts, L., & Tencza. (1992). *Mealtime challenges: Eating assistance for individuals with severe oral motor challenges*. Winter Park, FL: Oklahoma Department of Human Services by Therapeutic Concepts.

Bergstrom, N., Braden, B.J., Laguzza, A., & Holman, V. (1987). The Braden Scale for Predicting Pressure Sore Risk. *Nursing Research, 36*, 205–210.

Comfort, E. (2008). Reducing pressure ulcer incidence through Braden Scale risk assessment and support surface use. *Advances in Skin & Wound Care, 21*, 330–334.

Eyman, R.K., Grossman, H.J., Chaney, R., & Call, T. (1990). The life expectancy of profoundly handicapped people with mental retardation. *New England Journal of Medicine, 323*, 584–589.

Gavin-Dreschnack, D., & Barks, L. (2008a). Positioning guideline. In B. Ackley, G. Ladwig, B. Swan, & S. Tucker (Eds.), *Evidence-based nursing care guidelines: Medical-surgical interventions* (pp. 622-626). St. Louis: Mosby Elsevier.

Gavin-Dreschnack, D., & Barks, L. (2008b).

Wheelchair positioning guideline. In B. Ackley, G. Ladwig, B. Swan, & S. Tucker (Eds.). *Evidence-based nursing care guidelines: Medical-surgical interventions* (pp. 626–630). St. Louis: Mosby Elsevier.

Handmaker, S. (2005). Epidemiology of intellectual and developmental disabilities. In W. Nehring (Ed.), *Core curriculum for specializing in intellectual and developmental disability: A resource for nurses and other health care professionals* (pp. 33–54). Sudbury, MA: Jones & Bartlett.

Iwarsson, S., & Stahl, A. (2003). Accessibility, usability, and universal design: Positioning and definition of concepts describing person-environment. *Disability Rehabilitation, 25*, 57–66.

Nelson, A., & Baptiste, A. (2004). Evidenced-based practices for safe patient handling and movement. *Online Journal of Issues in Nursing, 9(3)*.

The National Institute for Occupational Safety and Health. (1997). *Musculoskeletal disorders and workplace factors: A critical review of epidemiologic evidence for work-related musculoskeletal disorders of the neck, upper extremity, and low back*. Cincinnati, OH: U.S. Department of Health & Human Services.

Potter, P., & Perry, A. (2009). *Fundamentals of nursing*. St. Louis: Mosby Elsevier.

Rubin, I.L., & Crocker, A. (Eds.). (2006). *Medical care for children & adults with developmental disabilities*. Baltimore: Paul H. Brookes Publishing Co.

Ryvlin, P., Montavant, A., & Kahane, P. (2006). Sudden unexplained death in epilepsy: From mechanisms to prevention. *Current Opinion in Epilepsy, 19*, 194–199.

Seirawan, H., Schneiderman, J., Greene, V., & Mulligan, R. (2008). Interdisciplinary approach to oral health for persons with developmental disabilities. *Special Care in Dentistry, 28*, 43–52.

Story, M. (1998). Maximizing usability: The principles of universal design. *Assistive Technology, 10*, 4–12.

CHAPTER 9

Nursing Care Approaches

Clinical and Practical Considerations

Cecily L. Betz and Martha Wilson Jones

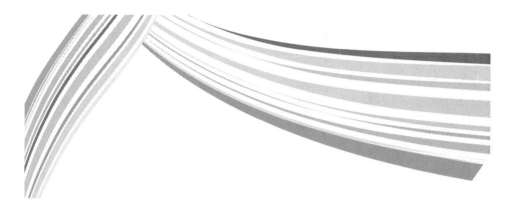

Nurses who specialize in the field of intellectual and developmental disabilities (IDD) can be found in a wide range of care settings providing nursing care to individuals across the life span, ranging from the newborn whose earliest life experience is spent in the neonatal intensive care unit to the elderly individual living in a group home. Unlike other nursing specialties, nurses who provide care to individuals with IDD may be expected to work with a broad range of clients, ranging from infants and children to the elderly.

This chapter provides a description of practices and concepts important to nursing practice. The discussion of the nursing care process includes assessment, outcome identification, planning and implementation, and medication administration that nurses can apply to the care of individuals with IDD. Other topics covered in the chapter include information about nursing standards of care pertinent to IDD nursing care. The chapter concludes with the discussion of roles that nurses who specialize in IDD may be involved in as a collaborator with other interdisciplinary partners, delegator of nursing tasks to ancillary personnel, and researcher as a member of a research team or as a principal investigator.

THE NURSING PROCESS

The nursing process serves as the framework for providing care to individuals with IDD across the life span in a variety of settings, such as the nurse practitioner in an inpatient hospital setting or in a school as the nursing consultant. The unique features of the application of the nursing process as it pertains to assessment, outcome identification, planning and implementation, and medication administration are highlighted in this section.

Assessment

Nursing assessment involves a variety of methods to collect data to identify the nursing needs of the individual with IDD. These methods include the collection of data from agency charts, observation of an individual's behavior in a variety of settings, the use of standardized assessment tools, and interviews with significant members of the individual's circle of support and social network (Betz & Sowden, 2008; Nehring et al., 2004).

The process of assessment is typically different from the assessment conducted for individuals without IDD who are provided care in primary, secondary, and tertiary settings. The individual with an IDD may have difficulties sharing pertinent information about current health status and history because of memory problems, articulation difficulties, or other physical, sensory, or motor difficulties. Individuals with IDD may be unable to understand questions or statements directed to them. Individuals with sensory difficulties present unique challenges for obtaining data. For example, individuals with auditory impairments may require an interpreter who can sign (see Chapter 17). Individuals with articulation difficulties due to cerebral palsy (CP) (see Chapter 13) or other neurodevelopmental conditions may need to communicate using a communication board or language-adapted computer (Betz & Sowden, 2008).

When caring for individuals with IDD, the nursing professional may have to rely more heavily on obtaining data from other people who are knowledgeable about the individual's needs and use other methods of data collection, such as observation and assessment and screening tools. Often, the nurse may collaborate with other members of the interdisciplinary team to collect data, such as assessment of cognitive functioning conducted by the psychologist, hearing evaluation performed by the audiologist, and pedigree data from the genetic counselor (Nehring et al., 2004).

The goal of nursing assessment is to assess the individual's response to the current health care problem and, in relevant circumstances, activities of daily living (ADL) that are impacted by their IDD. The collection of data by the nursing professional includes the individual's identification of their current need for services, as well as the identification of need as described by the individual's family members, caregiver(s), and/or provider(s). The health history information that contains the pertinent long-term issues associated with the current need and recent changes in health status are presented in Table 9.1 (Betz, 2007; Betz & Sowden, 2008; Nehring et al., 2004). The nursing assessment of the clinical needs of individuals with IDD is organized by conducting a review of systems, which are presented in the following sections.

General Health Assessment

Accurate measurement of height and weight is an important parameter because it indicates the process of growth in children and youth. Growth measurement has been described as the proxy for the child's health status (Tanner, 1986, 1992). According to the American Academy of Pediatrics (AAP, 2008), length/height and weight measurements should be performed across the life span of children at infancy (at birth, 3–5 days, then 1, 2, 4, 6, and 9 months), early childhood (at 12, 15, 18, 24, and 30 months, then 3 and 4 years), and annually during the middle childhood and adolescent period. Preterm or standard growth charts can be used with children born less than 37 weeks gestation.

Table 9.1.   Components of the health history

Information to be gathered from individual and support networks	Information to be gathered from interdisciplinary sources
• Individual's identification of current need for services • Family's identification of individual's need for services • Family health history • Community provider's identification of individual's service needs • Individual's current understanding of the health and health-related problem(s) • Individual's health history including current changes in health, emotional and mental status, recent illnesses, hospitalizations, medications, therapies, and health complications • Individual's, family's, and community provider's perceptions of long-term and recent limitations affecting self-care, receptive and expressive language, learning, mobility, self-direction, capacity for independent living, and economic self-sufficiency • List of health care providers, including usual schedule for visits • Individual's and family's cultural beliefs and practices • Individual's and family's health literacy • Individual's perceptions of his or her strengths and limitations • Family's perceptions of individual's/family's strengths and limitations	• Referral reports from medical specialists • Interdisciplinary team reports • Recent laboratory and diagnostic testing for medical problems • Interdisciplinary assessment and screenings (i.e., occupational therapy, audiology, speech and language) • School records including individualized education program and individualized health plan • Agency records such as individualized plan for employment • Individual's, family's, and community provider's perceptions of long-term and recent limitations affecting self-care, receptive and expressive language, learning, mobility, self-direction, capacity for independent living and economic self-sufficiency (Developmental Disabilities Assistance and Bill of Rights Act of 2000, PL 106-402) • Health literacy assessed by valid and reliable instruments • Assessment of individual's strengths and limitations based on professional observations and assessed by valid and reliable instruments • Assessment of individual's strengths and limitations based on professional observations and assessed by valid and reliable instruments

Sources: Betz and Sowden (2008), Nehring et al. (2004).

If the standard growth charts are used, corrected or adjusted age is used rather than chronological age until the age of 24 months (Centers for Disease Control and Prevention, n.d.). If the child has hip or knee flexion contractures or spinal problems (e.g., kyphosis, lordosis, scoliosis), other measurement methods adapted to these special needs should be used, such as handlebars for individuals with stability issues or for those who use wheelchairs (Akron Health Department, 2004; Lipman, Euler, Markowitz, & Ratcliff, 2009; Lipman et al., 2000).

Some children with IDD present challenges for obtaining accurate height and weight measurements. For example, the use of the National Center on Health Statistics (2007) growth charts for specific groups of individuals with IDD would be inappropriate for tracking growth patterns. Growth charts have been developed for use with infants and children with Down syndrome (DS) from birth to 18 years of age (Cronk et al., 1988). The growth pattern of children and youth with DS varies considerably from typically developing children, which is most apparent during the periods of infancy and adolescence (Cronk et al., 1988; Maguid, El-Kotoury, Abdel-Salam, El-Rudy, & Afifi, 2004). Other factors have been identified that can affect the growth patterns of children with DS, including the presence of moderate to severe congenital heart disease and living in an institutional setting (Cronk et al., 1988). Slight variations in the patterns of growth were found in international studies of children with DS attributable to differences associated with geographic regions and culture (Maguid et al., 2004). The AAP recommended that ongoing evaluation of the child's growth pattern using growth charts that have been adapted for children with DS be included with the health supervision visits at 2, 4, 6, 9, 12, 15, and 18 months and annually beginning at 2 years of age (AAP, 2001a). Charts have been designed especially for children with Williams syndrome and CP (AAP, 2001b, 2004; Stevenson, 1995; Stevenson et al., 2006). See Chapter 12 for additional information on DS.

The monitoring of height and weight of individuals with CP warrants special consideration because modified methods to obtain accurate assessments are required. Individuals with CP may be unable to stand or lie in a recumbent position to obtain an accurate measure of stature due to spasticity and abnormal posturing of the limbs. Adapted measurement methods include segmental measurements of the tibia and upper arm lengths and knee height (AAP, 2004; Stevenson, 1995; Stevenson et al., 2006). Growth charts for children and youth with moderate to severe levels of CP have been reported (Krick, Murphy-Miller, Zeger & Wright, 1996; Stevenson et al., 2006). See Chapter 13 for additional information on CP.

The AAP recommends that head circumference be measured until 2 years of age because it corresponds to a critical period of developing brain size and growth. Deviations from established norms of measurement may be indicative of a neurological problem (AAP, 2008; Mraz, Green, Dumont-Mathieu, Makin, & Fein, 2007). *Microcephaly* refers to head circumference that is 2 standard deviations (*SD*) below the mean, whereas *macrocephaly* refers to head circumference that is 2 *SD* above the mean (Purugganan & Adam, 2006). Neurologic impairment is associated with 3 *SD* above or below the normal range of the head circumference measurement. Microcephaly occurs with children who have genetic diagnoses, such as Cornelia de Lange syndrome, fetal alcohol syndrome, and trisomy disorders. Macrocephaly is associated with the diagnoses of hydrocephalus and fragile X syndrome (FXS) (Purugganan & Adam, 2006; Zahl & Wester, 2008). Accelerated brain growth has been reported in studies of infants later diagnosed with autism (Chiu et al., 2007; Mraz et al., 2007).

The individual's ability to engage in ADL is impacted by the extent of physical impairment and intellectual disability, as well as the ability to interact with others. See Chapter 13 for discussion of ADL and use of adaptive equipment.

Hearing and Vision Screening   Hearing and vision screening should begin in infancy to detect hearing and visual impairments. Some states, like California, mandate infant hearing screening prior to discharge from the nursery, which increases the potential for early detection of hearing loss (California Department of Health Care Services, 2007). If screening examinations indicate a possible impairment, then more intensive evaluations are needed. In states without this mandate, hearing evaluations are indicated if the child has a speech delay.

Individuals with IDD will benefit from periodically scheduled hearing and visual examinations because both hearing and vision may decline with age. Individuals who are unable to communicate or who are dependent on assistive technology for communication are at risk for having unmet health care needs, including screenings, preventive care, and health maintenance services. Individuals unable to communicate needs may experience prolonged discomfort, pain, and complications due to delayed treatment.

Auditory screening is particularly important for children with DS because they have an increased risk for hearing loss (75%) and otitis media (50–70%) (AAP, 2001a). Approximately 90% of children diagnosed with Williams syndrome have hypersensitivity to sound and approximately 50% have chronic otitis media. The AAP recommends that children with Down and Williams syndromes be screened for auditory issues during routine health assessments (AAP, 2001b). Infants with DS require screening for strabismus, cataracts, and nystagmus by 6 months of age. About 50% of children with DS have significant refractive errors and should be evaluated annually by a pediatric ophthalmologist with special needs expertise (AAP, 2001a).

Across the life span, individuals with IDD are at higher risk for dental caries due in part to limited access to dental care and inadequate dental hygiene (Pearlman & Sterling, 2006). Individuals with Down and Williams syndromes are at risk for a number of dental problems, including microdontia (Capone, Roizen, & Rogers, 2008; Menon, 2008). Individuals with FXS, DS, and CP have high arched palates, which create problems in feeding and articulation (Phalen, 2005). Individuals with CP warrant special attention to dental care due to disordered oral motor movements, increased gag reflex, and problems with swallowing food in their mouth. Other dental problems of individuals with CP and DS include bruxism, enamel hypoplasia and mouth breathing (AAP, 2001c; Pearlman & Sterling, 2006). See Chapters 12 and 13 for more information on DS and CP, respectively.

Cardiovascular Assessment   Individuals with limited or no mobility are at risk for developing thrombophlebitis. Dependent edema may be observed due to multiple factors of insufficient cardiac functioning, inadequate venous valve functioning, and immobility of the lower limbs. Decreased circulation to the extremities may result in varying degrees of cyanosis and cool skin temperatures of the hands and feet. Secondary conditions associated with cardiac problems noted in individuals with IDD include mitral valve prolapse (FXS), septal defects and endocardial cushion defects (DS), and supravalvular aortic stenosis (Williams Syndrome) (AAP, 2001b; Betz & Sowden, 2008; Phalen, 2005). The AAP recommended that infants born with Down or Williams syndrome be evaluated by a pediatric cardiologist because they are at higher risk for congenital cardiac defects (50%) (AAP, 2001a).

Pulmonary Assessment   Individuals with IDD are at increased risk for respiratory infections. They are at higher risk due to physiologic and environmental factors. Individuals who live in congregate settings, such as group homes wherein they live in close proximity to others, are particularly at risk, because transmission of viral and bacterial microorganisms can be more easily transmitted. Physical limitations causing inadequate respiratory effort due to insufficient respiratory muscle strength, abnormal chest size, and swallowing problems can lead to increased risk for food aspiration and decreased resistance to pulmonary infections (Waltz & Katz, 2006). See Chapter 13 for additional information on factors that can impact pulmonary functioning.

Gastrointestinal Assessment   Swallowing problems, overweight, obesity, and immobility are risk factors for developing gastrointestinal (GI) problems. Individuals who have swallowing problems are at risk for aspirating food consumed and developing aspiration pneumonia (AAP, 2001c; Betz & Nehring, 2007; Waltz & Katz, 2006). In addition, gastroesophageal reflux disease is a potential GI problem that makes feeding in children and eating in adults difficult and painful and thus results in weight loss, failure to thrive (in infants), respiratory distress, heartburn, and gastric fistula. Dietary and mechanical modifications, medications, and surgical interventions requiring the placement of a gastrostomy tube may be implemented to control symptoms and treat the disease (Betz & Sowden, 2008; Whitman, 2008). Constipation can be a problem for individuals with reduced capacity to maintain adequate hydration and lower levels of physical activities (AAP, 2004). GI problems of diarrhea and constipation are evident in nearly 50% and more of children with autism (AAP, 2007a). Infants with DS have a higher risk for Hirschsprung disease and GI atresias (AAP, 2001a). Infants with Williams syndrome who present with GI problems need to be evaluated for failure to thrive, colic, or gastroesophageal reflux. About 70% of children with Williams syndrome have feeding difficulties (AAP, 2001b; Betz & Nehring, 2007). See Chapter 17 of the Core Curriculum (Barks & Sheppard, 2005) for further information.

Other comorbid conditions can contribute to GI problems, such as impaired respiratory functioning, that making eating difficult. Many genetic conditions are associated with enzyme deficiencies (e.g., phenylkeytonuria) or neuromuscular deterioration (e.g., Tay-Sachs disease) that will adversely affect GI functioning (Betz & Sowden, 2008). Constipation may occur because of the inadequate intake of fluids and high-fiber foods or insufficient gastric motility (AAP, 2001c).

Idiosyncratic food behaviors are associated with IDD, such as autism spectrum disorders (ASD), Prader-Willi syndrome (PWS), and FXS. Individuals with FXS may demonstrate obsessive food behaviors that require close monitoring. Individuals with PWS may have a compulsive need to eat or pica behaviors (Whitman, 2008). Methods to control this insatiable appetite require environmental measures, such as locking the refrigerator and cabinets where food is stored. Highly limited food choices and aversions characterize the eating behaviors of individuals with ASD. As mentioned in discussion of general health, the monitoring of growth (height and weight) is essential to address the clinical concerns of underweight (failure to thrive in infants), overweight, and obesity. See Chapters 15 and 16 for additional information on risk factors related to GI functioning for children with ASD and FXS, respectively.

Endocrine Assessment   Children with DS are at increased risk for thyroid disease (15%), including congenital hypothyroidism (1%). The AAP recommends that children and youth with DS be screened during the neonatal period; at 6, 12, 15, and 18 months; and annually beginning at 2 years of age (AAP, 2001a). Hypothyroidism is a medical problem associated with Williams syndrome; screenings should be conducted during the neonatal period and every 2 years beginning at school age. Approximately 50% of children with Williams syndrome experience early pubertal changes (AAP, 2001b).

Individuals with PWS are of short stature due to insufficient levels of growth hormones. Treatment with supplemental growth hormone has been effective. Obesity is a significant problem in individuals with PWS because of a number of contributing factors. Although the underlying cause of hyperphagia in individuals with PWS is not known, it is speculated that hypothalamic dysfunction may be accountable. Hyperphagia and short stature together with abnormal body composition (higher proportion of fat to lean mass) contribute to problems of obesity (Whitman, 2008).

The clinical presentation in infants with inborn errors of metabolism may not be readily apparent. Their symptoms may not become noticeable until months following birth. Instead, the child may exhibit elevated or lowered laboratory values and clinical symptoms such as recurrent illnesses with no evident etiology, loss of motor skills, or growth failure. Additional metabolic testing will be necessary to appropriately identify the diagnosis (AAP, 2007b; Betz & Sowden, 2008).

Genitourinary and Reproductive Assessment

Urinary continence may be problematic if bladder functioning is impaired due to compromised sphincter control, lack of or decreased nerve innervations to the genitourinary tract, or altered muscle tone. Incontinence assessment includes determining the extent of the problem and its pattern (e.g., whether the individual is incontinent during the day, night, or both). Data are also gathered on the methods used to deal with incontinence, including the establishment of a toileting schedule, the use of adaptive equipment or diapers, clean intermittent catheterization, and care of cutaneous ureterostomy. Gathering data on the current baseline of bladder functioning and program is needed for determining the individual's needs for care.

Reproductive concerns and issues are sensitive areas of discussion. Parents of newborns with a readily identifiable IDD or genetic condition will need information not only on their own reproductive options about having additional children, but also on their children's future as well (Sherman, Allen, Bean, & Freeman, 2007). Full comprehension of the reproductive and genetic implications of their child's IDD diagnosis will require the continuous attention to ensure their needs for information are being met.

During preadolescence and adolescence when pubertal development occurs, the emergence of secondary sex characteristics can be monitored using the Tanner scale (Tanner, 1986, 1992). Depending on the IDD, genital development may differ. For example, adult males with FXS will have macroorchidism, whereas a higher incidence of cryptorchidism exists in males with CP. For young girls, the onset of menarche may pose challenges to their ability to understand and communicate their needs to others. A young girl with an IDD may be unable to communicate feelings of discomfort or pain associated with menses, which requires the caregiver to observe nonverbal behaviors that indicate distress. Girls and women with intellectual disabilities may not understand the physiologic explanations for the monthly menstrual cycles, so developmentally appropriate answers for a chronologically younger age may be required. In addition, the ability to engage in self-care of menses will be problematic unless these individuals receive developmentally appropriate instruction.

Later in adulthood, annual prostate screenings, pelvic examinations, Pap tests, and mammograms should be conducted according to established standards of care. Individuals with limited mobility will require accommodations, such as padded hydraulic stirrups, accessible examination tables, and wheelchair accessible spaces (Centers for Disease Control, National Center for Birth Defects and Developmental Disabilities, 2005). Individuals with intellectual disabilities may require behavioral supports prior to and during pelvic examinations, mammograms, and Pap tests. Ongoing needs for reproductive and contraceptive counseling that are developmentally appropriate remain a component of health assessment.

Skin Assessment   Foremost in the assessment of skin integrity is the observation for reddened areas and decubitus ulcers in various stages of formation on the skin surface. Particular attention should be directed to areas that are subjected to increased pressure associated with wearing of splints, use of assistive devices, use of wheelchair or walker, and immobility. Other causes of skin breakdown are urine and bowel incontinence, decreased blood flow to the extremities due to vascular disease and diabetes, and poor nutritional intake (Betz & Sowden, 2008; Gray, Radcliff, & Donovan, 2002). The factors contributing to the development of skin breakdown and decubitus ulcers require assessment of individual and environmental factors. The individual factors include the use of assistive devices, diet, the individual's level of mobility, extent of knowledge to prevent and treat skin breakdown, and level of intellectual functioning. Environmental factors include available caregiving assistance, the living environment, access to care for treatment, available supplies, and the condition of durable equipment used (Betz, 2007).

Neurological Assessment   Assessment of neurological status involves gathering data on the existence of seizures, sensory function, level of consciousness, vital signs with papillary reactions, and in infants, head circumference including fontanelles. If the individual has a seizure disorder, then data are gathered on the history, type, and current treatment effectiveness (Betz & Sowden, 2008). The diagnosis of seizures in individuals with IDD may be made as a secondary diagnosis to the primary diagnosis. The prevalence of seizures in individuals with ASD has been reported to vary from 11% to 39%, with higher prevalence rates associated with individuals who also have severe intellectual disabilities (Myers & Johnson, 2007). Seizures are reported to occur in 10% to 20% of individuals with FXS, attributed to a deficiency of fragile X mental retardation protein (Berry-Kravis, 2002; Phalen, 2005).

An overlooked area of assessment in individuals with IDD is determination of the existence of pain. The source of pain can be due to a number of different causes including muscle spasms, spasticity, and secondary conditions, such as decubitus ulcer, urinary tract infections, gastroesophageal reflux disease, esophagitis, dental problems, colitis, and ill-fitting splints on the arms and legs (AAP, 2004; Breau, Camfield, McGrath, & Finley, 2004).

Musculoskeletal Assessment   The musculoskeletal assessment involves the evaluation of gross and fine motor functioning. Gross motor functioning includes assessment of muscle tone for spasticity, range of motion, and hypotonia (i.e., decreased muscle tone). Spasticity, as observed in CP and other neurogenerative conditions, is manifested by exaggerated deep tendon reflexes, scissoring of the legs, abnormal posture, and clonus.

Fine motor functioning refers primarily to hand and finger movement, which can be assessed by observing the individual's ability to manipulate objects and use hands with small movements. For infants and children, it requires monitoring of their fine motor skills using developmental screening tools; for adults, it requires observation of their abilities to be functionally independent with ADL and in the community, whether in the school or work environments (AAP, 2001c).

Other areas of assessment include posture control, which is the ability to maintain an upright position. Individuals with IDD who have spasticity are at increased risk for posture control problems and may require the use of braces or specially designed walkers for treatment (AAP, 2004). Posture control becomes more problematic as individuals age, such as has been noted with individuals who have CP. Hips are assessed for presence of abduction or adduction. Hip adduction and flexion are found in individuals with CP. Abnormal spinal curvatures of scoliosis, kyphosis, and lordosis may also be present, particularly in individuals with CP and neuromuscular conditions (AAP, 2004). See Chapter 8 and Chapter 13 for additional information on issues pertaining to individuals with CP.

Outcome Identification

Based upon the assessment data, the nurse—in consultation with the individual and family—should identify and prioritize the expected and achievable outcomes of care (Nehring et al., 2004). The expected outcomes should be crafted in measurable terminology that can be verified by both objective and subjective methods. Measurable outcomes should be composed of the targeted behavior change, the methods by which the outcome will be measured, and the date by which the change is anticipated. Examples of outcomes written for nursing care plans include the following:

- The parent will demonstrate the ability to independently operate the oxygen equipment as evidenced by the following actions prior to her child's discharge from the NICU.
- The child will learn to independently dress himself before going to school by the end of the summer.
- The individual will obtain a bus pass, use a bus independently from home to work, and demonstrate understanding of rider safety rules following the completion of mobility training.

This process may be integrated with the outcomes identified by the interdisciplinary team to coordinate care. The benchmark for determining the achievement of the outcome is a component of the evaluation. The progress in achieving the identified outcome is compared to the baseline behaviors targeted (Nehring et al., 2004).

Planning and Implementation

Based on the identification and prioritization of the outcomes of care for the individual, the nurse should develop a plan of care. This plan of care may be based solely on nursing actions or developed in conjunction with an interdisciplinary team of professionals. The nursing approaches that may be chosen to achieve anticipate outcomes are coordination of care, health teaching and promotion, consultation, and prescriptive authority and treatment (Nehring et al., 2004).

As a coordinator of care, the nurse assures that the interdisciplinary recommendations are reviewed, understood, and accepted by the individual and (when appropriate) family members. In the role of the coordinator of care, the nurse serves as the primary resource for family members to consult with about care issues, have their questions answered, generate referrals made by interdisciplinary team members, and serve as the individual's and/or family's advocate. Nurses play an important role in instructing the individual and family on health matters using terminology and instructional materials that are appropriate to their learning needs and their health literacy levels. Importantly, the nurse will continually reassess the extent to which the information and/or skills have been learned, and by necessity, make the adjustments needed to facilitate learning.

As a consultant, the nurse may provide episodic assistance to the individual and family or other members of the interdisciplinary team, particularly when the nurse does not serve as the coordinator of care. In other circumstances, nurses provide direct care to individuals with IDD in a variety of clinical settings. The nursing professional may be a nurse practitioner who has prescriptive authority to generate medication prescriptions based upon the identified physiologic need. The nurse who practices in the hospital setting is responsible for ensuring that the prescribed plan of care is implemented, providing gastrostomy feedings, administering medications, and performing pulmonary toilet. This process of care is evaluated in terms of its effectiveness to facilitate the individual's and family's achievement of anticipated outcomes. Depending on the extent to which outcomes were achieved, the plan may have to be revised to generate new or alter current care approaches using the aforementioned structured nursing process approach (Betz, 2007; Betz & Sowden, 2008; Nehring et al., 2004; Nehring, 2005).

Medication Administration

A nursing issue of particular concern is the administration of medication. There are a number of physiologic, cognitive, and psychological factors to consider when administering medications to individuals with IDD. For example, individuals who are unable to communicate or have articulation difficulties may be at risk for over-medication (Florida Department of Juvenile Justice, 2006). The assessment of these factors will determine whether the individual is capable of self-medication administration; self-administration with physical assistance, such as helping the individual to dislodge a pill from safety packaging; assistance with medication administration pertaining to providing a verbal prompt as to the timing for taking the medication; and medication administration by licensed nursing staff or unlicensed assistive personnel (UAP) in circumstances when the individual with an IDD is unable to perform this self-care task (New Mexico Department of Health, 2006).

Physiologic factors often affect medication administration, especially dysphagia (i.e., the inability to swallow due to weak gag reflex and neck muscles). Administration of oral medications under these circumstances necessitates the following steps:

1. Determine if another form of the medication exists (e.g., liquid, per rectum, per inhalation)

2. Determine if the medication can be crushed and mixed with food or formula

3. Position the individual to facilitate administration in an upright or side lying position

4. Administer the medication via another route, such as nasogastrically or using a gastrostomy tube

Some seizure medication may cause daytime drowsiness in the individual, suggesting the need to reconsider altering the administration schedule to nighttime hours. Nonallergic (e.g., vomiting, diarrhea, hypotension, tinnitus) and allergic reactions should be observed for following administration of medications. Typically, both types of reactions will occur hours to days following ingestion of the medication. Allergic reactions ranging from minor to life threatening usually occur within an hour after the medication is taken; the life-threatening allergic reaction of anaphylaxis requires immediate emergency treatment (American Academy of Allergy, Asthma, & Immunology, 2007).

Adverse effects of medications may not be fully recognized or anticipated when used in individuals with IDD. For example, benzodiazepines (e.g., lorazepam, diazepam), which used in the treatment of anxiety by stimulating the production of gamma-aminobutyric acid in the limbic system, can increase the risk of falls in elderly individuals with IDD and those with motor difficulties (California State Board of Pharmacy, 2003; Skidmore-Roth, 2009).

An important consideration for nurses is polydrug use. An individual with IDD should be carefully monitored for the number and type of medications prescribed. Adverse effects may occur with certain drug interactions. For example, several anticonvulsant medications (e.g., phenobarbital, phenytoin) can decrease the mechanism of action of oral contraceptives (Skidmore-Roth, 2009).

The nurse should be fully informed as to action, uses, appropriate dosages, side effects, pharmacokinetics, interactions, and nursing considerations when administering medications to individuals with IDD (Duncan & Corcoran, 2007; Skidmore-Roth, 2009). Practice guidelines for administrating medications adhere to the six rights of medication administration (Bowden & Smith-Greenberg, 1998; Duncan & Corcoran, 2007):

1. Right patient
2. Right medication and dose
3. Right route
4. Right frequency
5. Right time
6. Right approach based on developmental level

DEVELOPMENTAL DISABILITIES NURSING STANDARDS

Professional nurses who work in the specialty field of IDD base their practice on the standards of practice set forth by their professional associations and as developed by nursing experts, referred to as *Intellectual and Developmental Disabilities Nursing Standards* (IDDNS). Standards were developed and published jointly by the Nursing Division of the American Association on Intellectual and Developmental Disabilities and the American Nurses Association (Nehring et al., 2004); they provide the template for the standards of practice and professional performance for nurses in the field of IDD. The practice standards are listed in Table 9.2.

IDDNS provide the framework for nursing clinicians, educators, and administrators to formulate the practice standards. IDDNS can be applied to develop and implement the practice and educational standards for use in clinical settings wherein primary, acute, or rehabilitative care is provided; they can also be used in

Table 9.2.   Standards of practice for nurses who specialize in intellectual and developmental disabilities (IDD)

Standard	Scope
Standard 1: Assessment	The nurse who specializes in IDD collects comprehensive data pertinent to the patient's health or the situation.
Standard 2: Diagnosis	The nurse who specializes in IDD analyzes the assessment data to determine the diagnoses or issues.
Standard 3: Outcome identification	The nurse who specializes in IDD assists identifying expected outcomes for the individual, family, and community.
Standard 4: Planning	The nurse who specializes in IDD develops a plan that prescribes strategies and alternatives to attain expected outcomes.
Standard 5: Implementation	The nurse who specializes in IDD implements interventions identified in the plan of care.
Standard 5a: Coordination of care	The nurse who specializes in IDD coordinates care delivery.
Standard 5b: Health teaching and health promotion	The nurse who specializes in IDD employs strategies to promote health and a safe environment.
Standard 5c: Consultation	The advanced practice registered nurse who specializes in IDD provides consultation to influence the identified plan, enhance the abilities of others, and effect change.
Standard 5d: Prescriptive authority and treatment	The advanced practice registered nurse who specializes in IDD uses prescriptive authority, procedures, referrals, and treatments in accordance with state and federal laws and regulations.
Standard 6: Evaluation	The nurse who specializes in IDD evaluates the individual's, family's, and community's progress toward attainment of outcomes.
Standard 7: Quality of practice	The nurse who specializes in IDD systematically evaluates the quality and effectiveness of nursing practice involving individuals with IDD.
Standard 8: Practice evaluation	The nurse who specializes in IDD evaluates one's own nursing practice in relation to professional practice standards and guidelines, relevant statutes, rules, and regulations.
Standard 9: Education	The nurse who specializes in IDD attains knowledge and competency that reflects current nursing practice.
Standard 10: Collegiality	The nurse who specializes in IDD interacts with and contributes to the professional development of peers and colleagues.
Standard 11: Collaboration	The nurse who specializes in IDD collaborates with the individual with IDD, family, and others in the conduct of nursing practice.
Standard 12: Ethics	The nurse who specializes in IDD integrates ethical provisions in all areas of practice.
Standard 13: Research	The nurse who specializes in IDD integrates research findings into practice.
Standard 14: Resource utilization	The nurse working in the field of IDD considers factors related to safety, effectiveness, cost, and impact on practice in the planning and delivery of nursing services to individuals with IDD.
Standard 15: Leadership	The nurse who specializes in IDD provides leadership in the profession and the professional practice setting.

From Nehring, W.M., Roth, S.P., Natvig, D., Betz, C.L., Savage, T., & Krajicek, M. (2004). *Intellectual and developmental nursing: Scope and standards of practice.* Silver Spring, MD: American Nurses Association and Nursing Division of the American Association on Mental Retardation; reprinted by permission.

community-based settings to enable the provision of care in the home, employment, or school settings.

COLLABORATION

Given the complexity of service needs that individuals with IDD require across the life span to function independently, inclusively, and productively in the community, it is essential that nurses collaborate not only with interdisciplinary members of specialized health care teams, but also with interagency providers in the community. Collaboration with interdisciplinary and interagency colleagues is key to the development, implementation, and evaluation of a comprehensive, person- or family-centered plan that is based on the individualized needs, interests, and preferences of the individual. For example, an Individualized Family Service Plan that includes an infant with DS and is based on a family-centered approach would be inadequate if interdisciplinary members from occupational therapy, speech and language, and pediatrics were not included in the team of professionals to provide comprehensive services (see Chapter 3 for more information about comprehensive services for children with disabilities). Collaboration with interagency adult providers representing health, vocational rehabilitation, housing, and transportation will be necessary to ensure that the adolescent with IDD successfully transitions to adulthood and adult services (Betz & Nehring, 2007; Nehring, 2005).

Collaboration with interdisciplinary and interagency professionals will require knowledge and understanding of the array and profile of services, supports, and programs available in the community for individuals with IDD. This is necessary for nurses to effectively coordinate services and make the appropriate referrals for individuals with IDD and their families. For additional information about community resources and the system of care for individuals with IDD, see Chapters 3, 4, and 5.

CULTURAL DIVERSITY

One of the goals of Healthy People 2010 is to eliminate health disparities, defined as "differences that occur by gender, race or ethnicity, education or income, disability, geographic location, or sexual orientation" by ensuring access to care and improved outcomes of care for culturally diverse populations (U.S. Department of Health and Human Services, 2000, p. 11). Individuals with IDD who are ethnically and culturally diverse are at risk for poorer health outcomes as they have less access to health care. A Surgeon General's report recommended that training content and clinical opportunities be provided to interdisciplinary health care professionals to raise their awareness and further their understanding of individuals with IDD who are ethnically and racially diverse. In addition, clinical services should be offered in the communities where individuals with IDD who are ethnically and racially diverse live (U.S. Department of Health and Human Services, 2002).

Limited information exists on the needs of individuals with disabilities who are ethnically and racially diverse. Findings from some surveillance reports (Besser, Shin, Kucik, & Correa, 2007; Centers for Disease Control and Prevention, 2001,

2006, 2007a, 2007b) indicate that prevalence patterns of IDD differ in racially and ethnically diverse individuals with IDD from non-Hispanic whites. However, more research is needed to better understand the factors that contribute to these differences and to learn what role culture may have in the access to services, allocation of resources, and family's and individual's understanding of and understanding towards attitudes of the IDD and its treatment.

For care to be culturally sensitive, it is important for the nurse to assess the extent to which the individual's lifestyle (or identity) is affected by a particular culture. This can be determined by learning the following:

1. The individual's and family's country of origin

2. The languages spoken in the home

3. Immigration and migration experiences

4. Cultural attitudes towards health, illness, and Western medicine

5. Alternative health practices and providers

Based upon this approach, information is gathered from the individual (and possibly family members and/or caregivers) about the network of support available. It is important to discover what assistance the individual has access to during times of need, both ongoing and episodic (Kagawa-Singer & Kassim-Lakha, 2003).

Culturally sensitive care is predicated on the synthesis of the information gathered and the nurse's knowledge of cultural practices and beliefs. Today, schools of nursing and health care organizations direct instructional efforts to educate nursing students and professionals about the cultural practices and beliefs of the diverse groups of individuals they serve. Nursing has been in the forefront of recognizing the importance of providing nursing care that is sensitive of the individual's and family's cultural beliefs and practices, as evidenced by the nursing literature on the influence of culture in the provision of nursing care (Betz, 2003; Nehring, 2007).

DELEGATION

Contemporary nursing practice in the field of IDD has evolved with the service needs of individuals. When the deinstitutionalization movement began in the 1970s, the practice of nurses changed dramatically at the urging of consumer groups and advocates (see Chapter 1). Innovative approaches are now required to respond to the growing need for nurses as the shortage of nursing professionals becomes more problematic (National Council of State Boards of Nursing [NCSBN], 2005). A strategy to address the public health needs with a shrinking nursing workforce is the use of UAPs, who provide selected care delegated by and under the supervision of registered nurses (American Nurses Association [ANA] & NCSBN, 2008).

UAPs have been used to perform delegated tasks to individuals requiring in home and health assistance, including individuals with IDD. *Delegation* is defined as "the process for a nurse to direct another person to perform nursing tasks and activities" (ANA & NCSBN, 2008, p. 1). The tasks and activities a UAP is allowed to perform are dependent upon state regulations as prescribed by the state boards of nursing and as recommended by professional nursing organizations, such as the

ANA and NCSBN (ANA & NCSBN, 2008; National Association of School Nurses, 2006; NCSBN, 2005; Oregon Department of Health Services, 2007).

In Washington, registered nurses supervise nursing assistants who work in the Medicaid program providing care to individuals with IDD in family homes. The tasks nursing assistants are allowed to provide include blood glucose monitoring and administration of medications (Washington State Department of Health and Human Services, n.d.). In Oregon, the UAP role is defined by the performance of basic nursing tasks. Basic nursing tasks refer to UAP care that assists individuals (including those with IDD) with ADL and the administration of medication—with restrictions (Oregon Department of Health Services, 2007). For example, the UAP can help the individual "with one or more steps in the process of taking medications... such as opening the medication container, reminding the client of the proper time to take the medication, and giving medication," but the UAP does not actually administer the medication (Oregon Department of Health Services, 1998, p. 2). However, in highly specified emergency situations, the UAP may administer medications.

Efforts have been directed to defining the role and responsibilities of the registered nurse as the supervisor (or delegator) of the UAP (or delegate). Numerous professional nursing organizations and nearly every state board of registered nursing have developed guidelines and regulations to guide the registered nurse with the supervision of an UAP (ANA & NCSBN, 2008; NCSBN, 2005). Specified criteria describing the five rights of delegations have been published, which are designed to provide professional guidelines for nurses in situations wherein they are responsible to supervise an UAP (NCSBN, 1995; ANA, 2005):

1.   Right task, referring to tasks that are specified in state regulations

2.   Right circumstances, meaning the delegate is certified to undertake the task

3.   Right person, referring to the appropriate licensed and unlicensed (certified) personnel involved in the task

4.   Right directions and communication, implying that the UAP tasks are clearly delineated and understood prior to being implemented

5.   Right supervision and evaluation, meaning that a process for monitoring and evaluating the UAP's performance is in place

ACCESSIBILITY

Accessible health care for individuals with IDD (U.S. Department of Health and Human Services, 2005) is impacted by a number of factors, including widespread erroneous societal attitudes as to what constitutes health and lack of professional expertise in providing health care to individuals with IDD. The negative societal attitudes towards individuals with IDD are based upon the belief that having a disability of any type is equated with an illness state and dysfunctional level of functioning. The negative societal attitudes contribute to the discriminatory attitudes of diminished expectations in all aspects of functioning, including the need for health services that extend beyond crisis and acute care needs, such as the provision of preventive and long-term rehabilitation services.

Another major factor negatively impacting the access to health care services by individuals with IDD is the lack of professional expertise available to provide needed services. Often, individuals with IDD have difficulties finding the services they need: "Individuals with disabilities often encounter professionals unprepared to identify and treat their primary and secondary conditions and any other health and wellness concerns" (U.S. Department of Health and Human Services, 2005, p. 11). The health and mental health problems experienced by individuals with IDD have been described as due in part to the lack of health care professionals available to provide care as exemplified by the phenomenon of *diagnostic overshadowing*, referring to the underdiagnosis of mental health problems in this group of individuals (Reiss, Levitan, & Szysko, 1982). Other problems that receive inadequate attention by health care providers are obesity, dental care, women's health problems (e.g., dysmenorrhea), routine mammograms and pelvic examinations, cancer surveillance, and osteoporosis. Treatment for hypertension and musculoskeletal problems associated with overuse syndrome and the acceleration of aging also are not always adequately addressed by health care providers (Centers for Disease Control and Prevention, 2004; Pearlman & Sterling, 2006; U.S. Department of Health and Human Services, 2000).

The problems with accessibility will require a multifaceted approach as advocated by a Surgeon General's report (U.S. Department of Health and Human Services, 2005). The goals and recommended action steps to achieve improved health care for individuals with IDD are presented in Table 9.3.

RESEARCH

Many advanced practice nurses in IDD are involved in research activities—as users, data collectors, project directors, and principal investigators. Nurses who participate in any one or all of these roles contribute to promoting to the science, practice, and art of nursing care for individuals with IDD. Today, there is recognition and support to base nursing care upon the available scientific evidence rather than solely on the opinions of clinical experts, advocacy groups, and special interests.

Nurses have conducted research on many topics that have contributed to the science of IDD. A partial listing of studies conducted by nurse researchers involving individuals with IDD is listed in Table 9.4. As is evident by the listing of studies, research emphasis has focused on the essence of nursing practice: "The protection, promotion, and optimization of health and abilities, prevention of illness and injury, alleviation of suffering through the diagnosis and treatment of human response, and advocacy in the care of individuals, families, communities, and populations" (ANA, 2004, p. 7). Investigations examining issues pertaining to living with an IDD in inclusive community-based settings reflect a growing trend by other disciplines to conduct research in naturalistic settings about individuals with IDD and their life experiences (Stoneman, 2007).

When conducting research with individuals with IDD, it is important for nurses to ensure that the individual's rights and welfare are protected. According to federal guidelines, institutional review boards (IRBs) of the researcher's affiliating institution are to give special consideration and ensure special provisions are in place in studies involving children, minors, individuals with intellectual disabilities, pregnant women, and individuals who are considered to be economically and educationally disadvantaged. These groups of research subjects are considered to be special classes of vulnerable research subjects, according to fed-

Table 9.3. Goals and strategies of *The Surgeon General's Call to Action to Improve the Health and Wellness of Persons with Disabilities*

Goals	Strategies
Goal 1—People nationwide understand that persons with disabilities can lead long, healthy, productive lives	• Promote the use of language to describe persons with disabilities that emphasizes the individual, not the disability first. This use of "people first" language that refers to persons with disabilities recognizes that individuals with disabilities are—first and foremost—persons with inherent value, individuality, dignity and capabilities and helps raise awareness of and reduce stigma and discrimination against persons with disabilities
	• Consider health literacy when making health and wellness information about persons with disabilities available to the public
	• Enhance understanding and acceptance of persons with disabilities of all ages nationwide by improving the content and dissemination of educational information in community programs, schools, faith-based programs, workplaces and at home about how persons with disabilities can lead long, healthy lives
	• Encourage the entertainment industry to increase its portrayal of realistic characters with disabilities and their challenges and successes in maintaining good health
	• Encourage the print and electronic media to increase coverage of disability-related issues and expand current health and wellness reporting to include ramifications for persons with disabilities
	• Continue to include age and specific disability status as demographic indicators in health surveys or surveillance systems
	• Encourage persons with disabilities to join as partners in public health initiatives and include them on advisory committees as services are being planned by federal, state, tribal and local governments
Goal 2—Health care providers have the knowledge and tools to screen, diagnose and treat the whole person with a disability with dignity	• Encourage health care and wellness service providers to relate to persons with disabilities in ways that recognize their value, dignity and capabilities, whether communicating in person, electronically, or in writing
	• Educate health care providers of persons with disabilities in an ongoing manner about state-of-the-art health services and supports that should be available to the patients with disabilities
	• Ensure that both clinical and health services research include persons with disabilities across the life span, particularly in areas in which health disparities in risk, access and outcome exist
	• Increase in an ongoing manner health care provider awareness of and compliance with laws designed to protect the rights of individuals with disabilities
	• Identify currently available disability-oriented training curricula and programs for health care providers, assess if the training curricula are evidence-based and delineate the next steps necessary to advance the adoption of evidence-based training curricula focused on persons with disabilities in professional and other service provider training and continuing education
	• Promote development and use of medical equipment and devices that allow universal access to all recommended screening and diagnostic tests and treatments
	• Enhance and broaden the content and expand the use of educational and training materials for health care providers that focus on the health care and wellness needs of persons with disabilities, including secondary conditions
	• Create a series of provider handbooks that include best practices and current resources to educate health professionals and service providers about the value of wellness promotion for persons with disabilities

(continued)

Table 9.3. (*continued*)

Goals	Strategies
Goal 2–(*continued*)	• Promote practical experiences with persons with disabilities in health and service provider training and continuing education, which includes information regarding civil rights and disability and the health care ramifications of the Americans with Disabilities Act
	• Promote researcher experiences with persons with disabilities in health care research training programs
	• Promote the development of research to enhance the evidence base for best practices in clinical service delivery for persons with disabilities
	• Promote interdisciplinary collaboration in scientific pursuits and to improve clinical research networks to advance better prevention, early diagnosis, and treatment of disabilities and secondary conditions
	• Analyze the content and diffusion of information about persons with disabilities that is used in health care settings
Goal 3–Persons with disabilities can promote their own good health by developing and maintaining healthy lifestyles	• Conduct health research to identify and support effective health promotion programs for persons with disabilities
	• Educate persons with disabilities, their families and advocates in an ongoing manner about state-of-the-art wellness and prevention activities
	• Consider health literacy when making health and wellness information accessible to persons with disabilities
	• Provide increased health promotion and wellness training opportunities specifically for persons with disabilities, their family members, personal attendants, and advocates, ensuring that both focus on the whole individual and not just the disability
	• Encourage health systems to use all media, computer-based, Internet, and other adaptive or assistive technologies when planning and developing health information for persons with disabilities
	• Encourage health systems to include materials that will be accessible to individuals with limited English proficiency
	• Include persons with disabilities in all stages of health care and wellness promotion communication research, including formative research, message development and testing, identification of appropriate communication strategies and channels, and evaluations of effectiveness
	• Identify evidence-based best practices for health promotion among persons with disabilities by developing, implementing, evaluating, and disseminating strategies to translate into practice the results of research

Goal 4—Accessible health care and support services promote independence for persons with disabilities

- Develop and implement surveys to assess the full range of health needs of persons with disabilities, including whether and how those needs are being met by providers and facilities in communities nationwide
- Advance accountability by all health service delivery programs, including clinical and community preventive services, to ensure that persons with disabilities have full access to their services
- Bring inventors, clinicians, and industry together through more effective incubator and development programs to collaborate efficiently and effectively to enhance research and development of assistive technology for all types of disabilities
- Encourage research efforts that collaborate and partner with integrated community-based provider networks to include individuals with disabilities in those efforts
- Continue to develop community-based, public-private partnerships to facilitate coordinated, integrated care of persons with disabilities. Include collaboration with transportation, education and wellness providers. Include communication between all providers and the disability community about the benefits of wellness resources
- Encourage the development of integrated, multidisciplinary service teams to provide one-stop health care for persons with disabilities
- Encourage or develop partnerships to facilitate coordinated, integrated care for populations identified as traditionally underserved, including persons with disabilities who are members of racial or ethnic groups
- Promote and disseminate the adoption of new treatments, models of care and adaptive or assistive technologies (e.g., making available specialized, adaptive cognitive and psychiatric research applications of assistive technology for individuals with communication deficits as well as a mental disorder)
- Identify key elements of best practices in health service delivery for persons with disabilities and, among existing health service delivery programs for this population, identify highlighted models that are using the key element and assess why they are successful
- Identify and implement in community-based care evidence-based best practices in health service delivery for persons with disabilities

---

From U.S. Department of Health and Human Services (2005). *The Surgeon General's call to action to improve the health and wellness of persons with disabilities*. Washington DC: Author.

Table 9.4.   Developmental disabilities studies conducted by nurse researchers, 2002–2007

Benderix, Y., & Sivberg, B. (2007). Siblings' experiences of having a brother or sister with autism and mental retardation: A case study of 14 siblings from five families. *Journal of Pediatric Nursing: Nursing Care of Children and Families, 22,* 410–418.

Betz, C.L., Baer, M.T., Haddad, Y., Nwarhuken, G., Poulsen, M., Vahanvaty, U., et al. (2004). Secondary analysis of primary and preventive services accessed and perceived service barriers by children with developmental disabilities and their families. *Issues in Comprehensive Pediatric Nursing, 27,* 83–106.

Betz, C.L., & Redcay, G. (2005). An exploratory study of future plans and extracurricular activities of transition-age youth and young adults. *Issues in Comprehensive Pediatric Nursing, 28,* 33–61.

Brosig, C.L., Mussatto, K.A., Kuhn, E.M., & Tweddell, J.S. (2007). Neurodevelopmental outcome in preschool survivors of complex congenital heart disease: Implications for clinical practice. *Journal of Pediatric Health Care, 21,* 3–12.

Escumalha, M., Cunha, M., Machado, M., Gouveia, C., & Vale, F. (2005). Pediatric ethics, issues, & commentary. Neonatal morbidity and outcome of live born premature babies after attempted illegal abortion with misoprostol. *Pediatric Nursing, 31,* 228–231.

Garro, A. (2004). Coping patterns in mothers/caregivers of children with chronic feeding problems. *Journal of Pediatric Health Care, 18,* 138–144.

Giarelli, E., Souders, M., Pinto-Martin, J., Bloch, J., & Levy, S.E. (2005). Intervention pilot for parents of children with autistic spectrum disorder. *Pediatric Nursing, 31,* 389–399.

Katz, S., & Kessel, L. (2002). Grandparents of children with developmental disabilities: Perceptions, beliefs, and involvement in their care. *Issues in Comprehensive Pediatric Nursing, 25,* 113–128.

Kuster, P.A., Badr, L.K., Chang, B.L., Wuerker, A.K., & Benjamin, A.E. (2004). Factors influencing health promoting activities of mothers caring for ventilator-assisted children. *Journal of Pediatric Nursing: Nursing Care of Children and Families, 19,* 276–287.

Little, L. (2002). Differences in stress and coping for mothers and fathers of children with Asperger's syndrome and nonverbal learning disorders. *Pediatric Nursing, 28,* 565–570.

Little, L. (2002). Middle-class mothers' perceptions of peer and sibling victimization among children with Asperger's syndrome and nonverbal learning disorders. *Issues in Comprehensive Pediatric Nursing, 25,* 43–57.

Little, L., & Clark, R. (2006). Wonders and worries of parenting a child with Asperger syndrome and nonverbal learning disorder. *MCN: The American Journal of Maternal/Child Nursing, 31,* 39–44.

Nehring, W.M., & Faux, S.A. (2006). Transitional and health issues of adults with neural tube defects. *Journal of Nursing Scholarship, 38,* 63–70.

Rehm, R.S., & Bradley, J.F. (2006). Social interactions at school of children who are medically fragile and developmentally delayed. *Journal of Pediatric Nursing: Nursing Care of Children and Families, 21,* 299–307.

Sanders, C.L., Kleinert, H.L., Free, T., Slusher, I., Clevenger, K., Johnson, S., et al. (2007). Caring for children with intellectual and developmental disabilities: Virtual patient instruction improves students' knowledge and comfort level. *Journal of Pediatric Nursing: Nursing Care of Children and Families, 22,* 457–466.

Shtayermman, O. (2007). Peer victimization in adolescents and young adults diagnosed with Asperger's Syndrome: A link to depressive symptomatology, anxiety symptomatology and suicidal ideation. *Issues in Comprehensive Pediatric Nursing. 30,* 87–107.

Sullivan, M.C., & Msall, M.E. (2007). Functional performance of preterm children at age 4. *Journal of Pediatric Nursing: Nursing Care of Children and Families, 22,* 297–309.

Van Riper, M. (2007). Families of children with Down syndrome: Responding to "a change in plans" with resilience. *Journal of Pediatric Nursing: Nursing Care of Children and Families, 22,* 116–128.

eral regulations. Nurses who intend to conduct research with individuals with IDD can consult with the institutional IRB, federal guidelines (Penslar, 1993), and the professional literature for additional guidance as they prepare for and implement research studies.

CONCLUSION

This chapter provided an overview of nursing considerations in the specialty of IDD as they pertain to practice and the role itself. Nurses who work in the field of IDD encounter many professional challenges. Many of the settings where nurses practice employment are not typical health care settings. As a result, there are many opportunities to work independently as a nursing practitioner and as an interdisciplinary team member in developing plans of care and service, training, and research programs. The topics addressed in this chapter highlighted the range of clinical practice and professional issues that nurses encounter as a provider of care to individuals with IDD.

REFERENCES

Akron Health Department. (2004). *Growth issues for children with disabilities.* Retrieved on June 29, 2009, from http://www.ci.akron.oh.us/Health04/Nutrition/growth.htm.

American Academy of Allergy, Asthma, & Immunology. (2007). *Tips to remember: Adverse reactions to medications and drug allergy.* Retrieved on August 7, 2008, from http://www.aaaai.org/patients/publicedmat/tips/adversereactions.stm.

American Academy of Pediatrics. (2001a). Health supervision for children with Down syndrome. *Pediatrics, 107,* 442–449.

American Academy of Pediatrics. (2001b). Health care supervision for children with Williams syndrome. *Pediatrics, 107,* 1192–1204.

American Academy of Pediatrics. (2001c). Developmental surveillance and screening of infants and young children. *Pediatrics, 108,* 192–196.

American Academy of Pediatrics. (2004). Providing a primary care medical home for children and youth with cerebral palsy. *Pediatrics, 114,* 1106–1113.

American Academy of Pediatrics (2007a). Management of children with autism spectrum disorders. *Pediatrics, 120,* 1163–1182.

American Academy of Pediatrics (2007b). Clinical genetic evaluation of the child with mental retardation or developmental delays. *Pediatrics, 115,* 2304–2316.

American Academy of Pediatrics. (2008). *Recommendations for preventive pediatric health care.* Retrieved July 30, 2008, from http://practice.aap.org/popup.aspx?aID=1625.

American Nurses Association. (2003). *Nursing's social policy statement* (2nd ed.). Washington, DC: Author.

American Nurses Association. (2004). *Nursing: Scope and standards of practice.* Washington, DC: Author.

American Nurses Association. (2005). *Principles for delegation.* Retrieved on August 5, 2008, from http://www.safestaffingsaveslives.org/WhatisSafeStaffing/SafeStaffingPrinciples/PrinciplesofDelegation.aspx.

American Nurses Association & National Council of State Boards of Nursing. (2008). *Joint statement on delegation: American Nurses Association (ANA) and the National Council of State Boards of Nursing (NCSBN).* Retrieved on August 5, 2008, from https://www.ncsbn.org/Joint_statement.pdf.

Barks, L.S., & Sheppard, J.J. (2005). Eating and swallowing disorders (dysphagia) in adults and children. In W.M. Nehring (Ed.), *Core curriculum for specializing in intellectual and developmental disability: A resource for nurses and other health care professionals* (pp. 271–290). Sudbury, MA: Jones & Bartlett.

Berry-Kravis, E. (2002). Epilepsy in fragile X syndrome. *Developmental Medicine & Child Neurology, 44,* 724–728.

Besser, L.M., Shin, M., Kucik, J.E., & Correa, A. (2007). Prevalence of Down syndrome among children and adolescents in metropolitan Atlanta. *Birth Defects Research, 79,* 765–774.

Betz, C.L. (2003). Nurse's role in promoting health transitions for adolescents and young adults with developmental disabilities. *Nursing Clinics of North America, 18,* 1–19.

Betz, C.L. (2007). Facilitating the transition of adolescents with developmental disabilities: Nursing practice issues and care. *Journal of Pediatric Nursing, 22,* 103–115.

Betz, C.L., & Nehring, W.M. (2007). *Promoting health care transition planning for adolescents with special health care needs and disabilities.* Baltimore: Paul H. Brookes Publishing Co.

Betz, C.L., & Sowden, L. (2008). *Pediatric nursing reference* (6th ed.). St. Louis: Mosby Elsevier.

Bowden, V., & Smith-Greenberg, C. (1998). *Pediatric nursing procedures* (2nd Ed.). Philadelphia: Lippincott Williams & Wilkins.

Breau, L., Camfield, C., McGrath, P., & Finley, G. (2004). Risk factors for pain in children with severe cognitive impairments. *Developmental Medicine & Child Neurology, 46,* 364–371.

California Department of Health Care Services. (2007). *California newborn hearing screening program overview.* Retrieved on August 10, 2008, from http://www.dhcs

.ca.gov/services/nhsp/Pages/NHSPPrgOv erview.aspx.

California State Board of Pharmacy (2003). *Consumer Education and Communication Committee Health notes: Care of children and adults with developmental disabilities.* Retrieved on August 6, 2008, from http://www.dds.ca.gov/Publications/docs/healthnotes_developdisabled.pdf.

Capone, G.T., Roizen, N.J., & Rogers, P.T. (2008). Down syndrome. In P.J. Accardo (Ed.), *Capute & Accardo's neurodevelopmental disabilities in infancy and childhood. Volume II: The spectrum of neurodevelopmental disabilities* (3rd ed., pp. 285–308). Baltimore: Paul H. Brookes Publishing Co.

Centers for Disease Control and Prevention (n.d.). *Overview of CDC growth charts.* Retrieved on June 29, 2009, from http://www.cdc.gov/nccdphp/dnpa/growthcharts/training/modules/module2/text/intro.htm

Centers for Disease Control and Prevention. (2001). Racial disparities in median age at death of persons with Down syndrome—United States, 1968–1997. *Morbidity and Mortality Weekly Report, 50,* 463–465.

Centers for Disease Control and Prevention. (2004). *Summary health statistics for the U.S. population, National Health Interview Survey, 2002. National Vital Health Statistics Reports 10.* Atlanta, GA: Centers for Disease Control and Prevention.

Centers for Disease Control and Prevention. (2006). Prevalence of four developmental disabilities among children aged 8 years. Metropolitan Atlanta Developmental Disabilities Surveillance Program, 1996 and 2000. *Morbidity and Mortality Weekly Report, 55,* 1–9.

Centers for Disease Control and Prevention. (2007a). Prevalence of autism spectrum disorders—autism and developmental disabilities monitoring network, six sites, United States, 2000. *Morbidity and Mortality Weekly Report, 56,* 1–11.

Centers for Disease Control and Prevention (2007b). Prevalence of autism spectrum disorders-autism and developmental disabilities monitoring network, 14 sites, United States, 2002, *Mortality and Morbidity Weekly Report, 56,* 12–28.

Centers for Disease Control, National Center for Birth Defects and Developmental Disabilities. (2005). *Women with disabilities: Access to health.* Retrieved on June 30, 2009, from http://www.cdc.gov/ncbddd/women/access.htm.

Chiu, S., Wegelin, J.A., Blank, J., Jenkins, M., Day, J., Hessl, D., et al. (2007). Early acceleration of head circumference in children with fragile X syndrome and autism. *Journal of Developmental and Behavioral Pediatrics, 28,* 31–35.

Cronk, C., Crocker, A.C., Pueschel, S.M., Shea, A.M., Zackai, E., Pickens, G., et al. (1988). Growth charts for children with Down syndrome: 1 month to 18 years of age. *Pediatrics, 81,* 102–110.

Duncan, J., & Corcoran, J. (2007). *Pediatric high-alert medication: Evidence-based safe practices for nursing professionals.* Marblehead, MA: HCPro.

Florida Department of Juvenile Justice (2006). *Health services manual: Youth with developmental disabilities.* Retrieved on August 6, 2008, from http://www.djj.state.fl.us/manuals/approvedmanuals/health_services/Chapter_20_Developmental_Disabilities.pdf.

Gray, M., Radcliff, C., & Donovan, A. (2002). Perineal skin care for the incontinent patient. *Advances in Skin and Wound Care, July/August.* Retrieved on June 30, 2009, from http://findarticles.com/p/articles/mi_qa3977/is_200207/ai_n9115677/?tag=content;col1.

Krick, J., Murphy-Miller, P., Zeger, S., & Wright, E. (1996). Pattern of growth in children with cerebral palsy. *Journal of the American Dietetic Association, 96,* 680–685.

Lipman, T.H., Euler, D., Markowitz, G.R., & Ratcliff, S.J. (2009). Evaluation of linear measurement and growth plotting in an inpatient pediatric setting. *Journal of Pediatric Nursing, 24,* 323–329.

Lipman, T.H., Hench, K., Logan, J.D., Difaxio, D.A., Hale, P.M., & Singer-Granick, C. (2000). Assessment of growth by primary health care providers. *Journal of Pediatric Health Care, 14,* 166–171.

Maguid, N.A., El-Kotoury, A.I.S., Abdel-Salam, G.M.H., El-Rudy, M.O., & Afifi, H.H. (2004). Growth charts of Egyptian children with Down Syndrome (0-36 months). *Eastern Mediterranean Health Journal, 10,* 108–115.

Menon, D. (2008). Williams syndrome. In P.J. Accardo (Ed.), *Capute & Accardo's neurodevelopmental disabilities in infancy and childhood. Volume II: The spectrum of neurodevelopmental disabilities* (3rd ed., pp. 353–362). Baltimore: Paul H. Brookes Publishing Co.

Mraz, K.D., Green, J., Dumont-Mathieu, T., Makin, S., & Fein, D. (2007). Correlates of head circumference growth in infants later diagnosed with autism spectrum disorders. *Journal of Child Neurology, 22,* 700–713.

Myers, S.M., & Johnson, C.P. (2007). Management of children with autism spectrum disorders. *Pediatrics, 120,* 1162–1182.

National Association of School Nurses. (2006). *Delegation.* Retrieved on August 11, 2008, from http://www.nasn.org/Default.aspx?tabid=349.

National Center on Health Statistics. (2007). *CDC growth charts: United States.* Retrieved on January 7, 2009, from http://www.cdc.gov/nchs/about/major/nhanes/growthcharts/background.htm.

National Council of State Boards of Nursing. (1995). *The five rights of delegation.* Retrieved on August 5, 2008, from https://www.ncsbn.org/323.htm#The_Five_Rights_of_Delegation.

National Council of State Boards of Nursing. (2005). *Working with others. A position paper.* Retrieved on August 5, 2008, from https://www.ncsbn.org/Working_with_Others(1).pdf.

Nehring, W.M. (Ed.). (2005). *Core curriculum for specializing in intellectual and developmental disability: A resource for nurses and other health care professionals.* Sudbury, MA: Jones & Bartlett.

Nehring, W.M. (2007). Cultural considerations for children with intellectual and developmental disabilities. *Journal of Pediatric Nursing, 22,* 93–102.

Nehring, W.M., Roth, S.P., Natvig, D., Betz, C.L., Savage, T., & Krajicek, M. (2004). *Intellectual and developmental nursing: Scope and standards of practice.* Silver Spring, MD: American Nurses Association and Nursing Division of the American Association on Mental Retardation.

New Mexico Department of Health. (2006). *Medication administration and delivery policy.* Retrieved on August 6, 2008, from http://www.nmhealth.org/DDSD/regulationsandstandards/documents/MedAdmAssessPolicy8012006.pdf.

Oregon Department of Health Services. (1998). *Developmental disabilities nursing manual. Division 47. Standards for registered nurse delegation and assignment of nursing care tasks to unlicensed persons. Rule summary, statement of purpose and intent. 851-047-0000.* Retrieved on August 5, 2008, from http://www.oregon.gov/DHS/spd/provtools/dd/nursing_manual/division_47.pdf.

Oregon Department of Health Services. (2007). *Nursing manual: Delegation, assignment and teaching for emergencies for delegation.* Retrieved on August 5, 2008, from http://www.oregon.gov/DHS/spd/provtools/dd/nursing_manual/delegation.shtml.

Pearlman, J., & Sterling, E. (2006). Dentistry. In I.L. Rubin & A.C. Crocker (Eds.), *Medical care for children and adults with developmental disabilities* (2nd ed., pp. 435–449). Baltimore: Paul H. Brookes Publishing Co.

Penslar, R.L. (1993). *Institutional review board guide book: Chapter VI: Special classes of subjects.* Retrieved on August 4, 2008, from http://www.hhs.gov/ohrp/irb/irb_chapter6.htm#g3.

Phalen, J.A. (2005). Fragile X syndrome. *Pediatrics in Review, 26,* 181–182.

Puruganan, O.H., & Adam, H.M. (2006). Abnormalities in head size. *Pediatrics in Review, 27,* 473–476.

Reiss, S., Levitan, D., & Szysko, J. (1982). Emotional disturbance and mental retardation: Diagnostic overshadowing. *American Journal of Mental Deficiency, 86,* 567–574.

Sherman, S.L., Allen, E.G., Bean, L.H., & Freeman, S.B. (2007). Epidemiology of Down syndrome. *Mental Retardation & Developmental Disabilities Research Reviews, 13,* 221–227.

Skidmore-Roth, L. (2009). *Mosby's nursing drug reference* (22nd ed.). St. Louis: Mosby.

Stevenson, R.D. (1995). Use of segmental measures to estimate stature in children with cerebral palsy. *Archives of Pediatrics & Adolescent Medicine, 149,* 658–662.

Stevenson, R.D., Conaway, M., Chumlea, C., Rosenbaum, P., Fung, E.B., Henderson, R.C., et al. (2006). Growth and health in children with moderate-to-severe cerebral palsy. *Pediatrics, 118,* 1010–1018.

Stoneman, Z. (2007). Disability research methodology. In S.I. Odom, R.H. Horner, M.E. Snell, & J. Blacher (Eds.), *Handbook of developmental disabilities* (pp. 35–54). New York: Guilford Press.

Tanner, J.M. (1986). Normal growth and techniques of growth assessment. *Clinics in Endocrinology & Metabolism, 15,* 411–451.

Tanner, J.M. (1992). Growth as a measure of the nutritional and hygienic status of a population. *Hormone Research, 38,* 106–115.

U.S. Department of Health and Human Services. (2000). *Healthy People 2010: Understanding and improving health* (2nd ed.). Washington, DC: Author.

U.S. Department of Health and Human Services. (2002). *Report of the surgeon general's conference on health disparities and mental retardation.* Washington DC: Author.

U.S. Department of Health and Human Services. (2005). *The Surgeon General's call to action to improve the health and wellness of persons with disabilities.* Washington DC: Author.

Waltz, D.A., & Katz, E.S. (2006). Pulmonology. In I.L. Rubin & A.C. Crocker (Eds.), *Medical care for children and adults with developmental disabilities* (2nd ed., pp. 325–342). Baltimore: Paul H. Brookes Publishing Co.

Washington State Department of Health and Human Services. (n.d.). *Nurse delegation program: Getting started as an RND.* Retrieved on August 5, 2008, from http://www.aasa.dshs.wa.gov/Professional/ND/start.htm.

Whitman, B.Y. (2008). Prader-Willi syndrome. In P.J. Accardo (Ed.), *Capute & Accardo's neurodevelopmental disabilities in infancy and childhood. Volume II: The spectrum of neurodevelopmental disabilities* (3rd ed., Vol. II, pp. 308–329). Baltimore: Paul H. Brookes Publishing Co.

Zahl, S.M., & Wester, K. (2008). Routine measurement of head circumference as a tool for detecting intracranial expansion in infants: What is the gain? A nationwide survey. *Pediatrics, 121,* e416–e420.

CHAPTER 10

Genetics

Felissa R. Lashley

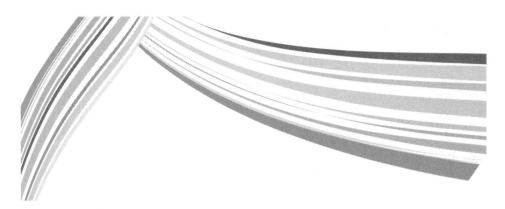

T he knowledge that has rapidly accumulated since the 1970s has elucidated the relationship between genetics and various aspects of behavior and intel- lect. This association involves both hereditary and nonhereditary aspects. Many intellectual and developmental disabilities (IDD) have been found to have a genetic basis, either as a primary cause or less directly from a genetic susceptibility to effects from environmental agents (e.g., microbes, chemicals). Thus, the nurse must have a basic understanding of the principles of genetic transmission.

Many advances in technology—largely through the impetus of the Human Genome Project—have allowed the identification of subtle genetic changes that result in specific conditions, including IDD, where previously no specific variation could be found (Driessnack, 2009). For example, although a chromosomal test for fragile X syndrome was developed by Lubs in 1969, it was not until the early 1990s that the exact genetic defect was identified so that a precise molecular test could be developed (Abrahms, 2009; Lubs, 1969). With such advances, appropriate ge- netic testing and counseling is now offered to relatives of individuals with IDD, al- lowing for realistic reproductive and life planning. Many people with IDD are also being retested due to the advent of much more accurate chromosomal and de- oxyribonucleic acid (DNA) tests.

CATEGORIES OF GENETIC DISORDERS

Genetic disorders can be characterized in various ways. *Genetic* is not synonymous with *inherited,* although many genetic variations are inherited. The traditional method of categorizing genetic disorders is as follows:

- Chromosome abnormalities
- Single-gene disorders
- Multifactorial, polygenic, or complex disorders
- Others

With increasing knowledge, however, this method has proved to be somewhat simplistic because there is more overlap than formerly appreciated. For example, many chromosomal disorders involve changes in multiple genes. Single-gene errors are influenced by the precise variation present, variations present in other genes, and environmental factors. In addition, environmental agents such as microbes, certain chemicals and drugs, and other agents may damage genetic material in the fetus, especially if exposure takes place during certain vulnerable periods in pregnancy. Some researchers also include a category of somatic genetic disease (Mueller & Young, 2001).

GENETIC DISEASE ACROSS THE LIFE SPAN

Although genetic disorders may first appear at any point in the life span, the majority of severe disorders are recognized at birth, in infancy, or in childhood. However, others are either first manifested or first recognized later in life, even into late adulthood. For example, some types of inherited biochemical disorders, such as Tay-Sachs disease (a genetic lipid storage disorder), have a severe infantile form, a less severe juvenile form appearing in childhood, and a milder form manifesting in adulthood. These different forms occur because variants in the genetic mutation result in a specific disorder. Other disorders become evident when the developmental function that would normally occur does not occur or is flawed. However, the genetic mutation is present since fertilization and can often be detected if there is reason to test for a specific condition.

AN INTRODUCTION TO GENETICS

Human somatic (body) cells aggregate together to form tissues and organs. Humans have approximately 25,000 genes, which are the units of heredity. In nearly all somatic cells, there are 46 chromosomes, or the diploid (2N) number. In gametic cells (the sperm and egg), there are 23 chromosomes, or the haploid (N) number. When the sperm and egg unite to form the zygote, the diploid number of 46 chromosomes is restored and the embryo has the genetic information for development. This DNA set is known as the *genome*.

Within the cells—mainly in the nucleus and mitochondria—are genes. Genes are composed of DNA sequences of four types of nucleotides. Each nucleotide is made up of a nitrogenous base, a sugar, and a phosphate to form nucleic acid. Nucleic acids may be either ribonucleic acid (RNA) or DNA. The bases in DNA are adenine, guanine, cytosine, and thymine. RNA contains adenine, guanine, cytosine, and uracil instead of thymine. Certain arrangements of these four bases into triplets (known as *codon*s) comprise the genetic code. These codons specify a specific amino acid and ultimately provide instructions for making polypeptides and proteins.

Very simplistically, genetic information is transcribed from DNA to messenger RNA (mRNA). The mRNA undergoes posttranscriptional processing and leaves the nucleus for the cytoplasm, where it is translated into polypeptides and protein through various interactions with ribosomes and transfer RNA. The final polypeptide product may also undergo posttranslational modification and transportation to its appropriate location. For further details, see Lashley (2007) and Mueller and Young (2001).

In mitosis (i.e., somatic cell division for growth and repair), each daughter cell typically ends up with the same chromosome complement as the parent. During oogenesis and spermatogenesis, meiosis (i.e., reduction division of 2N germ cells) typically results in gametes with the haploid chromosome number. Nondisjunction can occur in anaphase 1 or 2 of meiosis or in anaphase of mitosis.

If nondisjunction occurs in meiosis, the chromosomes fail to separate and migrate properly into the daughter cells. When this occurs both chromosomes of a pair end up in the same daughter cell, leading to some gametes with 24 (N + 1) chromosomes and some with 22 (N − 1) chromosomes. When such gametes are fertilized by a normal gamete, trisomic or monosomic zygotes result, such as in trisomy 21 or Turner syndrome, respectively. DNA also undergoes self-replication each time a cell divides (National Center for Biotechnical Information, 2009a; National Institutes of Health, Eunice Kennedy Shriver Institute of Child Health and Development, n.d).

CHROMOSOMES AND GENES

Chromosomes are microscopic structures in the cell nucleus that are composed of chromatin. Chromatin is mostly composed of DNA, RNA, histones (a basic protein), and nonhistone (acidic) proteins. Genes are located on chromosomes, each normally in a specific place or locus. Each chromosome can be individually identified by means of its size, staining qualities, and morphological characteristics. Each chromosome has a centromere, which is a region in the chromosome that can be seen as a constriction. Telomeres are specialized structures on the end of chromosomes.

The normal human chromosome number in most somatic (body) cells and in the zygote is 46. Humans normally have 46 chromosomes, 44 of which are autosomes (nonsex chromosomes common to both sexes) and 2 of which are sex chromosomes. The sex chromosomes of females are two X chromosomes, whereas those of males are one X and one Y chromosome. Chromosomes occur in pairs. Normally one of each pair is derived from the individual's mother and one from the father. Gametes (ova and sperm) each contain one member of a chromosome pair for a total of 23 chromosomes (22 autosomes and 1 sex chromosome)—the haploid number, or one chromosome set. When the fusion of male and female gametes during fertilization occurs, the diploid number of chromosomes (46) is restored to the zygote. For more details on the basic principles of cell division of the somatic cells (mitosis) and germ cells (meiosis), during which chromosomes and genes are transmitted to descendants, see Lashley (2007).

Genes are arranged in a linear fashion on a chromosome, each with its specific locus (place). Those that are close together on the chromosome (within 50 map units) are said to be linked. There are large areas of DNA that are not known to contain gene-coding sequences. Autosomal genes are those whose loci are on one of the autosomes (nonsex chromosomes). Each chromosome of a pair (homologous chromosomes) normally has the identical number of arrangement of genes, except for the X and Y chromosomes in the male. Nonhomologous chromosomes are members of different chromosome pairs. Only one copy of a gene normally occupies its given locus on the chromosome at one time, except for the X and Y chromosomes of the male or certain structural abnormalities of the chromosome.

Genes at corresponding loci on homologous chromosomes that govern the same trait may exist in slightly different forms or alleles. Alleles are alternative forms or variations of a gene at the same locus, which may or may not produce a change in the gene product or a visible effect. Variations that occur in 1% or more of the population are known as *polymorphisms.* Those variations that occur less frequently often include *mutations,* a term often used to refer to those variations that are harmful. A change in a single base pair, which is known as a *single nucleotide polymorphism,* has become increasingly important in understanding human variation. This variation may or may not result in disease, but may determine various predispositions and susceptibility. Polymorphisms have an elaborate system of nomenclature, which has not yet been agreed upon internationally (International Standing Committee on Human Cytogenetic Nomenclature, 2005).

CHROMOSOME VARIATIONS AND DISORDERS

More than 1,000 different chromosome abnormalities have been described in live births. Changes in both chromosome number and in chromosome structure can result in various disorders. The majority of spontaneous abortions or miscarriages (about 50%–60%) are the result of chromosomal abnormalities, particularly if they occur early. Approximately 0.8% of live-born infants have been estimated to have chromosome abnormalities using usual cytogenetic detection methods (Sharkey, Maher, & Fitzpatrick, 2005). Some chromosome variations, especially if they involve the sex chromosomes, are not detected until childhood, adolescence, or adulthood. An example is traditional Turner syndrome, in which one X chromosome is absent. Females with Turner syndrome have 45 chromosomes (typically written as 45, X). If not detected at birth because of findings such as lymphedema, this syndrome may be recognized in childhood due to the characteristic short stature or around puberty when secondary sex characteristics and menarche do not occur.

Factors Influencing Chromosomal Disorders

A variety of factors influence the transmission of chromosomes. The most common of these are increased maternal age, mosaicism, nondisjunction, and anaphase lag during cell division. The increased risk for trisomy 21 (Down syndrome) and other trisomies with advancing maternal age has long been known (Heffner, 2004). This effect begins to become more important at about age 35 years, which is the reason for the inclusion of maternal age of 34 years of age and older as one of the indications for prenatal diagnosis.

As discussed earlier, there are two types of cell division—mitosis and meiosis. If nondisjunction occurs in meiosis, the chromosomes fail to separate and migrate properly into the daughter cells. Both chromosomes of a pair end up in the same daughter cell, leading to some gametes with 24 (N + 1) chromosomes and some with 22 (N – 1) chromosomes. When such gametes are fertilized by a normal gamete, trisomic or monosomic zygotes result, such as in trisomy 21 or in Turner syndrome, respectively. Offspring resulting from such fertilization generally have a single abnormal cell line. If nondisjunction occurs in the first meiotic division, only abnormal gametes result; if it occurs in the second division, half of the gametes will be normal. Anaphase lag, in which the chromosomes of a pair separate and one member is lost, leads to monosomy. If this occurs in meiosis, it affects the gamete.

The occurrence of these errors during mitosis results in mosaicism in somatic cells, except in the first zygotic division, which results in tetrasomy. An individual who is mosaic possesses two or more cell populations, each with a different chromosome constitution that (in contrast to a chimera) arises from a single zygote during somatic cell development. The number of cells that will have an abnormal chromosome makeup depends on how early in the division of the zygote the error occurs. The earlier it occurs, the higher the percentage of abnormal cells there will be. Chromosome abnormalities resulting from errors in mitosis are only seen in descendants of the initial cell with the error. If the person with mosaicism has some cells with a normal constitution, then their genetic variation is often phenotypically milder.

Analyzing Chromosomes

Chromosome analysis may be performed for diagnosis of a person's condition, prenatal diagnosis, determining the parental origin of a particular chromosomal variation, or relating specific changes to treatment plans and prognosis, especially in certain cancers.

Analysis for chromosome abnormalities has advanced considerably (Tartaglia, Hansen, & Hagerman, 2007). The standard conventional chromosome studies used G-banded karyotyping for analysis (National Center for Biotechnical Information, n.d.). After metaphase chromosomes were stained, microscopy was used to arrange them according to size and location of the centromere in an internationally standardized way. These techniques advanced in sophistication to include high-resolution G-banded karyotypes and fluorescence in situ hybridization. Array comparative genomic hybridization is a relatively new technique that can detect submicroscopic gains and losses of genetic material. The use of various types of array comparative genomic hybridization has allowed the identification of new chromosomal submicroscopic deletion, duplication, and rearrangement syndromes, including chromosome 17q21.31 deletion and duplication. These techniques have allowed an actual diagnosis in many individuals with IDD for whom diagnosis was formerly not possible, as well as the identification of hitherto unrecognized microdeletion syndromes (Slavotinek, 2008).

Standardized terminology is used to refer to the karyotype: The normal male is written as 46, XY and the normal female as 46, XX. Other terminology of particular interest is the use of p to refer to the short arm of a particular chromosome and q to refer to the large arm. Detailed information on terminology may be found in Shaffer, Slovak, and Campbell (2009) and Lashley (2007).

Numerical Changes

An alteration in the number of chromosomes is called *aneuploidy*. Most large numerical changes in chromosomes result in multiple genes being affected with the corresponding result. These large changes can result in such observable effects as congenital anomalies, IDD, and behavioral difficulties. When an entire chromosome is absent, the condition is referred to as *monosomy*. To date, autosomal monosomies have been incompatible with life. Turner syndrome, in which one of the X chromosomes of a female is absent, is the only viable sex chromosome monosomy. When an extra chromosome is present, the condition is known as *trisomy*. In addition, there may be two or three extra X or Y chromosomes present. Examples are tetrasomy X (48, XXXX) or pentasomy X (49, XXXXX), both of which are rarely seen.

Down syndrome (trisomy 21 or 47, XX) is the most common autosomal trisomy. The chromosomal material of an extra chromosome 21 is present as a free chromosome, in which case 47 chromosomes may be seen. It may also occur if a translocation of chromosome 21 occurs, in which case the overall chromosome number may be normal. Chromosome analysis is very important because the parent may be a balanced translocation carrier. Children with Down syndrome have a constellation of clinical features including hypotonia, certain dysmorphic features (e.g., epicanthic folds, flat nasal bridge, transverse palmer crease, clinodactyly), Brushfield spots, short stature, protruding tongue with high arched palate, varying degrees of intellectual disability, congenital heart defects, hearing impairment, gastrointestinal problems, ocular problems, orthopedic problems, thyroid problems, hypogonadism in males and reduced fertility in females, a pattern of aging that may resemble Alzheimer's disease, and an elevated risk for transient newborn myeloproliferative leukemia and acute lymphocytic leukemia in childhood (Nehring, 2008; 2010). For more information, see Chapter 12.

Edwards syndrome (trisomy 18) is the second most common autosomal trisomy. Individuals with Edwards syndrome typically have a small jaw, recessed chin, "rocker bottom" feet, intellectual disability, severe congenital heart disease, and other malformations. Death usually occurs by 1 month of age, but a few children live longer, especially if mosaicism is present (Papp et al., 2007). Patau syndrome (trisomy 13) consists of severe external malformations, such as cleft lip and palate, eye defects, and polydactyly as well as congenital heart disease, renal and reproductive tract abnormalities, intellectual disability, and a "punched-out" scalp. Most individuals with Patau syndrome die within the first year of life, but some children survive into adulthood.

Sex chromosome variations tend to be milder than those of the autosomes. Early studies emphasized more abnormalities than have been described now that more cases have been identified. A common trisomy of the sex chromosomes is Klinefelter syndrome (47, XXY). Males with Klinefelter syndrome have an extra X chromosome, which may not be recognized until adolescence or adulthood. Hypogonadism may be seen and infertility is common. Some males may show tall stature, clumsiness, passivity, overweight with a fat distribution resembling females, or certain difficulties in specific areas of speech and language. Other men with this variation have few noticeable signs.

With triple X syndrome (47, XXX), females have an extra X chromosome. This variation is often not detected until adulthood, if ever. These individuals may have menstrual or learning difficulties (although this is highly variable), but often they do not show any noticeable signs. Males (47, XYY) have an extra Y chromosome. Early studies associated this variation with criminal behavior, but that has not been proven. Most individuals with this variation have no physical symptoms, although some have learning difficulties. They tend to be tall and fertility appears normal (Gotz, Johnstone, & Ratcliff, 1999).

Structural Changes

The major types of changes in structure of chromosomes are deletions, duplications, translocations, and inversions. Each type is described in this section, with the karyotypic abbreviation indicated in parentheses.

In deletions (del), part of a chromosome is missing. It can be in the middle (interstitial) or at the end (terminal). A minus sign (–) may be used to describe a particular situation. Thus, a rare chromosomal disorder in which there is deletion of part of the long arm of chromosome 18 could be indicated by 18 q deletion syndrome, 18q–, or del(18q) syndrome. More details regarding the specific bands and sub-bands may also be given to describe the exact problem.

In duplications (dup), there is extra chromosomal material present. A plus sign (+) may be used to refer to this condition. An inversion (inv) is an alteration in which two breaks have occurred in the chromosome, and the piece between them is rotated and reinserted. A translocation (t) involves transfer of a chromosome segment to another chromosome after breakage has occurred. In reciprocal translocations, two chromosomes exchange pieces. In a balanced translocation, no genetic material was thought to be added or lost, but it now appears that submicroscopic pieces may be added or lost.

Translocation trisomy 21 (Down syndrome) may result from the presence of 46 chromosomes that includes a translocation chromosome, such as t(14;21) or t(14q21q), so that the genetic material of 47 chromosomes with genetic material of 3 chromosomes 21 are present. There is a normal chromosome 14, two normal chromosomes 21, and a translocation chromosome consisting of the second chromosome 14 and an extra chromosome 21. Other translocations may also be seen.

A ring chromosome is formed when a segment at the end(s) of one of a pair of chromosomes is lost and fuses to form a circular structure, but these tend to be rare. An example is ring chromosome 14, which is associated with psychomotor delay, intellectual disability, and dysmorphic craniofacial features (Genetic Home Reference, 2009a).

SINGLE-GENE/INHERITED BIOCHEMICAL DISORDERS

For any given gene under consideration, if the two gene copies or alleles are identical, the genes are said to be *homozygous*. If one gene copy or allele differs from the other, the genes are said to be *heterozygous*. The term *genotype* is most often used to refer to the genetic makeup of a person when discussing a specific gene pair. *Genome* refers to a person's total genetic makeup or constitution. *Phenotype* refers to the observable expression of a specific trait or characteristic that can either be visible or biochemically detectable. Examples of phenotypic features are brown eyes and blood type B.

A trait or characteristic is considered to be dominant if it is expressed or phenotypically apparent when one copy or dose of the gene is present. A trait is considered to be recessive when it is expressed only when two copies or doses of the gene are present or if one copy is missing, such as with X-linked recessive traits in males. Codominance occurs when each one of the two alleles present are expressed when both are present, as in the case of the AB blood group. Genes located on the X chromosome (X linked) are present in two copies in females but only one copy in males, because males only have one X chromosome. Therefore, in the male, the genes of his X chromosome are expressed for whatever trait they determine. In the female, a process known as *X inactivation* occurs so that there is only one functioning X chromosome in each somatic cell. Very few genes are known to be located on the Y chromosome, but they are only present in males.

The group of single-gene errors is often called *inherited biochemical disorders* or *Mendelian errors* (National Center for Biotechnical Information, 2009b). These disorders are caused by a heritable permanent change (mutation) occurring in the DNA, usually resulting in alteration of the gene product. Gene products are usually polypeptide chains that form all or part of substances, such as structural proteins, membrane receptors, regulatory proteins, coagulation factors, and enzymes. The gene product may be changed to be absent, deficient, defective, or not have an effect that is observed. There are other factors that are important in gene expression and function such as penetrance, variable expression, parental age, the effects of other genes and environmental factors, X inactivation, epigenetic factors, and more. Further, some genes are limited to one sex or are affected by sex. Penetrance, variable expression, and parental age are discussed briefly in the following paragraphs. For more information, see Lashley (2005, 2007).

Penetrance is the percentage of people known to possess a certain mutant gene who actually show the trait. Incomplete or nonpenetrance occurs when a person is known to have a specific gene and shows no phenotypic manifestations of that gene. Incomplete penetrance is a frequent finding in the autosomal dominant disorders. Estimates of penetrance have been calculated for certain autosomal dominant genes so that they can be used in calculating risks for genetic counseling (Lashley, 2005, 2007). One of the effects of incomplete penetrance is that the gene appears to skip a generation. This characteristic can be responsible for errors in genetic counseling if care is not exercised, although the use of molecular diagnostic techniques allows greater precision. The risk for a person to manifest a specific disorder is equal to the risk for inheriting the gene multiplied by the penetrance.

Variable expressivity occurs when an individual has the gene in question and is clinically affected, but the degree of severity of the manifestations of the mutant gene varies. As a simple example, in the case of polydactyly, the extra digit present may be full size or just a finger tag. Such variation may occur within a single family and may be caused by the influence of other factors on the major defective gene. It is most obvious in autosomal dominant disorders. Careful examination or testing is necessary before deciding that someone is free of the manifestations of a genetic disorder. The extent of severity of a disorder in one family member is not related to its severity in another. Therefore, if a parent is mildly affected with only minor manifestations of a disorder, the parent's offspring may be severely, moderately, or mildly affected. The severity cannot be predicted reliably by the gene's expression in another family member.

The frequency of some gene mutations in offspring increases with parental age, especially paternal age, whereas some chromosome abnormalities are associated with advanced maternal age of 34 and older. Information related to older fathers is clearest for autosomal dominant mutations; men age 40 years and older are usually excluded from gamete donation (Bray, Gunnell, & Smith, 2006).

The traditional knowledge regarding transmission of genetic disorders is still basically correct. Typical Mendelian patterns of inheritance of mutations in single genes are autosomal recessive, autosomal dominant, X-linked recessive, X-linked dominant, and Y. In addition to typical Mendelian patterns and multifactorial inheritance, recognition of mitochondrial disorders due to mitochondrial inheritance has been relatively recent (Lashley, 2005, 2007). There has also been recognition of nontraditional methods of inheritance, including epigenetic factors, uniparental disomy, genomic imprinting, unstable or expanding triplet repeat mutations, and gonadal mosaicism (Genetic Home Reference, 2009a; Lashley, 2005, 2007).

Autosomal Recessive Inheritance

The major characteristics of autosomal recessive inheritance are

- The mutant gene is located on an autosome.
- Males and females are affected in equal numbers.
- The affected person usually inherits one copy of the same mutant gene from each heterozygous (Aa) carrier or parent, and is thus homozygous (aa) at that locus.
- There are usually no sex differences in clinical manifestations.
- Vertical family history is usually negative.
- Other people in the same generation may be affected.
- Consanguinity is more likely to be present than in other types of inheritance.
- New gene mutations are rare.
- Age of onset tends to be relatively early.
- Enzyme defects are common.

In the most typical clinical situations, an affected child has two carrier parents. Occasionally, a rare recessive disorder is manifested in a child when only one parent is a carrier, because of one of the two following reasons:

1. There was a small deletion of the chromosome segment involving the normal gene, thus allowing expression of the mutant gene on the other chromosome of the pair.

2. The person inherited two copies of the same chromosome from the parent with the mutant gene (uniparental disomy).

Because normal gene function is dominant to the altered function of the mutant recessive gene, the heterozygote usually shows no obvious phenotypic manifestations but may show biochemical differences. Enzyme defects and deficiencies are frequent. Most people carry a number of mutant recessive genes in single copy. Various ethnic groups have certain autosomal recessive diseases in higher frequency, such as Tay-Sachs disease in people of Eastern European (Ashkenazi) Jewish origin and sickle-cell disease in African Americans. This knowledge is used for targeted carrier screening and prenatal detection (National Institute of Neurological Disorders and Strokes, 2007).

If a couple has had a child with an autosomal recessive disorder, the family history for the genetic disease may be completely negative, either because of a smaller family size or simply because two copies of a rare gene were needed in order to be affected. If there are other affected individuals, they are usually members of the same generation. If the parents of the affected child are related to each other by blood (consanguinity), this suggests autosomal recessive inheritance but does not prove it. For more about the mechanics of transmission of autosomal recessively inherited genes, see Lashley (2005, 2007).

The most common autosomal recessive situation is when both parents are heterozygotes (carriers) of a gene. The theoretical risks for their offspring, regardless of sex, are therefore

- Affected with the disorder (aa): 25%
- Carriers like their parents (Aa): 50%
- Normal, without inheriting the mutant gene (AA): 25%

Of the phenotypically normal offspring (AA and Aa), two thirds will be carriers. These risks hold true for each pregnancy. Because "chance has no memory," each pregnancy is independent of the others; the outcome of a past pregnancy has no effect on a future one. Within an individual family at risk with two carrier parents, the actual number of affected children can range from none to all. This is a point that individuals often need clarified and reinforced, so nurses should be able to understand it and to explain it. If two carriers have had three unaffected children in three sequential pregnancies, it does not mean that their next child will be affected. Each prior event has no bearing on the outcome of the next pregnancy in autosomal recessive inheritance (Lashley 2005, 2007).

Because of advances in diagnosis and treatment in certain autosomal recessive diseases, such as sickle-cell anemia and cystic fibrosis, individuals who would have formerly died in childhood now are reaching young adulthood and having their own children, creating obligatory transmission of the mutant gene to all of their offspring (Betz & Sowden, 2008). If the affected person mates with someone who does not carry the same mutant gene, then all of their children, regardless of sex, will be carriers but none will be affected. If the affected person mates with someone who is a carrier for the same recessive gene, then there is a 50% risk for having an affected child and a 50% risk for having a child who is a heterozygous carrier, regardless of sex for each pregnancy. This risk is most likely to materialize for disorders such as cystic fibrosis, for which the frequency of carriers is about 5% for Caucasians, or for sickle-cell disease, for which the frequency of carriers in the African American population is 7%–9% (Betz & Sowden, 2008).

Autosomal Dominant Inheritance

The major characteristics of autosomal dominant inheritance are (Lashley 2005, 2007)

- The gene is located on an autosome.
- One copy of the mutant gene is needed for effects.
- Males and females are affected in equal numbers on average.
- There is no sex difference in clinical manifestations.
- Vertical family history through several generations may be seen.
- There is wide variability in expression.
- Penetrance may be incomplete (i.e., gene can appear to "skip" a generation).
- Increased paternal age effect may be seen.
- Fresh gene mutation is frequent.

- Later age of onset is frequent.
- Male-to-male transmission is possible.
- Normal offspring of an affected person will have normal children, grandchildren, and so forth.
- Structural protein defect is often involved.

In general, autosomal dominant disorders tend to be less severe than autosomal recessive disorders. Only one copy of the dominant gene is necessary for the detrimental effects to be evident. The affected individual is heterozygous; there is no carrier status. It is believed that in most autosomal dominant disorders, homozygous individuals who have inherited two genes for an autosomal dominant disorder are so severely affected that they die in utero or in infancy. Autosomal dominant disorders are usually less life threatening than autosomal recessive ones, although they may involve more evident physical malformations (Lashley 2005, 2007).

The recognition of an autosomal dominant disorder in a child may indicate the presence of that disorder in one of the parents as well. When the parents appear to be unaffected, several possibilities exist:

- The gene may be present but nonpenetrant.
- The gene expression may be minimal and not have been detected by the practitioner.
- The disorder can be caused by a new mutation.
- The child is not the natural offspring of both parents.

Careful examination of both parents is extremely important. In one of my cases, a child was brought for counseling with full-blown Waardenburg syndrome (deafness, heterochromic irises, partial albinism, and broad facial appearance) before subgrouping of this syndrome was known. No evidence was at first seen in either parent. If the disorder was actually caused by a new mutation, then the risk for those parents to have this syndrome appear in another child would be negligible. If, however, one of the parents actually had the syndrome, then the risk for recurrence in another child would be 50%. Upon further examination, the only manifestation that the mildly affected mother had was a white forelock of hair, which she usually dyed. Thus, simply looking at the couple would not have revealed the situation. This case is an example of variable expression in which the parent was only mildly affected but the child had severe manifestations. Such cases represent a challenge to the practitioner. In this case, the counselor, knowing the full constellation of the syndrome, specifically asked the mother if anyone in the family had prematurely white hair. If not directly asked, such information may not have been discovered.

When one partner is affected and one is normal, the risk for their child to inherit the gene, and therefore the disorder (except in disorders with less than 100% penetrance), is 50%, regardless of sex. The chance for an unaffected child is also 50%. This holds true for each pregnancy, regardless of the outcomes of prior pregnancies. Unless nonpenetrance has occurred, those truly unaffected individuals run no greater risk than the general population of having an affected child or grandchild of their own. Risk calculations that include the possibility of nonpenetrance can be made by the geneticist. If a woman was an affected heterozygote for a rare autosomal dominant disorder with 60% penetrance and was planning a family with an unaffected man, the risk for each child to both inherit the mutant gene and to manifest the disorder is as follows:

> The risk to inherit the mutant gene from each parent (50% from the mother and the population mutation rate from the father, which in this case is disregarded because of rarity) is multiplied by the penetrance (60%), or

$$0.5 \times 0.6 = 0.3$$

Therefore, the risk for the child to inherit the gene is 50%. The risk to both inherit the gene and manifest the disorder is 30%.

   If two individuals affected with the same autosomal dominant disorder have children—for example, with achondroplasia (a type of dwarfism)—then for each pregnancy the chance is 25% for having a child who is an affected homozygote, 50% for having an affected heterozygote like the parents, and 25% for having a normal child without a mutant gene. The homozygote is usually so severely affected that the condition is lethal in utero.

X-Linked Inheritance

In both dominant and recessive X-linked disorders, the mutant gene is located on the X chromosome. Males have only one X chromosome and there is no counterpart for its genes. In males, therefore, any gene located on the X chromosome is expressed when present in one copy, regardless of whether it is dominant or recessive in females. Males cannot be carriers; they will show the effects of the gene in question. A female receives one X chromosome from each of her parents for a normal sex constitution of XX. A male receives his single X chromosome from his mother and his Y chromosome from his father for a normal sex constitution of XY.

   X-Linked Recessive Inheritance   Major characteristics of X-linked recessive inheritance are

- The mutant gene is on the X chromosome.
- One copy of the mutant gene is needed for phenotypic effect in males (hemizygous).
- Two copies of the mutant gene are usually needed for phenotypic effect in females.
- Males are more frequently affected than females.
- Unequal X inactivation can lead to a manifesting heterozygote in female carriers.
- Transmission is often through heterozygous (carrier) females.
- All daughters of affected males will be carriers if the mother is normal.
- All sons of affected males will be normal if mother is normal.
- There is no male-to-male transmission.
- There are some fresh gene mutations.

   The most common pattern of X-linked transmission is that in which the female partner is a heterozygous carrier for the mutant gene. If her partner is normal, then for each pregnancy the couple runs an equal chance for the offspring to be one of the following:

- A female carrier like the mother: 25%
- A normal female without the mutant gene: 25%
- A normal male without the mutant gene: 25%
- A male who is affected with the disease in question: 25%

The risk for a male offspring to be affected is therefore 50%. As in the other types of single gene inheritance, the outcome of one pregnancy does not influence the others; these odds remain the same. The carrier female usually shows no obvious clinical manifestations of the mutant gene unless X inactivation is skewed. In such an instance, she may be a manifesting heterozygote. For example, if the mutant gene was for Duchenne muscular dystrophy, a carrier female might demonstrate muscle weakness, enlarged calves, and moderately elevated serum creatine kinase levels. If the mutant gene was for hemophilia A, the woman may demonstrate prolonged bleeding times. Females with X chromosome abnormalities, such as even submicroscopic deletions, may also manifest X-linked recessive disorders if the normal gene on the counterpart chromosome is deleted.

Because better treatment has increased the life span for many individuals with X-linked recessive disorders, such as hemophilia, affected males are now reproducing. If the female is normal in such a mating, all of their female children will be carriers and all the males will be normal. In other words, the theoretical risk for each pregnancy is that there is a 50% chance that the offspring will be carrier females and a 50% chance that they will be normal males. If the male is affected and the female is a carrier for the same disorder, as may occur in the very common X-linked recessive disorders such as glucose-6-phosphate dehydrogenase deficiency, then with each pregnancy there is a theoretical risk of 25% each for the birth of an affected female, a carrier female, a normal male, or an affected male.

X-Linked Dominant Inheritance

X-linked dominant inheritance is less frequently seen than the other modes of inheritance discussed. Major characteristics are

- The mutant gene is located on X chromosome.
- One copy of the mutant gene is needed for phenotype manifestation.
- X inactivation modifies the gene effect in females.
- It is often lethal in males, and so transmission may be seen only in the female line.
- Affected families usually show excess of female offspring (2:1).
- An affected male transmits the gene to all of his daughters and to none of his sons.
- Affected males have affected mothers (unless new mutation).
- There is no male-to-male transmission.
- There is no carrier state.
- Disorders are relatively uncommon.

Affected females are more likely to transmit the gene to their offspring because the gene is less severe in females due to X inactivation. If a female's mate is not affected, the theoretical risk for each pregnancy to her offspring is an equal chance for each of the following:

- An affected female: 25%
- An affected male: 25%
- A normal female: 25%
- A normal male: 25%

Therefore, there is a 50% chance that the offspring of each pregnancy will be affected without considering sex.

The gene is often lethal in males because males have no normal gene counterpart. Therefore, the mating of an affected male and normal female is uncommon. An example of this type of genetic disorder is incontinentia pigmenti, which is usually prenatally lethal in males; has abnormalities of skin, hair, and nails; and may result in intellectual disabilities because of defects in the NF-kappa-β essential modulator gene (Smahi et al., 2000).

Y-Linked (Holandric) Inheritance   Few genes are known to be located on the Y chromosome, so this type of inheritance has little clinical significance. Most Y-linked genes have to do with male sex determination. Y-linked genes manifest their effect with one copy, and show male-to-male transmission exclusively.

MULTIFACTORIAL/POLYGENIC INHERITANCE

Multifactorial refers to the interaction of several genes (often with additive effects) with environmental factors. Sometimes the terms *multifactorial* and *polygenic* are used synonymously, but the latter does not imply any environmental component. Many morphologic features and developmental processes are believed to be under multifactorial control, with minor differences determining variability in the characteristic they determine. The spectrum ranges from different degrees of normal to abnormal outcomes. The concept of this gene–environment interaction is well illustrated by the interruption of the development of the palate, leading to a cleft.

Some disorders, often including a variety of congenital malformations, do not follow a single-gene inheritance pattern and are not known to be due to a chromosomal abnormality (although with the newer precise techniques, this might change). Many of the common complex disorders, such as certain cancers, are considered to be the result of multiple mutant genes in combination with certain environmental factors. Understanding the role of multiple mutant genes in the development of a specific cancer, for example, is the focus of much attention.

MITOCHONDRIAL INHERITANCE

As described earlier, genes are also present in the mitochondria of cells. Mitochondria (Mt) are cell organelles that use oxygen in the process of energy production. Mitochondria are essentially transmitted along maternal lines (matrilinear). An mtDNA mutation can be present in all mtDNA copies (homoplasmy) or in some (heteroplasmy). The percent of mtDNA mutations necessary to cause dysfunction is believed to vary depending upon the type of tissue affected, and even among cells in the same tissue (Egger & Wilson, 2002; Lashley, 2005, 2007). Cells with high energy demands, such as nerve and muscle, have many more mitochondria present than others. Most nuclear gene defects resulting in mitochondrial disorders are associated with abnormalities of oxidative phosphorylation. Diseases due to mtDNA mutations often involve tissues dependent on large amounts of adenosine triphosphate, such as the skeletal and heart muscles, central nervous system, kidney, liver, pancreas, and retina. Sensorineural hearing loss is frequent.

Mitochondrial diseases can result from

- Mutations in the mtDNA
- Defects in nuclear DNA that affect mitochondrial function, such as defects of the Krebs cycle (these are becoming better understood and defined)
- Defects in communication between mtDNA and nuclear DNA
- Nonhereditary defects of mtDNA, such as those resulting from zidovudine (an antiretroviral drug)

During division of cells containing both mutant and normal mtDNAs, individual cells can accumulate varying proportions of each. A mother with a homoplasmic mtDNA mutation can transmit only that mutant mtDNA to her offspring, whereas a mother with varying levels of mutated mtDNA may not always transmit mutated mtDNA, depending on the percentage of mutated mtDNA present. However, above a certain level, it is likely that all children will receive some mutated mtDNA. Susceptibility of specific tissue types to impaired mitochondrial function as a result of an mtDNA mutation, the proportion of mutated mtDNA in a given cell or tissue type, and the severity of the specific mutation determine the phenotype. This may explain why some disorders show a childhood form with rapid early-onset progression and multiple organ effects, whereas others lead to an adult form with slower late-onset slower progression and effects mainly confined to the nervous and muscular systems.

Accumulating damage to mtDNA in somatic tissues over time appears important in aging and in Parkinson's disease development. Like mutations in nuclear DNA, those in mtDNA may be sporadic or inherited. Some disorders due to mitochondrial mutation include Leber optic neuropathy, Leigh syndrome, mitochondrial myopathy with encephalopathy, lactic acidosis and stroke-like episodes, and myoclonic epilepsy with ragged red fibers. Mutations in certain nuclear genes may predispose to mtDNA aberrations and thus result in mitochondrial disorders. Characteristics of mitochondrial inheritance are

- Mutant gene is located in the mitochondrial DNA.
- Each mitochondrion contains multiple DNA molecules.
- Cells contain multiple mitochondria.
- Normal and mutant mitochondrial DNA for the same trait can be in the same cell (heteroplasmy).
- Inheritance is through the maternal line.
- Males and females are affected in equal numbers on average.
- Variability in clinical expression is common.
- There is no transmission from a father to his children.

Disorders are relatively uncommon.

NONTRADITIONAL INHERITANCE

A number of assumptions underlie the basic tenets of patterns of inheritance. While these are correct in the majority of instances, there are exceptions to those assumptions: epigenetics, differential gene expression, uniparental disomy, imprinting, gonadal mosaicism, and unstable mutations involving expanding repeats that often include the phenomenon of anticipation. Epigenetics may be described as "heritable changes in gene expression that are not due to any alteration in the DNA sequence" (Esteller, 2008, p. 1148). DNA methylation and histone regulation are examples of the epigenetic ways in which gene expression is controlled and regulated.

Uniparental Disomy

In the normal course of events, a child inherits one of each pair of genes and chromosomes from the mother and one from the father. In uniparental disomy, both chromosomal homologues are inherited from the same parent instead of inheriting one copy of each chromosome pair from the mother and the father (e.g., two paternal chromosome 9 homologues and no maternal chromosome 9 homologues). The child has a normal total number of chromosomes. Uniparental disomy may apply to all or part of a chromosome. If all the genes involved are normal, then this may occur without being recognized, although sometimes growth restriction and other effects may result. However, if a mutant allele for an autosomal recessive disorder is present on one parental chromosome that was inherited, then it now will be present in two copies and be manifested. Uniparental disomy was first recognized in a person who had inherited two maternal copies of chromosome 7 and came to attention with cystic fibrosis, short stature, and growth hormone deficiency (Genetic Home Reference, 2009b).

Genomic Imprinting

Another nontraditional inheritance mechanism is genomic imprinting, also called *parental imprinting* and *genetic imprinting*. Normally, one of an identical pair of alleles from one parent is expressed in the same way as the other of the pair from the other parent. In imprinting, the alleles of a given pair of genes are not expressed in an equivalent manner depending upon the parent of origin. A gene is said to be maternally imprinted if the allele derived from the mother is the one that is silenced, turned off, repressed, or inactivated, and paternally imprinted if it is the allele contributed by the father that is turned off or inactivated. This may be accomplished via the regulation of DNA methylation. Thus, certain genes may be expressed from either the maternal or paternal chromosome, depending on imprinting.

Clinically, uniparental disomy and imprinting have been predominantly recognized in disorders of growth and behavior. One of the best known examples of differential gene expression due to parent of origin effects uniparental disomy and imprinting is Angelman syndrome. One of the causes is the presence of two paternally derived chromosomes 15. Angelman syndrome (AS) is marked by severe intellectual disability, inappropriate laughter, decreased pigmentation, speech impairments, ataxia and jerky arm movements, and seizures.

Unstable Repeat Expansions

Present throughout the human genome are short repeated segments usually in tandem that contribute to polymorphism. The most common repeats associated with disease to date are repeated units of 3 nucleotides that are arrayed contiguously and known as *triplet repeats* or *trinucleotide repeats*. Usually, there are less than

20–40 of any given repeat. When these nucleotides become unstable and expand or lengthen, usually during meiosis, they may cause disease. Some of the diseases so far known to be associated with this type of mutation at specific sites include fragile X syndrome, Huntington disease, and myotonic dystrophy (Abrahms, 2009).

Gonadal (Germline) Mosaicism

Gonadal or germline mosaicism occurs when one parent has a mutant allele that results from mutation in the gonads, which occurs after fertilization and results in mosaicism. Clinical manifestations in that parent may not be seen because the mutation occurs in the cells of the developing gonad in either the male or the female; it may be present in few, if any, somatic cells. Thus, some germ cells may be normal and others may carry the specific mutation. Gonadal mosaicism may occur in both autosomal dominant and X-linked inheritance. One example is the case in which a clinically normal father had two children with osteogenesis imperfecta by two different women.

NURSING IMPLICATIONS

Understanding the potential role that genetics plays in IDD is important for nurses. Even when it appears that the origin of a particular person's condition is unknown, the discovery of new knowledge and the development of new diagnostic techniques mean that diagnosis may be possible in the near future. A family history over three generations may be conducted by the nurse, who should be aware of the essential elements in such a history. Nurses may also conduct a history of the pregnancy, as well as developmental assessment. Nurses should ensure that individuals with IDD have a comprehensive evaluation that includes review by a qualified geneticist. Reasons for establishing an etiology and diagnosis include the elimination of further unnecessary testing; planning for treatment and management; the short- and long-term outlook and prognosis, as well as challenges that might be anticipated; the opportunity for genetic counseling with estimates of recurrence risk; realistic life and reproductive planning for family members; and the availability of additional community support for people with certain diagnoses. Nurses, with the appropriate education, should also be able to assist families to understand the genetic etiology and recurrence risks, as well as guide them through the processes of diagnosis and counseling (Lashley, 2005, 2007). Moeschler (2008) stated that an additional benefit is enabling the family to once more have a sense of control.

CONCLUSION

Major advances are occurring in the understanding of the contribution of genetics to a wide variety of disorders. This contribution may be a major, primary, direct one, or it may involve multiple genes or susceptibility to damage. Advances in diagnostic technology have allowed identification of subtle genetic defects resulting in disorders, such as submicroscopic chromosomal deletions. Thus, a person who has had comprehensive genetic testing even a few years ago may benefit from re-evaluation and the use of the most current techniques. It is vital that nurses understand the various genetic mechanisms by which IDD may occur, as well as be prepared to work with families affected by genetic disease.

REFERENCES

Abrahms, L.J. (2009). *Summary of fragile X syndrome*. Retrieved on July 2, 2009, from http://www.fragilex.org/html/summary.htm.

Betz, C.L., & Sowden, L. (2008). *Pediatric nursing reference* (6th ed.). St. Louis: Mosby Elsevier.

Bray, I., Gunnell, D., & Smith, G.D. (2006). Advanced paternal age: How old is too old? *Journal of Epidemiology and Community Health, 60,* 851–853.

Driessnack, M. (2009). Growing up at the intersection of the genomic era and the information age. *Journal of Pediatric Nursing, 24,* 189–193.

Egger, J., & Wilson, J. (2002). Mitochondrial inheritance in a mitochondrially mediated disease. *New England Journal of Medicine, 347,* 208–2082.

Esteller, M. (2008). Epigenetics in cancer. *New England Journal of Medicine, 358,* 1148–1159.

International Standing Committee on Human Cytogenetic Nomenclature. (2005). *An international system for human cytogenetic nomenclature.* Basel, Switzerland: Author.

Genetic Home Reference. (2009a). *Ring chromosome 14 syndrome.* Retrieved on July 2, 2009, from http://ghr.nlm.nih.gov/condition=ringchromosome14syndrome.

Genetic Home Reference. (2009b). *What are genomic imprinting and uniparental disomy?* Retrieved on July 2, 2009, from http://ghr.nlm.nih.gov/handbook/inheritance/updimprinting.

Gotz, M.J., Johnstone, E.C., & Ratcliff, S.G. (1999). Criminality and antisocial behavior in unselected men with sex chromosome abnormalities. *Psychological Medicine 29,* 953–962.

Heffner, L. (2004). Advanced maternal age —How old is too old? *New England Journal of Medicine, 351,* 1927–1929.

Lashley, F.R. (2005). *Clinical genetics in nursing practice* (3rd ed.). New York: Springer.

Lashley, F.R. (2007). *Essentials of clinical genetics in nursing practice.* New York: Springer.

Lubs, H.A. (1969). A marker X chromosome. *American Journal of Human Genetics, 21,* 231–244.

Moeschler, J.B. (2008). Genetic evaluation of intellectual disabilities. *Pediatric Neurology, 15,* 2–9.

Mueller, R.F., & Young, I.D. (2001). *Emery's elements of medical genetics.* New York: Churchill Livingstone.

National Center for Biotechnical Information. (2009a). *Down syndrome.* Retrieved on July 2, 2009, from http://www.ncbi.nlm.nih.gov/entrez/dispomim.cgi?id=190685.

National Center for Biotechnical Information. (2009b). *Online Mendelian inheritance in man.* Retrieved on July 2, 2009, from http://www.ncbi.nlm.nih.gov/omim/.

National Center for Biotechnical Information. (n.d.). *Gene tests.* Retrieved on July 2, 2009, from http://www.ncbi.nlm.nih.gov/sites/GeneTests/?db=GeneTests.

National Institutes of Health, Eunice Kenney Shriver Institute of Child Health and Development (n.d.). *Genetic features of Turner syndrome.* Retrieved on July 2, 2009, from http://turners.nichd.nih.gov/genetic.html.

National Institute of Neurological Disorders and Strokes. (2007). *Tay Sachs disease information page.* Retrieved on July 2, 2009, from http://www.ninds.nih.gov/disorders/taysachs/taysachs.htm.

Nehring, W.M. (2008). Down syndrome. In C.L. Betz & L.A. Sowden (Eds.), *Mosby's pediatric nursing reference* (6th ed., pp. 149–161). St. Louis: Mosby Elsevier.

Nehring, W.M. (2010). Down syndrome. In P. Jackson Allen, J.A.Vessey, & N.A. Schpiro (Eds.), *Primary care of the child with a chronic condition* (5th ed., pp. 447–469). St. Louis: Mosby Elsevier.

Papp, C., Ban, Z., Szigeti, Z., Csaba, A., Beke, A. & Papp, Z. (2007). Role of second trimester sonography in detecting trisomy 18: A review of 70 cases. *Journal of Clinical Ultrasound, 35,* 68–72.

Shaffer, N., Slovak, M.L, & Campbell, L.J., (Eds.). (2009). *ISCN 2009: An international systemfor human cytogenetic nomenclature (2009): Recommendations of the international standing committee on human cytogenetic nomenc.* Basel: Karger.

Sharkey, F.H., Maher, E., & Fitzpatrick, D.R. (2005). Chromosome analysis: What and when to request. *Archives of Disease in Childhood, 90,* 1264–1269.

Slavotinek, A.M. (2008). Novel microdeletion syndromes detected by chromosome microarrays. *Human Genetics, 124,* 1–17.

Smahi, A., Courtois, G., Vabres, P., Yamaoka, S., Heuretz, S., Munnich, A., et al. (2000). Genomic rearrangement in NEMO impairs NF-kappaB activation and is a cause of incontinentia pigmenti. *Nature, 405,* 466–472.

Tartaglia, N.R., Hansen, R.L., & Hagerman, R.J. (2007). Advances in genetics. In S.L. Odom, R.H. Horner, M.E. Snell, & J. Blacher (Eds.), *Handbook of developmental disabilities* (pp. 98–128). New York: Guilford Press.

Intellectual and Developmental Disabilities

Sandra A. Faux and Wendy M. Nehring

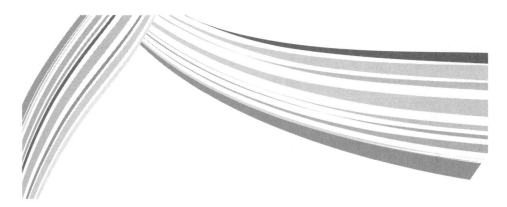

Mental retardation (MR) is a relatively common, general term used to designate a lifelong condition in which there is diminished cognitive and adaptive functioning caused by various biological and/or social etiologies. The term has been used for decades and is still currently used, although it has been considered to be pejorative. Therefore, in some countries the term is often replaced by such terms as *learning disability* (LD), *intellectual disability* (ID), intellectual and developmental disability (IDD), mentally challenged, developmentally delayed, or mental disability, deficiency, or handicap (Shea, 2006; World Health Organization [WHO], 2007). Currently, in the United States, ID and IDD are used. Whatever term is used, it is essential for the health care provider to provide clear explanations of the implications for and prognosis of the individual (Shea, 2006).

MR is part of the language and is written into laws, which protect and support individuals with this diagnosis. However, the term *IDD* will be used interchangeably with *MR* in this chapter. MR will be used when it is appropriate to the literature being cited. The common definitions of IDD, epidemiology, etiology and symptoms, screening and diagnosis, general treatment approaches (including alternative and complementary treatments), and principles of family-centered, culturally appropriate nursing care are reviewed here.

DEFINITION

The criteria and terms used to define IDD have evolved over the last several decades. The three most commonly used are those developed by the American Association on Intellectual and Developmental Disabilities (AAIDD), the American Psychological Association, and the American Psychiatric Association (2000). Traditionally, MR has been described using IQ scores based on a population normal of 100, with 15 points representing 1 standard deviation (*SD*) on standardized tools for measuring intelligence (Shea, 2006). Thus, MR refers to scores that are 2 or more *SD* below the mean. There are four commonly used levels of severity: mild (50–70 IQ, 2–3 *SD*); moderate (40–54 IQ, 3–4 *SD*); severe (25–39 IQ, 4–5 *SD*), and profound (<25 IQ, >5 *SD*).

The definition of IDD in the United States varies by organization. According to the AAIDD, it is "a disability (not a diagnosis) characterized by significant limitations in intellectual functioning and in adaptive behavior as expressed in conceptual, social and practical adaptive skills . . . [and that] originates before age 18" (Luckasson et al., 2002, p. 19). In addition to these three core components, it is essential to assess age, culture, language, and environment, and to identify strengths, limitations, and support needs. For additional information on the history of the terms used to describe IDD across time in the United States, see Chapter 1.

EPIDEMIOLOGY

The most generally accepted prevalence of MR is 1%, although in some cohorts it is found to be 2%–3%, with rates as high as 9.7% in a recent study of 10 to 14 year olds (Murphy, Boyle, Schendal, Decoufle, & Drews, 1998; Shea, 2006). It has been estimated that 85%–95% of individuals with ID have a mild form, which is fairly common and is usually detected in kindergarten and early elementary school (Acharya & Msall, 2008). Moderate to severe MR usually occurs in individuals with genetic syndromes; it is estimated to occur in 5 per 1,000 children in developed countries (Leonard & Wen, 2002). Murphy, Yeargin-Allsopp, Decoufle, and Drews (1995) documented an overall prevalence of 12 per 1,000 children for MR, with mild MR in 8.4 per 1,000 and severe MR in 3.6 per 1,000 children.

The observed prevalences of MR differ due to population variables, such as age, sex, and socioeconomic status. Some of the variation is also due to methodological issues, such as definitions, case findings, and analytic techniques. MR prevalence is usually at its highest between 10 and 14 years of age, probably due to increased diagnosis of children with mild MR detected in educational settings rather than new occurrences. It has been extensively documented that a higher proportion of males have MR due in part to incidence of X-linked conditions (e.g., fragile X syndrome). The male-to-female ratio of MR is 1.5:1 in the United States (Leonard & Wen, 2002), 1.8:1 in Sweden, to 1.4:1 in the Netherlands (Yeargin-Allsopp, Drews-Botsch, & Van Naarden Braun, 2008). This trend also occurs with severe MR, with a 1.2:1 ratio. The overrepresentation of males with mild MR may be due to the greater attention paid to boys' behaviors. In addition, there is an inverse relationship between socioeconomic status and MR. Mild MR is highly correlated with lower socioeconomic status. These data have led to the postulation that there are two types of MR: a mild form influenced primarily by social and demographic factors and a more severe form related to biological or pathological factors (Drews, Yeargin-Allsopp, Decoufle, & Murphy, 1995).

Racial and ethnic differences have been documented in the U.S. population. Children who are African American, Hispanic, and Asian have higher rates of MR than Caucasian children. The higher prevalence, particularly for mild MR in African American children has been attributed to potentially inadequate IQ testing; environmental conditions (e.g., poverty, poor nutrition); growing up in racially segregated, disadvantaged communities; and higher rates of maternal biologic conditions (e.g., hypertension, anemia, preterm births, diabetes, sickle-cell anemia) (Bhasin, Brocksen, Achen, & Van Naarden Braun, 2006).

Bhasin et al. (2006, p. 3) documented an "overall prevalence of 15.5 per 1,000 children in 1996 and 12.0 per 1,000 in 2000" in 8-year-old children from Atlanta. Although the prevalence decrease was seen in all racial groups, the highest decrease was found among boys and black children. Prevalence for ID was higher among males than females and twice as high for black as white children. Prevalence of mild MR was found to be 3–4 times higher in black than white males.

Other risk factors for IDD include maternal age and educational level; etiology; family history; and prenatal, perinatal, and postnatal events. Teenage mothers have a higher risk of having a child with mild IDD, while mothers age 40–44 years have a greater risk of having a child with a moderate to severe IDD. Mothers who never finished high school are 4 times more likely to have children with mild IDD than those mothers who did finish (Batshaw, Shapiro, & Farber, 2007). About 75% of children with severe IDD have an identified cause of their disability, whereas only about 40% of children with mild IDD have an identified etiology. It has been noted that over 500 genetic diseases cause IDD, with Down syndrome, fragile X syndrome, and Prader-Willi syndrome accounting for the majority of all genetic causes of IDD. Down syndrome, fragile X syndrome, and fetal alcohol syndrome together account for one third of the causes of moderate to severe IDD. There is a 3%–9% risk of reoccurrence of IDD in families with one child with severe IDD (Batshaw et al., 2007).

ETIOLOGY

It is important to know the cause of a child's IDD. This information may assist in finding associated health issues, determining early treatment that may improve cognitive outcomes, highlighting genetic implications for the children and their families, helping families to understand their child's problems, and facilitating access to support systems (Shea, 2006). There are multiple known causes of MR. However, in 50% of children with mild MR there is no identifiable causation; these children are often identified after age 5 when they encounter difficulties on entering the educational system. In contrast, 75% of children with severe MR have an identified cause of their disabilities and are identified before age 6 (Leonard & Wen, 2002; Yeargin-Allsopp et al., 2008). Known causes of IDD are classified by time of occurrence: prenatal, perinatal, and postnatal.

Prenatal Etiologies

Prenatal etiologies include teratogens; maternal nutrition, drinking, and smoking; maternal phenylketonuria; intrauterine infections (e.g., rubella, human immunodeficiency virus, herpes virus, cytomegalovirus); low birth weight; preterm delivery; intrauterine growth restriction; twins and other multiple births; maternal medications (e.g., anticonvulsants); and medical conditions (e.g., thyroid problems). Prenatal alcohol exposure is believed to be the most common single cause of IDD. Genetic defects and syndromes are the most common cause of moderate to severe IDD, with one quarter of individuals with IDD having a chromosome abnormality (e.g., Down syndrome, Klinefelter syndrome, Prader-Willi syndrome, Angelman syndrome, Williams syndrome) (Batshaw et al., 2007).

Perinatal Etiologies

Perinatal etiologies include complications of delivery (e.g., birth trauma, preeclampsia, eclampsia), complications of prematurity (e.g., intracranial bleeds, hypoglycemia), perinatal asphyxia and perinatal infections (e.g., group B *Streptococcus*, herpes simplex virus). However, these conditions are no longer major causes of IDD due to increased screening and preventative measures (Yeargin-Allsopp et al., 2008).

Postnatal Etiologies

About 3%–15% of postnatal etiologies are of known causation and are preventable. These etiologies include environmental exposure (e.g., lead, methylmercury, pollutants), accidental injuries (e.g., near drowning, falls, motor vehicle collisions), nonaccidental injuries (e.g., abuse, maltreatment), traumatic brain damage, and postnatally acquired infections (e.g., meningitis/encephalitis, malnutrition, environmental deprivation). The two most common causes are shaken baby syndrome and bacterial meningitis (Handmaker, 2005).

GENETICS

Chromosomal abnormalities are found in about 40%–50% of individuals with moderate to severe IDD. These genetic defects are categorized as chromosomal, single gene, and multifactorial/polygenic (Handmaker, 2005); examples are shown in Table 11.1. As previously noted, Down syndrome is the most common chromosomal disorder causing IDD; fragile X syndrome is the most common single-gene disorder causing IDD (see Chapters 10, 12, and 16).

COMORBIDITIES

Comorbidities are common in individuals with IDD. They include health risks specific to a syndrome. Individuals with Down syndrome, for example, may exhibit the following comorbidities (Batshaw et al., 2007; Shea, 2006):

- Hearing and visual problems (55%)
- Autism (20%–30%)
- Attention-deficit/hyperactivity disorder (9%–15%)
- Sensory impairments (2%–11%)
- Cerebral palsy (8%–30%)
- Psychiatric and behavioral problems (25%–80%)
- Seizure disorders (11%–21%)
- Sleep disorders (15%–60%)

PATHOPHYSIOLOGY

As stated earlier in this chapter, the known causes of IDD include genetic abnormalities, infections, exposure to toxins and teratogens, malnutrition, trauma, neglect, and lack of stimulation. Genetic causes of IDD have been divided into two

Table 11.1. Genetic causes of intellectual and developmental disabilities

Categories	Examples
Chromosomal	Autosomal trisomy: Down syndrome (trisomy 21)
	X chromosomal: Klinefelter syndrome, Turner syndrome, syndromes with more than three X chromosomes
	Microdeletions: Prader-Willi syndrome, Angelman syndrome, Williams syndrome, Smith-Magenis syndrome
	Translocations, inversions, duplications
Single gene (Mendelian)	X-linked recessive: fragile X syndrome, Duchenne muscular dystrophy, Lesch-Nyhan syndrome
	Autosomal recessive: metabolic disorders (phenylketonuria, hypothyroidism, galactosemia), neurodegenerative disorders (Tay-Sachs)
	Autosomal dominant: neurofibromatosis, tuberous sclerosis
Polygenic/multifactorial	Spina bifida

Source: Handmaker (2005).

groups: "syndromic with specific clinical, radiological, metabolic, or biological features and nonsyndromic or nonspecific MR in which intellectual impairments are the only manifestation of the disease" (Chelly, Khelfaoui, Francis, Cherif, & Bienvenu, 2006, p. 702). Some phenotype and genotype studies have found that nonspecific forms could be syndromic as more syndromes are being identified (Chelly et al., 2006).

The developing brain, whether in the prenatal or postnatal period, can be damaged during all stages of brain development. Interruption of the cell formation involved in the development of the central and peripheral nervous systems and the brain will ultimately impair normal learning, memory, and adaptive behavior (Chelly et al., 2006). The primary dysfunctions are localized in the cortical structures (e.g., hippocampus, medial temporal cortex). The majority of individuals with significant IDD have no structural brain abnormalities. Approximately 10%–15% of children with IDD have such central nervous system malformations (e.g., neural tube defects, hydranencephaly, microcephaly). Alcohol and other chemicals (e.g., cocaine, nicotine, prescription drugs) can affect fetal brain development.

Chelly et al. (2006, p. 708) have noted that

> Defects in synaptogenetic and synaptic activities, as well as plasticity, especially in postnatal stage during learning and acquisition of intellectual performances and emotional behavior, are perhaps crucial cellular processes that underlie cognitive impairment resulting from mutations in some MR related genes.

These synaptic structure and neuronal connectivity deficiencies are postulated to "hamper the brain to process information" (Chelly et al., 2006, p. 708).

SYMPTOMS

Infants and children who have not achieved "age-appropriate neurodevelopmental milestones in language, motor, and social-adaptive development" are evaluated by health care professionals for developmental disabilities, specifically IDD (Batshaw et al., 2007, p. 245). In fact, Shea (2006) has stated that IDD is really not a "diagnosis, but a symptom of neurologic dysfunction" (p. 262). The most common symptoms are exhibited in the areas of language, motor, and social-adaptive development. Infants born with congenital defects or a genetic syndrome are usually identified in the first year of life with symptoms specific to the defect or syndrome, whereas children with milder delays may not be identified until they enter kindergarten.

Symptom severity often reflects the level and severity of the possible IDD. For example, a child who is slow in motor development may have mild IDD whereas a child with moderate to severe IDD will have obvious delays in speech, mobility, and/or walking. When taking a history and conducting a physical in assessing for IDD, the nurse should not only be comprehensive, but also be aware of specific symptomatology that may indicate ID.

The nurse should look for hypotonia (i.e., low muscle tone overall or in extremities), delayed walking, clumsiness, seizures, growth delays (height and weight less than normal when plotted on age-appropriate growth charts), head circumference (either too small or too large), feeding and swallowing problems, and lethargy. In addition, major or minor abnormalities in any system, specifically the neurologic system, should be noted. Areas of abnormal findings that should be identified if present and referred to a physician for diagnosis include the following (Natvig, 2005):

1. **Head:** macro/microcephaly, frontal bossing, receding forehead, prominent or flat occiput, asymmetry

2. **Eyes:** upward or downward slanting, ptosis, hypertelorism, nystagmus/strabismus, microphthalmia, epicanthal folds

3. **Nose/mouth:** wide or depressed nasal bridge, short or bulbous nose

4. **Hair:** unusual eyebrow pattern or bushy eyebrows, low hairline, too little or excessive hair, scalp defect

5. **Mouth:** micrognathia, high arched palate, unusual mouth contour, large tongue, dental abnormalities

6. **Neck:** short, webbed

7. **Hands/feet:** fused fingers or toes, extra digits, laterally bent fingers, long or short fingers, abnormal thumbs

8. **Genitalia:** ambiguous, enlarged clitoris, small penis, bifid scrotum, undescended testicles

9. **Skin:** port wine stain, *café au lait* spots, telangiecasia

10. **Language:** delayed speech (often in contrast to a sibling's speech development), hearing and visual acuity problems

11. **Social/adaptive behavior:** hyperactivity, not interacting with others (e.g., lack of infant eye-to-eye contact with parents), other behavior problems

SCREENING/DIAGNOSIS

Parental concern is a primary reason for children to be screened for IDD. Children are referred for evaluation at a median age of 27 months (probably reflecting the most severe cases), whereas milder cases (which are the most amenable for treatment) are often not seen for referral (Sices, 2007). According to Daily, Ardinger, and Holmes (2000, p. 1060),

The most common reasons for delayed diagnosis of mental retardation in young children include believing that normal appearance and ambulation are not compatible with mental retardation, assuming that testing is not possible in young children, and failing to consider the diagnosis.

The majority of parents have concerns by the second year of life, but specialists' diagnostic assessments are often not done until 3–4 years of age (Sices, 2007). In addition to parental concerns, delayed speech, dysmorphic features (minor anomalies), generalized hypotonia or hypotonia of the extremities, and children's general inability to do things for themselves are often initial symptoms that require evaluation. Screening and diagnosis for IDD includes assessing for the information on symptoms presented in the previous section, as well as collecting the data as described in this section because "no single method is available for detecting all cases of intellectual disability" (Batshaw et al., 2007, p. 253).

History

History should include maternal gynecologic and obstetric background; maternal health during pregnancy, including use of alcohol, tobacco, and drugs; risk for sexually transmitted diseases; and other infections or illnesses. The child's history needs to include birth information (delivery, APGAR score, birth weight, length, and head circumferences), feeding or sleeping problems, extremes in temperament, presence of seizures, and developmental milestones. Information on the hospitalization during the neonatal period, admitting diagnoses, medical complications, and interdisciplinary treatments are gathered. Family history should be documented with a pedigree for three generations.

Physical Examination

A complete review of systems should focus on growth problems, history of seizures, lethargy, and developmental milestones. In addition, the nurse should note growth curves since birth, dysmorphic features (face, eyes, ears, hands, and feet; see Symptoms), behavioral phenotype, visual acuity, and hearing. The nurse should also look for features of the four common syndromes associated with IDD: Down, fetal alcohol, fragile X, and velocardiofacial.

Additional Testing

Further testing may include genetic, metabolic, and laboratory data; electroencephalogram; neuroimaging; vision and hearing screening; and specific developmental testing. Genetic/cytogenetic tests should be done with microcephaly, multiple anomalies, family history of disabilities or fetal loss, skin pigment anomalies, and suspected syndromes including fragile X, Prader-Willi, and Angelman. The studies should include chromosome studies with karyotype with expanded banding, expanded random mass spectroscopy, subtelemeric deletion, and methyl CpG binding protein 2 (MECP2 gene) for Rett syndrome.

Metabolic studies should be done when there is vomiting, lethargy, poor growth, seizures, unusual body odors, movement disorders, and/or retinal abnormalities. Testing may include newborn metabolic screening, amino acids, thyroid tests, urine organic acids, plasma ammonia, lactate, and capillary blood gases. Laboratory testing is ordered for assessing lead levels and assay for exposure to infectious agents. Electroencephalogram is indicated by a history of seizures. Neuroimaging is often done with cerebral palsy, craniofacial malformation, abnormal head size or shape, seizures, and loss of developmental skills (Daily et al., 2000, p. 1067). These tests include skull radiographs and cranial computerized tomography under sedation. Vision and hearing evaluation using audiology tests, consultation with ophthalmologist, and vision examination also should be performed.

Developmental Screening

Global developmental screening can be done using the Denver Developmental Screening Test II (Frankenburg & Dodds, 1990), the Kansas Infant Development Screen (Holmes & Hassanein, 1982), or other available tests that screen for IDD. Language and social delays should be explored with the parents using appropriate screening measures. Infants and children can then be referred for more specific developmental testing including intellectual measures. In particular, there should be an extensive exploration and detailed history of parental concerns (Acharya & Msall, 2008; Batshaw et al., 2007; Daily et al., 2000). See Table 11.2 for a description of commonly used tests.

The extent of testing for the cause of IDD is based on four factors (Batshaw et al., 2007):

1. What is the degree of IDD?
2. Is there a specific diagnostic path to follow?
3. Are the parents planning to have additional children?
4. What are the parent's wishes?

The screening test results need to be reviewed with the parents. The nurse should remember that data for infants are more variable and difficult to assess. How these results are presented to the parents by health care professionals will determine future relationships between families and the health care providers.

Developmental testing should be continued over time. In many instances, health care providers may take the "watch and wait" approach. However, once IDD is suspected, specialist referrals, evaluations, and early intervention programs should be explored. Once diagnosed with IDD, treating children and their families includes multimodal strategies that focus on many educational, social, and recreational activities of children and their families.

TREATMENT APPROACHES

Individuals with IDD must be cared for by an interdisciplinary team throughout their life span. These team members will change over time, but may remain the same throughout childhood, changing with the transition to adulthood. As each time period in an individual's life is reviewed below, it is important that the parents realize that they will be the child's primary advocate throughout their life.

If the etiology of IDD is biologic, then a physician is the first to inform the parents of the diagnosis; this usually occurs in the first months of life. Blood work and x rays may be necessary to confirm the diagnosis as mentioned previously; the child and parents will spend time navigating the health care system. The parents may also seek out counseling services to help them cope with the diagnosis. Genetic testing may be needed for knowledge of a familial link and/or for consideration of future children. Health care providers often inform the parents of local support groups, which can be very helpful. These groups are often part of national organizations that

Table 11.2. Developmental, intelligence, language, and behavioral screening tests

Screening tests	Age range	Description
Developmental		
Denver Developmental Screening Test II (Frankenburg & Dodds, 1990)	Birth–6 years	Cognitive, motor, language, adaptive/behavioral (personal/social)
Denver Prescreening Developmental Questionnaire II (Frankenburg & Bresnick, 1998)	Birth–30 months	Cognitive, motor, language, adaptive/behavioral (personal/social)
Bayley Scales of Infant Development, 2nd ed. (Bayley, 1993)	Birth–12 months	Cognitive, motor, language, adaptive/behavioral
Bayley Infant Neurodevelopmental Screener (Aylward, 1995)	3, 6, 9, 12, 18, 24 months	Cognitive, motor, language, adaptive/behavioral
Kansas Infant Development Scales (Holmes & Hassanein, 1982)	Birth–12 months	Cognitive, motor, language, adaptive/behavioral
Ages and Stages Questionnaires® (ASQ-3): A Parent-Completed, Child Monitoring System (3rd ed.) (Squires & Bricker, 2009)	Birth–48 months	Cognitive, motor, neurodevelopmental/neurological, language
Parents' Evaluation of Developmental Status (Glascoe, 2003)	Birth–8 years	Cognitive, motor, language, behavior/adaptive
Intelligence/cognitive		
Fagan Test of Infant Intelligence (Fagan & Detterman, 1992)	Birth–12 months	Communication, gross motor, fine motor, problem solving, personal/social
Weschler Intelligence Scale for Children IV Integrated (Kaplan, Fein, Kramer, Delis, & Morris, 2004)	6–16 years, 11 months	Expressive language and articulation, receptive language, fine motor, gross motor, behavior, social/emotional, self-help, academic progress
Stanford-Binet 5th edition (Roid, 2003)	2 years–adult	Intellectual development
Kaufman Brief Intelligence Test–2 (Kaufman & Kaufman, 2004)	4–9 years	Intelligence
Language		
Peabody Picture Vocabulary Test–4 (Dunn & Dunn, 2007)	2 years, 9 months–90 years	Receptive language
Early Language Milestone Scale 2 (Coplan, 1993)	Younger than 3 years	Receptive and expressive language, articulation
Preschool Language Scale 4 (Zimmerman, Steiner, & Pond, 2002)	1–36 months	Auditory comprehension, expressive communication, language
Adaptive/emotional		
Infant/Toddler Symptom Checklist (Degangi, Poisson, Sickel, & Wiener, 1999)	7–30 months	Sensory, attention, behavioral problems
Vineland SEEC: Vineland II–Social-Emotional Early Childhood Scales (Sparrow, Cicchetti, & Balla, 1998)	Birth–5 years, 11 months	Communication, daily living skills, socialization, motor skills
Pediatric Symptom Checklist (Jellinek, Murphy, & Burns, 1986)	4–16 years	Problem behaviors including conduct, depression, anxiety, adjustment

Sources: Aylward (1994); Glascoe (1999).

are excellent sources of information and conferences for up-to-date research results and best practices. In rare instances, the parents may decide that they cannot raise their child; the child then may be placed for adoption or entered into foster care. In some cases, the child's parenting is shared between the parents and the grandparents, especially if the mother is a single parent or the parent also has a disability.

In the first year of life, the child will continue to see a primary care provider for well-child care. The child may need to see a pediatric medical specialist for the care of the specific condition and any other associated problems or secondary conditions. Usually the specialist functions out of a clinic that employs nurses and may employ a pediatric nurse practitioner. The Maternal and Child Health Bureau and the American Academy of Pediatrics has advocated for the term *medical home* to represent a comprehensive philosophy of care (American Academy of Pediatrics, 2004). In addition, the child may be referred to an early intervention program to assist the child to enhance their developmental skills where needed. These programs are specified in Part C of the Individuals with Disabilities Education Improvement Act (IDEA) of 2004 (PL 106-448) (U. S. Department of Education, n.d.). In early intervention programs, the disciplines of physical therapy, occupational therapy, speech therapy, social work, education, nutrition, psychology, and nursing may be present. Such programs are found in most major cities; usually there is one in every county. These programs may be integrated with children without IDD, or they may be comprised of all children with special health care needs and IDD. An integral component of Part C, an individualized family service plan (IFSP), is developed and evaluated each year. The IFSP addresses the comprehensive needs of the child and family members for services. During this period of time, parents may still require informal or formal supports to assist them or other family members in caring for the child with IDD (Blann, 2005). Participation in parent support groups may continue. Finally, the parents may see a genetic counselor if they are planning additional children and the cause of their child's IDD is genetic.

Part B of IDEA provides for free education for the child with IDD between the ages of 3 to 21 years. Throughout these years, while in school, an individualized education program (IEP) is developed and evaluated each year. Preschool programs are available in most towns and may be integrated. These programs mainly involve early childhood educators, but may also include health care providers, psychologists, social workers, physical therapists, occupational therapists, speech therapists, and nutritionists. Health care providers can provide parents with a list of these programs. During these years, the child will continue to see their primary health care provider (who may be a nurse practitioner) for well-child care and a pediatric specialist and team for concerns specific to an illness or condition.

When the child begins school, the parents should interview the school personnel to see if the school will provide a good fit for their child. Ascertaining the principal's philosophy on providing education for children with special health care needs and IDD is important. Parents should identify the school personnel who will interact with the child during the school day, as well as determine if additional aides (individuals and/or equipment) will be needed, so that their child will be accommodated for an optimal learning environment.

Throughout the school years, health care services continue, as may counseling and other support services. Nurses may be instrumental in assisting a child to learn how to do certain self-management skills, such as self-catheterization. It is important that the child get involved in social and recreational activities if they are able. These activities could be school based, but may also be planned outside the home and school, such as scouts, clubs, music, and athletic activities. Special Olympics provides a wonderful opportunity for children with special health care needs and IDD to participate in individual/group sports activities and social events. Another opportunity for children with IDD is religious programs. Many churches provide adapted religious classes for children with special health care needs or they are integrated in developmentally relevant experiences.

In rare cases, a child with IDD may have additional behavioral and medical issues, such as uncontrollable seizures, which may precipitate placement in a residential setting. In such settings, the child is seen by health care professionals, including nurses.

As the child reaches adolescence, the need for well-child health care, specialty health care, physical and motor assists, education, and social supports continue, but now planning must begin for the transition to adulthood (Betz & Nehring, 2007). Besides the transition to adult health care providers, prevocational, educational, and residential choices must be made and planned for (Betz, 1999). The adolescent is now learning to prepare for a more independent lifestyle, making as many of their own choices as possible. Based on their level of cognitive delay, appropriate supports and realistic goals must be planned. Counseling may be needed again when an individual with IDD considers social relationships. Rejection can be very hard, so some additional help may be necessary. Often secondary conditions may begin to be more obvious depending on the condition; it is important that such symptoms not be ignored due to diagnostic overshadowing or belief that the symptoms are due to the condition that causes the IDD (Ailey, 2005). For example, a person diagnosed with depression may actually have a thyroid condition. For additional information, see Chapters 5, 12, and 14.

Once the individual with IDD reaches age 21, many things change as pediatric eligibility for programs terminate and there are less opportunities for adults, such as insurance, health care, and plans for the day. A social worker can be very helpful in assisting the family in determining what insurance plans are best for this individual. Primary health care providers will most likely change, as will the specialty providers. Now that this individual can no longer attend public school, decisions will have to be made as to whether this individual will attend life skills courses at a community college, begin a job, volunteer, or be connected with community programs. The decisions will be based on the individual's cognitive level as well as the individual's wishes. The court system may also be involved if a decision needs to be made on the level of this individual's competency.

Without school, social and recreational activities will need further planning. Often, a person with IDD cannot drive; therefore, transportation to such activities is limited. Individuals with IDD need to know of opportunities for mobility training and programs that offer education on using public transportation if available in the area where the individual lives and/or works. Depression may also occur, so efforts to involve the person with IDD in the everyday activities of the family are important. In addition, as parents begin to age, assistance by health care providers and social workers may be necessary to help plan for a residential placement according to needs of the person with IDD (Baker & Blacher, 2002).

As an older adult, a person with IDD continues to need health care, social supports, and residential care. The individual with IDD should live in the community with residential choices for as long as possible. When permanent placement is needed, the person's needs should be considered in making the decision about where to live. This decision should include a place where long-term placement can occur; often, people with IDD need structure and a change in familiar day-to-day activities can be devastating. This condition is known as *transfer anxiety* or *relocation stress;* it has been discussed in the literature concerning the transfer to a general unit from an intensive care unit in a hospital (Field, Prinjha, & Rowan, 2008).

ALTERNATIVE AND COMPLEMENTARY TREATMENTS

Individuals with IDD may choose to use a number of alternative therapies; however, there are no such therapies designed specifically for this population. Instead, alternative therapies have been discussed for specific conditions (e.g., Nehring, 2010a, 2010b; see Chapters 13 and 15). Some alternative therapies that might be used by individuals with IDD of all ages are nutritional supplements, dietary practices, exercise, use of environmentally friendly household cleaning products, massage, physical therapy, prayer, and aromatherapy (Barnes & Coulter, 2006). The therapies that individuals with IDD or their family members choose for them may be based on religious and/or cultural preferences. It is important that nurses, along with any health care providers, ascertain what alternative therapy practices a person uses when making a comprehensive assessment and planning for any health-related interventions, especially for any drug incompatibilities (Rehm, 2010).

NURSING CARE OF INDIVIDUALS WITH IDD

In this section, the characteristics of appropriate nursing care for and specific concerns of individuals with IDD are discussed. It is important to also review the information on any specific condition if an individual has a diagnosis. It is rare today for someone to be diagnosed with IDD of unknown etiology.

In general, the nursing care of individuals with IDD needs to be accessible, continuous, comprehensive, coordinated, compassionate, culturally effective, and family-centered (Williams, 2006). Each of these characteristics will be discussed in more detail in the following sections.

Accessibility

The nurse is often a source of information and support for individuals with IDD and their family members at a primary care provider location or a specialty clinic. It is important that families have a source of contact who is available at all times by either phone or email. The nurse can also assist the other members of the interdisciplinary team to make sure that the office area is accessible to accommodate any client needs.

Continuous, Comprehensive, and Coordinated Care

It is important that the nurse—particularly the pediatric nurse practitioner, if present—provides continuous, comprehensive, and coordinated service to a child with IDD. As the child ages, there is need for continuous and comprehensive well-child and condition-specific care, anticipatory guidance, and coordination with other areas of the child's life, such as the early intervention program, preschool, and school. The nurse can be part of the program plans for the early intervention and school programs as described earlier. When the child ages, the nurse or pediatric nurse practitioner plays an integral role in making sure that the transition to adult services is positive and comprehensive (Betz & Nehring, 2007).

Coordination is also accomplished between the primary care site nurse and the primary nurse at the specialty clinic. One of these nurses must be identified as the primary care coordinator so that efforts are not in conflict. For example, this primary nurse will coordinate the care associated with medication management with the school personnel, including the school nurse, and may be present at the child's IFSP and IEP meetings.

In the adult years, a nurse and perhaps an advanced practice nurse will be employed by the primary physician. This nurse will be involved in the coordination of referrals to specialty physicians and other health care professionals, such as therapists. The nurse may also get involved in helping individuals with IDD and their families in making decisions about employment, insurance, social opportunities, residential choices, and end-of-life care (Betz & Nehring, 2007).

Compassion

The nurse who works with individuals with IDD across the life span must be compassionate about this population. Their special needs may be challenging at times. For example, it may be difficult to communicate with individuals with IDD, so new strategies may need to be learned to be successful. For example, the nurse who specializes in IDD must continue to update knowledge and skills in this area (Graff et al., 2007).

Culturally Effective Care

Individuals with IDD form a culture of people with cognitive challenges. Historically, this culture has had a negative stigma. However, this stigma has lessened since the 1990s due to positive portrayals of people with IDD in popular literature, television, and movies, and overall integration in society (Nehring, 2007).

Many individuals with IDD are also members of different ethnic and racial cultures. Some conditions that result in IDD may occur with more frequency in some ethnicities (e.g., Lashley, 2005; Rehm, 2010). It is important for the nurse to understand what a person's ethnicity or race means to him or her, including the primary language used, favorite foods and music, and choice of health care providers.

McCallion, Janicki, and Grant-Griffin (1997) explored the impact of culture and acculturation on families of individuals with IDD. The strategies for culturally sensitive care fell into 10 categories:

1. Determine the meaning of the disability to the individual, each family member, and to the culture
2. Identify who makes up the family
3. Identify the primary caregiver
4. Identify who makes the decisions for the family
5. Determine the expectations for each family member (especially the person with IDD)

6. Identify the sources of support

7. Determine the reasons for moving to the United States

8. Determine the family's cultural values

9. Determine the primary language of the individual members of the family

10. Determine any issues that may impact full compliance with any treatment or intervention plan

The nurse can play an integral role in ascertaining this information and working with the team, including the individual and the family, to coordinate an appropriate and successful plan for care. The nurse should always respect the cultural values of the individual and the family. In addition, Rehm (2010) suggested that the nurse ascertain whether the individual with IDD and/or the family requests a translator, what home remedies are used, and the individual's and family member's views about health.

Another area that represents cultural value is a person's religion or spiritual beliefs. The nurse should ascertain the meaning of this religion or spiritual beliefs to the person with IDD and what their normal practices are in participating in the activities of this religion or spiritual beliefs (Williams, 2006). Also, the sexual orientation of the person with IDD should be identified, if applicable. Sexuality and sexual practices are often ignored in people with IDD. Appropriate age education based on developmental age is necessary across the life span; often, nurses are in a position to offer this information.

Family-Centered Care

It is essential that all care delivered to any individual is delivered with the family in mind. Family may mean more than someone who is biologically related; it may include those in the individual's circle of support. It is important for the nurse to ascertain who the individual with IDD considers to be family and then involve these people in care decisions. This is applicable across a person's lifetime.

SPECIFIC CONCERNS FOR PEOPLE WITH IDD

A person with IDD may experience a variety of specific concerns, including secondary health conditions, difficulty finding appropriate dental and mental health care (if necessary), and environmental concerns.

Secondary Health Conditions

A person with IDD often acquires secondary health conditions, such as pain, contractures, mental health concerns (most notably, depression), sleep issues (e.g., sleep apnea), bowel or bladder problems, fatigue, infections, cardiac problems, neurological sequelae, and social problems (e.g., lack of a social life, intimacy concerns) (Institute of Medicine, 2007; Kinne, 2008). Specific conditions have common secondary health conditions associated with them; this knowledge should be obtained by nurses (see other chapters in this book on specific conditions). It is important to be aware of the medications that an individual is taking to prevent any side effects due to adverse medication interactions. This is especially relevant in the case of an individual with IDD who may be seeing a number of specialists, but no one is monitoring the comprehensive intervention plan for that individual.

During the childhood years, anticipatory guidance for the developmental stages yet to be experienced is an integral part of well-child care. It is important that anticipatory guidance for the person with IDD be identified for the life span.

Difficulty Finding Appropriate Dental and Mental Health Care

Many families who have children with IDD have complained that they did not have adequate dental and mental health care (Reichard, Sacco, & Turnbull, 2004). It is important to identify appropriate professionals who have experience with individuals with IDD. Families can be provided with such a list for the geographical area in which they reside. There are also guidelines for oral care for individuals with IDD (National Institute of Dental and Craniofacial Research, 2007; see Chapters 7 and 14).

Environmental Concerns

In recent years, the effects of the environment on an individual's learning, communication abilities, and health has been brought to the attention of the public. Graff, Murphy, Ekvall, and Gagnon (2006) wrote of the deleterious effects of toxic chemical exposure on children with IDD. Specifically, the authors discussed the effects of lead, secondhand smoke, and mercury. Tyler, White-Scott, Ekvall, and Abulafia (2008) also discussed the effects of the same three environmental exposures, as well as alcohol. The authors of both articles provided suggestions for prevention and intervention for health care professionals. This area of study will continue to be explored as more information about additional toxins is learned.

CONCLUSION

IDD is a complex challenge for children, families, and health care providers. Discrepancies in documented prevalence of the disability and actual identification in childhood indicate that the problem is underidentified or identified later than the optimal period for initiating early intervention programs. Health care providers need education and encouragement to implement the American Academy of Pediatrics screening guidelines and developmental assessment tools in primary care settings. In addition, there needs to be continued development of high-quality screening tools and implementation of developmental screening needs to be extensively practiced (Sices, 2007). In addition to improved, more extensive screening, there need to be more resources available for children and their families to attain the most optimal developmental outcomes. These children become adolescents and adults, requiring continued health care and advocacy by health care professionals, as well as needing assistance with specific issues of sexuality and intimacy, jobs, social and functional independence, and in more severe situations, planning for assisted or custodial care, family responsibilities, or guardianship. There has been a great paradigm shift since the 1970s, with more opportunities for these individuals to become valued, visible, and contributing members of society. As part of this shift, health care professionals and families have become strong advocates for this unique population.

REFERENCES

Acharya, K., & Msall, M.E. (2008). The spectrum of cognitive-adaptive developmental disorders in intellectual disability. In P.J. Accardo (Ed.), *Capute & Accardo's neurodevelopmental disabilities in infancy and childhood* (3rd ed., pp. 241–259). Baltimore: Paul H. Brookes Publishing Co.

Ailey, S. (2005). Behavior management and mental health. In W.M. Nehring (Ed.), *Core curriculum for specializing in intellectual and developmental disability: A resource for nurses and other health care professionals* (pp. 291–304). Boston: Jones & Bartlett.

American Academy of Pediatrics, Medical Home Initiatives for Children with Special Needs Project Advisory Committee. (2004). The medical home. *Pediatrics, 113,* 1545–1547.

American Psychiatric Association. (2000). *Diagnostic and statistical manual of mental disorders DSM-IV-TR* (4th ed., text rev.). Washington, DC: Author.

Aylward, G.P. (1994). *Practitioner's guide to development and psychological testing.* New York: Plenum.

Aylward, G.P. (1995). *Bayley infant neurodevelopmental screener.* San Antonio, TX: The Psychological Corporation, Harcourt Brace & Company.

Baker, B.L., & Blacher, J. (2002). For better or worse? Impact of residential placement on families. *Mental Retardation, 40,* 1–13.

Barnes, L.L., & Coulter, D.L. (2006). Concepts of holistic care. In I.L. Rubin & A.C. Crocker (Eds.), *Medical care for children and adults with developmental disabilities* (2nd ed., pp. 645–656). Baltimore: Paul H. Brookes Publishing Co.

Batshaw, M.L., Shapiro, B., & Farber, M.L.Z. (2007). Developmental delay and intellectual disability. In M.L. Batshaw., L. Pellegrino, & N.J. Roizen (Eds.), *Children with disabilities* (6th ed., pp. 245–261). Baltimore: Paul H. Brookes Publishing Co.

Bayley, N. (1993). *Bayley scales of infant development* (2nd ed.). San Antonio, TX: The Psychological Corporation, Harcourt Brace & Company.

Betz, C.L. (1999). Adolescents with chronic conditions: Linkages to adult service systems. *Pediatric Nursing, 25,* 473–476.

Betz, C.L., & Nehring, W.M. (Eds.). (2007). *Promoting health care transitions for adolescents with special health care needs and disabilities.* Baltimore: Paul H. Brookes Publishing Co.

Bhasin, T.K., Brocken, S., Achen, R.N., & Van Naarden Braun, K. (2006). Prevalence of four developmental disabilities among children aged 8 years—Metropolitan Atlanta Developmental Disability Surveillance Program, 1996 and 2000. *Morbidity & Mortality Weekly Report, 55,* 1–9.

Blann, L.E. (2005). Early intervention for children and families with special needs. *Maternal Child Nursing, 30,* 263–267.

Bricker, D., & Squires, J. (with Mounts, L., Potter, L., Nickel, R., Twombly, E., & Farrell, J.) (1999). *Ages & stages questionnaires® (ASQ): A parent-completed, child-monitoring system.* (2nd ed.). Baltimore: Paul H. Brookes Publishing Co.

Chelly, J., Khelfaoui, M., Francis, F., Cherif, B., & Bienvenu, T. (2006). Genetics and pathophysiology of mental retardation. *European Journal of Human Genetics, 14,* 701–713.

Coplan, J. (1993). *Early language milestone scale (ELM Scale-2)* (2nd ed.). Austin, TX: PRO-ED.

Daily, D.K., Ardinger, H.H., & Holmes, G.E. (2000). Identification and evaluation of mental retardation. *American Family Physician, 61,* 1059–1070.

Degangi, G.A., Poisson, S., Sickel, R.Z., & Wiener, A.S. (1999). *Infant/toddler symptom checklist: A screening tool for parents.* San Antonio, TX: The Psychological Corporation, Harcourt-Brace Publishing.

Drews, C.D., Yeargin-Allsopp, M., Decoufle, P., & Murphy, C.C. (1995). Variation in the influence of selected sociodemographic risk factors for mental retardation. *American Journal of Public Health, 85,* 329–334.

Dunn, L.M., & Dunn, D.M. (2007). *Peabody picture vocabulary test (PPVT-4)* (4th ed.). Upper Saddle River, NJ: Pearson Education.

Fagan, J.F., & Detterman, D.K. (1992). The Fagan test of infant intelligence: A technical summary. *Journal of Applied Developmental Psychology, 13,* 173–193.

Field, K., Prinjha, S., & Rowan, K. (2008).

"One patient amongst many": A qualitative analysis of intensive care unit patients' experiences of transferring to the general ward. *Critical Care, 12,* R21.

Frankenburg, W.K., & Bresnick, B. (1998). *Denver II prescreening questionnaire (PDQ II).* Denver, CO: Denver Developmental Materials.

Frankenburg, W.K., & Dodds, J.B. (Eds.). (1990). *Denver developmental screening test II.* Denver, CO: Denver Developmental Materials.

Glascoe, F.P. (1999). Using parents' concerns to detect and address developmental and behavioral problems. *Journal of the Society of Pediatric Nurses, 4,* 24–35.

Glascoe, F.P. (2003). Parents' evaluation of developmental status: How well do parents' concerns identify children with behavioral and emotional problems? *Clinical Pediatrics, 42,* 133–138.

Graff, J.C., Barks, L., Nehring, W., Schlaier, J., Tupper, L., & Moore, M.K. (2007). Nursing support and nurse staffing: Guidelines to improve the health of people with intellectual and developmental disabilities. *International Journal of Nursing in Intellectual and Developmental Disabilities, 3.* Retrieved September 24, 2008, from http://journal.ddna.org.

Graff, J.C., Murphy, L., Ekvall, S., & Gagnon, M. (2006). In-home toxic chemical exposures and children with intellectual and developmental disabilities. *Pediatric Nursing, 32,* 596–603.

Handmaker, S.D. (2005). Etiology of intellectual and developmental disabilities. In W.M. Nehring (Ed.), *Core curriculum for specializing in intellectual and developmental disability: A resources for nurses and other health care professionals* (pp. 33–46). Boston: Jones & Bartlett.

Holmes, G.E., & Hassanein, R.S. (1982). The KIDS chart. A simple, reliable infant development screening tool. *American Journal of Diseases in Childhood, 136,* 997–1001.

Individuals with Disabilities Education Improvement Act (IDEA) of 2004, PL 108-446, 20 U.S.C. §§ 1400 *et seq.*

Institute of Medicine. (2007). *The future of disability in America.* Washington, DC: The National Academies Press.

Jellinek, M.S., Murphy, J.M., & Burns, B.J. (1986). Brief psychosocial screening in outpatient pediatric practice. *Journal of Pediatrics, 109,* 371–378.

Kaplan, E., Fein, D., Kramer, J., Delis, D., & Morris, R. (2004). *Wechsler intelligence scale for children (WISC-IV Integrated)* (4th ed. integrated). Upper Saddle River, NJ: Pearson Education.

Kaufman, A.S., & Kaufman, N.L. (2004). *Kaufman brief intelligence test (KBIT-2)* (2nd ed.). Upper Saddle River, NJ: Pearson Education.

Kinne, S. (2008). Distribution of secondary medical problems, impairments, and participation limitations among adults with disabilities and their relationship to health and other outcomes. *Disability and Health Journal, 1,* 42–50.

Lashley, F.R. (2005). *Clinical genetics in nursing practice* (3rd ed.). New York: Springer.

Leonard, H., & Wen, X. (2002). The epidemiology of mental retardation: Challenges and opportunities in the new millennium. *Mental Retardation and Developmental Disabilities Research Reviews, 8,* 117–134.

Luckasson, R., Borthwick-Duffy, S., Buntinx, W.H.E., Coulter, D.L., Craig, E.M., Reeve, A., et al. (2002). *Mental retardation: Definition, classification, and systems of support.* Washington, DC: American Association on Mental Retardation.

McCallion, P., Janicki, M., & Grant-Griffin, L. (1997). Exploring the impact of culture and acculturation on older families caregiving for persons with developmental disabilities. *Family Relations, 46,* 347–357.

Murphy, C.C., Yeargin-Allsopp, M., Decoufle, P., & Drews, C.D. (1995). The administrative prevalence of mental retardation in 10-year-old children in metropolitan Atlanta, 1985 through 1987. *American Journal of Public Health, 85,* 319–323.

Murphy, C., Boyle, C., Schendal, D., Decoufle, P., & Yeargin-Allsopp, M. (1998). Epidemiology of mental retardation in children. *Mental Retardation and Developmental Disabilities Research Reviews, 4,* 6–13.

National Institute of Dental and Craniofacial Research. (2007). *Practical oral care for people with mental retardation.* Bethesda, MD: National Oral Health Information Clearinghouse.

Natvig, D.A. (2005). Genetic concepts. In

W.M. Nehring (Ed.), *Core curriculum for specializing in intellectual and developmental disability* (pp. 57–80). Boston: Jones & Bartlett.

Nehring, W.M. (2007). Cultural considerations for children with intellectual and developmental disabilities. *Journal of Pediatric Nursing, 22,* 93–102.

Nehring, W.M. (2010a). Cerebral palsy. In P.L. Jackson & J.A. Vessey (Eds.), *Primary care of the child with a chronic condition* (5th ed., pp. 326–346). St. Louis: Mosby Elsevier.

Nehring, W.M. (2010b). Down syndrome. In P.L. Jackson & J.A. Vessey (Eds.), *Primary care of the child with a chronic condition* (5th ed., pp. 447–469). St. Louis: Mosby Elsevier.

Rehm, R.S. (2010). Family culture and chronic conditions. In P.L. Jackson, J.A. Vessey, & N.A. Shapiro (Eds.), *Primary care of the child with a chronic condition* (5th ed., pp. 90–99). St. Louis: Mosby Elsevier.

Reichard, A., Sacco, T.M., & Turnbull, H.R. (2004). Access to health care for individuals with developmental disabilities from minority backgrounds. *Mental Retardation, 42,* 459–470.

Roid, G.H. (2003). *Standford-Binet intelligence scales* (5th ed.). Rolling Meadows, IL: Riverside Publishing.

Shea, S.E. (2006). Mental retardation in children ages 6 to 16. *Seminars in Pediatric Neurology, 13,* 262–270.

Sices, L. (2007). *Developmental screening in primary care: The effectiveness of current practice and recommendations for improvement.* Boston: Commonwealth Fund.

Sparrow, S.S., Cicchetti, D.V., & Balla, D.A. (1998). *Vineland social-emotional early childhood scales.* Upper Saddle River, NJ: Pearson Education.

Tyler, C.V., Jr., White-Scott, S., Ekvall, S.M., & Abulafia, L. (2008). Environmental health and developmental disabilities: A life span approach. *Family and Community Health, 31,* 287–304.

U.S. Department of Education. (n.d.). *Building the legacy: IDEA 2004.* Retrieved February 13, 2009, from http://idea.ed.gov.

Williams, W. (2006). Advanced practice nurses in a medical home. *Journal for Specialists in Pediatric Nursing, 11,* 203–206.

World Health Organization. (2007). *Atlas global resources for persons with intellectual disabilities (Atlas-ID).* Geneva: Author.

Yeargin-Allsopp, M.M., Drews-Botsch, C., & Van Naarden Braun, K. (2008). Epidemiology of developmental disabilities. In M.L. Batshaw, L. Pellegrino, & N.J. Roizen (Eds.), *Children with disabilities* (6th ed., pp. 231–243). Baltimore: Paul H. Brookes Publishing Co.

Zimmerman, I.L., Steiner, V.G., & Pond, R.E. (2002). *Preschool language scale (PLS-4)* (4th ed.). Upper Saddle River, NJ: Pearson Education.

CHAPTER 12

Down Syndrome

Wendy M. Nehring and Cecily L. Betz

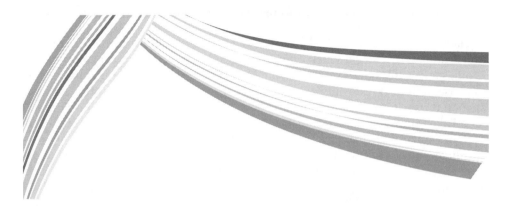

own syndrome is the most common chromosomal etiology of the intellectual disabilities. This condition was first identified in 1838 by Jean Etienne
Esquirol and later described in detail in 1866 by John Langdon Down, from
which the name of the syndrome is derived (Nehring, 2010). Lejeune, Gautier, and
Turpin (1959) were the first to identify the third copy of the 21st chromosome as
the chromosomal abnormality.

Down syndrome has an easily identifiable phenotype and genotype. The characteristic eyes, head, neck, hands, and feet are predominant features of this condition. The third copy of the 21st chromosome causes the intellectual limitation
and is readily apparent on the karyotype. Individuals with Down syndrome enjoy
full lives that are enhanced by family support, educational initiatives, health care
knowledge, diagnostic improvements, and employment and social opportunities.
In this chapter, the pathophysiology, epidemiology, secondary conditions, assessment and diagnosis, interdisciplinary and life-span approaches to care, and nursing considerations in care are fully explored.

PATHOPHYSIOLOGY

In this section, the genetic picture of Down syndrome is discussed, along with the
etiology and phenotypic features. The risk factors are discussed under each genetic
mechanism.

Chromosomal Outcomes in Down Syndrome

The 21st chromosome is composed of approximately 400 genes in the long arm.
This chromosome was the first to be fully mapped by deoxyribonucleic acid sequencing (Hattori et al., 2000). It is known that sets of these genes serve a function in metabolism, whereas others influence the central nervous system. These
latter genes, when abnormally expressed, may cause the onset of Alzheimer's disease in individuals with Down syndrome (Roizen, 2007; Roizen & Patterson,

2003). Only a segment of the full number of genes results in Down syndrome when altered. It is the region designated as 21q22 to 21qter, or the *Down syndrome critical region*. The complete pathology of Down syndrome will not be fully understood until all of the chromosomes and proteins in this region are identified and their functions explained (Roizen, 2007).

Down syndrome can result through three mechanisms: trisomy or nondisjunction (~95%), translocation (~4–5%), or mosaicism (~1-2%). The exact mechanism is apparent on the karyotype (Lashley, 2005; Roizen, 2007). Trisomy (nondisjunction) is found when 100% of the cells have an extra copy of the 21st chromosome. This situation is caused during anaphase 1 or 2 in meiosis or the anaphase of mitosis; it results in an unequal array of chromosomes. This nondisjunction is usually of maternal meiotic origin (90%) and is spontaneous without a familial origin. Thus, it takes the fertilization of the cell with 24 chromosomes to result in Down syndrome (see Figure 12.1). A paternal origin is found in approximately 8% of cases; it is often a result of paternal age greater than or equal to 55 years. Factors that can influence the incidence of nondisjunction are early menopause, maternal age, and gene polymorphisms that are affected by folate metabolism (Lashley, 2005; Roizen, 2007). Additional environmental risk factors include alcohol intake, smoking, fertility drugs, oral contraceptives, and low socioeconomic status. For a full literature review of these risk factors, see Sherman, Allen, Bean, and Freeman (2007).

The recurrence risk for nondisjunction is low at 1%. For mothers older than 35 years, the recurrence risk is 1% plus the risk percentage for the mother's age (Tolmie & MacFadyen, 2006). Translocation results from a total or partial exchange of two different chromosomes. This exchange can be balanced or unbalanced depending on whether the exchange of material is equal or unequal. In Down syndrome, the exchange is balanced and is usually an exchange between the 14th and 21st chromosome (14; 21), followed by both copies of the 21st chromosome (21; 21) or the 21st and 22nd chromosomes (21; 22). These are considered Robertsonian translocations because the exchange is between the long arms of the chromosomes. In translocation, there are still three copies of the 21st chromosome, but the extra copy is attached to the other chromosome so that the total chromosome count is 46. The cause of a translocation is multifactorial and is not influenced by parental ages (Lashley, 2005; Roizen, 2007), although a parent can be a carrier (Jones, 2006).

The phenotypes for nondisjunction and translocation are the same. The recurrence risk for translocation Down syndrome is higher than nondisjunction. For translocation 14; 21, the recurrence risk is 10% at the earliest maternal age and decreases across time. If the father is the translocation carrier, the risk is about 5%. The recurrence risk for translocation 21; 21 is 100% (Aitken, Crossley, & Spencer, 2002; Tolmie & MacFadyen, 2006).

The final mechanism for Down syndrome is mosaicism, or the finding that not all cells are trisomic for Down syndrome. When this occurs, it is usually caused by maternal meiotic nondisjunction. The phenotype for this form of Down syndrome is different from the other forms in that the symptomatology or phenotypic features are fewer (Lashley, 2005; Roizen, 2007). The risk for recurrence of mosaic Down syndrome is very rare. For more details on the genetic findings on Down syndrome, it is recommended that current genetics information be reviewed (Lashley, 2005).

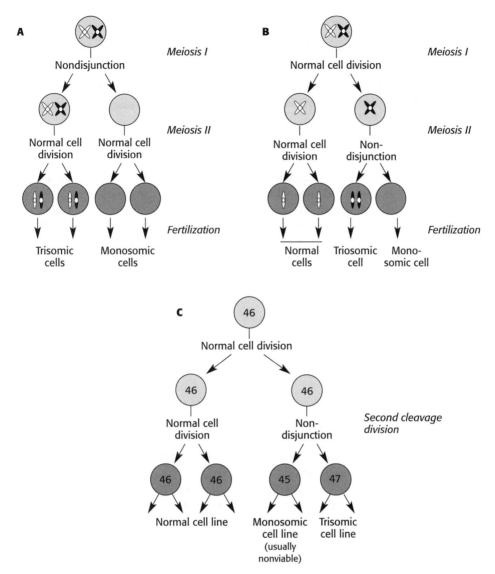

Figure 12.1. **A.** Nondisjunction during meiosis I. **B.** Nondisjunction during meiosis II. **C.** Nondisjunction following fertilization, during mitosis, resulting in mosaicism. (This figure was published in *Primary care of the child with a chronic condition*, [4th ed.], P. Jackson Allen & J.A. Vessey [Eds.], pp. 446, Copyright Mosby Elsevier [2004]; reprinted by permission.)

Etiology

Even with increased genetic knowledge, the exact cause of Down syndrome remains unknown. Most researchers agree that the cause is most likely multifactorial and more complicated than originally thought. Olson, Richtsmeier, Leszl, and Reeves hypothesized that the exact cause is most likely the result of "nonspecific small effects of many genes on chromosome 21" (2004, p. 687). Understanding the function of these genes will help in knowing how the clinical manifestations and secondary conditions result in individuals with Down syndrome. For example, it is speculated that the chromosomal alterations that occur in Down syndrome also result in physiological changes that create health problems (e.g., heart, brain, and intestinal malformations) (Roizen, 2007; Zigman & Lott, 2007). Additional causative hypotheses include autoimmunity, hormonal changes in women of advanced maternal age, chemical and environmental factors, diabetes in pregnancy, chromosomal damage, age of maternal grandmother, and frequency of intercourse (Coppede et al., 2007; Malini & Ramachandra, 2006).

Phenotypic Features

There are more than 75 physical features of Down syndrome that cover the entire body and together make the visual diagnosis fairly accurate (see Table 12.1). However, there is not a singular feature that is characteristic. Each individual with Down syndrome has a different set of features; many features, including the simian crease, can also be found in individuals without Down syndrome. Some of these features, such as Mongolian spots, may be common in Blacks and difficult to see (Nehring, 2008). Rex and Preus (1982) developed an index of physical features that predicted Down syndrome in 75% of cases:

1. Three dermatoglyphic patterns in the hands
2. Ear length
3. Brushfield spots
4. Excess skin at the back of the neck
5. Widely spaced first and second toes ("sandal gap")
6. Internipple distance

In Ireland, Devlin and Morrison (2004) examined the six physical signs of hypotonia, epicanthic folds, palpebral fissures, simian crease, sandal gap, and tongue protrusion. They found that they had accurate clinical diagnoses in 90% of nondisjunction, 100% of translocation, and 37.5% of mosaic Down syndrome cases when identifying one or more of these physical signs. They also found increased numbers of false-positive diagnoses. Regardless of the characteristic physical features, it is essential to complete a chromosomal analysis (Roizen, 2007).

EPIDEMIOLOGY

In this section, the incidence, prevalence, and survival rates for Down syndrome are discussed. The impact of improved systems of care are also highlighted.

Incidence

The incidence rate of Down syndrome in the United States is estimated at approximately 4,000 infants born each year (National Dissemination Center for Children with Disabilities, 2004). This rate has been influenced by the availability of prenatal diagnosis. The incidence of nondisjunction increases as the mother ages: It is approximately 1:1,667 live births for women in their 20s, increasing to 1:30 live births after age 45 (Hecht & Hook, 1996). The incidence of nondisjunction is also influenced by advanced paternal age (older than 55), as mentioned previously (Lashley, 2005). The incidence of translocation as noted previously is not dependent on age, but one third of cases of translocation Down syndrome are inherited from a carrier parent (Tolmie & MacFadyen, 2006).

Table 12.1.   Clinical manifestations in Down syndrome

SKULL
False fontanel
Flat occipital area
Brachycephaly
Separated sagittal suture
Hypoplasia of midfacial bones
Reduced interorbital distance
Underdeveloped maxilla
Obtuse mandibular angle

EYES
Oblique narrow palpebral fissures
Epicanthal folds
Brushfield spots
Strabismus
Nystagmus
Myopia
Hypoplasia of the iris

EARS
Small, shortened ears
Low and oblique implantation
Overlapping helices
Prominent antihelix
Absent or attached earlobes
Narrow ear canals
External auditory meatus
Structural aberrations of the ossicles
Stenotic external auditory meatus

NOSE
Hypoplastic
Flat nasal bridge
Anteverted, narrow nares
Deviated nasal septum

MOUTH
Prominent, thickened, and fissured lips
Corners of the mouth turned downward
High-arched, narrow palate
Shortened palatal length
Protruding enlarged tongue
Papillary hypertrophy (early preschool)
Fissured tongue (later school years)
Periodontal disease
Partial anodontia
Microdontia
Abnormally aligned teeth
Anterior open bite

NECK
Short, broad neck
Loose skin at nape

CHEST
Shortened rib cage
Twelfth rib anomalies
Pectus excavatum or carinatum
Congenital heart disease

ABDOMEN
Distended and enlarged abdomen
Diastasis recti
Umbilical hernia
Muscle tone and musculature
Hyperflexibility
Muscular hypotonia
Generalized weakness
Integument
Skin appears large for the skeleton
Dry and rough
Fine poorly pigmented hair

EXTREMITIES
Short extremities
Partial or complete syndactyly
Clinodactyly
Brachyclinodactyly

Upper Extremities
Short broad hands
Brachyclinodactyly
Single palmar transverse crease
Incurved short fifth finger
Abnormal dermatoglyphics

Lower Extremities
Short and stubby feet
Gap between first and second toes
Plantar crease between first and second toe
Second and third toes grouped in a forklike position
Radial deviation of the third to the fifth toe

PHYSICAL GROWTH AND DEVELOPMENT
Short stature
Increased weight in later life

OTHER FINDINGS SEEN IN NEWBORNS
Enlarged anterior fontanel
Delayed closing of sutures and fontanels
Open sagittal suture
Nasal bone not ossified, underdeveloped
Reduced birth weight

Gender differences in the incidence of Down syndrome also occur, depending on the mechanism. Nondisjunction Down syndrome is found in more boys (59%) than girls (41%), but there are more girls with translocation Down syndrome (74%) (Staples, Sutherland, Haan, & Clisby, 1991). Individuals with Down syndrome are found in all races and ethnicities. Khoshnood, Pryde, and Wall (2000) found that there are significantly higher rates of infants with Down syndrome born to Hispanic mothers and moderately higher rates of infants with Down syndrome born to Black mothers over the age of 35. They hypothesized that these differences may be due to differences in views on abortion, incidence of prenatal diagnosis, and participation in early prenatal care.

Prevalence

The prevalence rate for Down syndrome in the United States is approximately 1.3 per 1,000 live births (Centers for Disease Control and Prevention, 2006). This figure was the same for a sample of births of Down syndrome in metropolitan Atlanta in 2003 (Besser, Shin, Kucik, & Correa, 2007) and was slightly higher (1.365 per 1,000 live births) in a study of the United States by Canfield et al (2006). An Israeli study found a prevalence of 1.1 per 1,000 live births in 1997, but when terminated pregnancies were added to the equation, the prevalence was 2.32 per 1,000 (Merrick, 2000). The prevalence of Down syndrome varies by the mechanism, as noted previously in the discussion of nondisjunction, translocation, and mosaicism. Sherman et al. (2007) called for prevalence studies of adolescents and adults with Down syndrome in order to more accurately determine needed resources and services for adequate intervention.

Survival Rates

The quality of life of individuals with Down syndrome has greatly improved over the past half century due to parent support groups; increased knowledge of the condition; better educational opportunities; better health care management and treatments; improved diagnostics; and increased social, employment, and housing options and support systems. After a review of death certificates from 1983 to 1997 across the United States, Yang, Rasmussen, and Friedman (2002) found that the median age for death in Caucasians with Down syndrome was 49 years, although this number was lower for people of other races. They identified the primary causes of death as congenital heart disease, dementia, hypothyroidism, and leukemia.

A study of mortality in people with Down syndrome who died in California between the years 1988 to 1999 found higher mortality in Blacks at a younger age (Day, Strauss, Shavelle, & Reynolds, 2005). Fewer children also died from congenital heart disease than in earlier years. The primary causes of death in this study were circulatory diseases, congenital anomalies, leukemia, and respiratory diseases. An Australian study on mortality during the years from 1953 to 2000 found that heart defects were the most prevalent cause of death (Bittles, Bower, Hussain, & Glasson, 2007). Another Australian study found the median age at death for individuals with Down syndrome living in Western Australia was 58.6 years (Glasson et al., 2002). Rasmussen, Wong, Correa, Gambrell, and Friedman (2006) also stressed that socioeconomic status, health status, access to health care, and type of residence impacted mortality.

DIAGNOSTIC CRITERIA

Diagnosis of Down syndrome can be determined in the prenatal or postnatal period though chromosomal analysis. Prenatal diagnostic screening can be done through a blood test for chromosomal analysis between 16 to 18 weeks of pregnancy. It consists of two components: serum screening and ultrasound (nuchal translucency). Referred to as the *quadruple screen,* serum alpha-fetoprotein, human chorionic gonadotropin, unconjugated estriol, and dimeric inhibin A are used to screen for Down syndrome. It is followed by an ultrasound, called *nuchal translucency,* to measure the thickness of the back of the infant's neck. The results of these tests are calculated to determine the risk of having a child with Down syndrome. Its accuracy for detecting Down syndrome ranges from 82% to 87% (March of Dimes, 2008).

Later in the second trimester, another screen may be done if there were chromosomal problems with the first trimester screen. A triple screen measuring serum alpha-fetoprotein, human chorionic gonadotropin, and unconjugated estriol or a quadruple screen may be done (Newberger, 2000). The accuracy for detecting a child with Down syndrome in the second trimester is 95% (March of Dimes, 2008). More invasive testing can be done between 8 and 12 weeks using chorionic villi sampling, amniocentesis between 12 and 20 weeks, and percutaneous umbilical blood sampling after 20 weeks (National Association for Down Syndrome, n.d.). If no prenatal screening was done or a false-negative result was obtained, then a chromosomal analysis is done postnatally for an accurate diagnosis.

SECONDARY CONDITIONS

Secondary conditions can arise in every body system for individuals with Down syndrome. Some can be present at birth, whereas others will not be present until later in life. The severity of the condition also individually varies. Each system is described in detail.

Cardiac Anomalies

Between 40% and 50% of children with Down syndrome have congenital heart defects (Pierpoint et al., 2007). The most common cardiac defects are atrioventricular septal defects, atrial septal defects, patent ductus arteriosus, and ventricular septal defects (American Academy of Pediatrics [AAP], 2001; Cohen, 1999; Pierpoint et al. 2007). Atrioventricular septal defect is the most common cardiac defect; it affects one in five children with Down syndrome (Down Syndrome Center, 2007). Other defects affecting children with Down syndrome, in order of frequency as reported by the Atlanta Down Syndrome Project, are ventricular septal defects, isolated secundum atrial septal defect, isolated persistent patent ductus arteriosus, and tetralogy of Fallot (Freeman et al., 1998). Mitral value prolapse occurs in more than 50% of individuals with Down syndrome before entering adulthood (Geggel, O'Brien, & Feingold, 1993; National Institute of Dental and Craniofacial Research [NIDCR], 2009).

Respiratory Problems

Children with Down syndrome are predisposed to respiratory tract infections and pulmonary edema in high altitudes (Durmowicz, 2001). As such, the symptoms for these conditions should be monitored closely and medical attention should be sought earlier to prevent more severe exacerbations.

Neurodevelopmental Issues

Nearly all individuals with Down syndrome will have an intellectual disability, although the level will vary. Most individuals will be moderately affected; some will be severely affected and others, especially those with mosaic Down syndrome, will be mildly affected. In fact, some children with mosaic Down syndrome may not be identified as having an intellectual disability on standardized intelligence tests. Early intervention, the home environment, proper nutrition, and the individual health status will greatly affect intelligence. However, it is known that intelligence, as well as memory and social skills, decreases over time as a result of central nervous system and brain function changes; this often results in dementia or Alzheimer's disease (Roizen, 2007).

Behavioral issues may also arise during the school-age and adolescent years; these may include depression, inattention, hyperactivity, and aggression. The prevalence of behavioral issues in Down syndrome is approximately 18%–40% (Capone, Goyal, Ares, & Lannigan, 2006; Capone, Grados, Kaufmann, Bernad-Ripoll, & Jewell, 2005; Nicham et al., 2003; Visootsak & Sherman, 2007). When assessing for behavioral problems, physical etiologies should be ruled out and diagnostic overshadowing should not occur (see Chapter 14).

Musculoskeletal Problems

Orthopedic problems are common due to several underlying inherent conditions. Hypotonia and ligamentous laxity, which are speculated to be caused by an inherent defect of connective tissue, are associated with numerous orthopedic problems such as scoliosis, dislocated hips, muscle fatigue, and joint and muscle pain. Generalized hypotonia is evident in the neonate and requires ongoing monitoring for its manifestations (Concolino, Pasquzzi, Capalbo, Sinopoli, & Strisciuglio, 2006). Another orthopedic problem affecting 15% of children with Down syndrome is atlantoaxial instability, which refers to the excessive movement between C1 (atlas) and C2 (axis) that causes compression of the cervical nerves. Atlantoaxial instability can cause neck pain, torticollis, gait changes due to increasing spasticity, and urinary incontinence. This is a progressive disorder with slow manifestation of the symptoms, although life-threatening complications are rare (Alvarez, 2008).

Sensory Impairments: Vision and Hearing

Visual impairments are common problems, affecting approximately 60% of individuals with Down syndrome (Stephen, Dickson, Kindley, Scott, & Charleton, 2007). Visual problems identified include congenital cataracts, corneal and retinal anomalies, strabismus, and nystagmus. Other visual impairments reported are refractive errors (near- and farsightedness), keratoconus, and blepharitis (Merrick & Koslowe, 2001).

Hearing loss affects a significant proportion of individuals diagnosed with Down syndrome, ranging from 40% to 75% due to either conductive or sensory-neural hearing loss (Shott, 2006). Sensory-neural hearing loss is the more frequent type of hearing loss, affecting individuals with Down syndrome with an estimated incidence of 1 per 1,000. As individuals age, the hearing loss worsens due to the degenerative changes of the cochlear structure in the inner ear (Snashall, 2002). Conductive hearing loss is attributed to recurrent problems with otitis media exacerbated by the altered structure of the eustachian tube; it is shorter and narrower than in typical children (Shott, 2006). It is estimated that 66% to 89% of children with Down syndrome have hearing loss in at least one ear (Chen, 2007).

Gastrointestinal Anomalies

It is estimated that 5% of infants with Down syndrome are diagnosed with a range of gastrointestinal (GI) anomalies that include pyloric stenosis, Hirschsprung disease, duodenal or esophageal atresia, and imperforate anus (Roizen & Patterson, 2003). Other GI problems include tracheoesophageal fistula, omphalocele, and Meckel diverticulum (Chen, 2007). Celiac disease, a digestive problem that is the inability to digest gluten (an essential element of wheat and grains), is discussed in next section.

Immune System Deficiencies

Individuals with Down syndrome are at higher risk for autoimmune disorders, including celiac disease and thyroid problems. Each is discussed in more detail.

Celiac Disease   The most frequently occurring immune problem affecting individuals with Down syndrome is celiac disease, with estimates ranging from a low of 1.6% to a high of 16.9%. This estimated range of celiac disease is significantly higher than in the general population (Uibo et al., 2006; Wouters et al., 2009).

Thyroid Problems   Thyroid problems due to autoimmune diseases occur with greater frequency in individuals with Down syndrome as compared to the general population. Estimates of the prevalence of hypothyroidism range from 10% to more than 50% (Capone, Roizen, & Rogers, 2008; Dinani & Carpenter, 1990). Hyperthyroidism occurs far less frequently than hypothyroidism; however, some suggest that it may be underdiagnosed as well as underreported (Ali, Al-Busairi, & Al-Mulla, 1999). Type 1 diabetes mellitus occurs more frequently in children with Down syndrome when compared to their typical age mates. Type 2 diabetes occurs more often in adults with Down syndrome compared to adults without Down syndrome. The increased rates of type 2 diabetes are associated with higher prevalence of obesity in individuals with Down syndrome (National Congress of Down Syndrome, n.d.).

Dental Problems

Dental problems are a significant concern in individuals with Down syndrome. Delayed eruption of primary and permanent teeth is evident, with primary dentition completed by age 4–5 years and less frequently as late as 15 years of age (NIDCR, 2009). Individuals with Down syndrome have higher rates of malocclusion. Rates of malocclusion are among the highest when compared to other groups of individuals with disabilities (Chen, 2007; Winter, Baccaglini, & Tomar, 2008). Individuals with Down syndrome are more likely to have congenitally missing teeth compared to individuals without Down syndrome. The most common missing teeth are the laterals, third molars, and second bicuspids (NIDCR, 2009).

A compromised immune system makes individuals with Down syndrome more vulnerable to periodontal disease. This includes mouth ulcers, acute necrotizing ulcerative gingivitis, and *Candida* infections (NIDCR, 2009). One study found that gingivitis was prevalent in 91% and periodontitis in 33% of children and youth with Down syndrome (Loureiro, Costa, & da Costa, 2007). As a result of the increased incidence of periodontal disease, a greater number of adolescents with Down syndrome are likely to lose their permanent anterior teeth. Dental caries are found less frequently in children with Down syndrome due to the loss of permanent teeth and delayed eruption of both primary and permanent teeth. However, dental caries occur in adults with Down syndrome due to decreased saliva production causing dry mouth and the ingestion of foods that cause tooth decay such as sweets (NIDCR, 2009).

Leukemias

Children with Down syndrome are more likely to be diagnosed with acute myeloid leukemia (AML) and much more likely to be diagnosed with acute megakaryoblastic leukemia (AMKL) than children without Down syndrome (Vyas & Roberts, 2006). This is most likely due to having a trisomy, a mutation of GATA1, and other factors not yet known (Cushing et al., 2006; Vyas & Roberts, 2006). Children with AML experience a better outcome than children without Down syndrome with this form of leukemia; it is speculated that this is due to a higher sensitivity to the chemotherapeutic agents (Tomizawa et al., 2007). Children with Down syndrome with AMKL also have a better prognosis and respond to treatment better than children without Down syndrome with this form of leukemia (Vyas & Roberts, 2006).

Children with Down syndrome experience higher rates of acute lymphatic leukemia (ALL) and transient leukemia (TL) than children without Down syndrome. In most cases, children with Down syndrome with ALL survive at about the same rate as children without Down syndrome with ALL (Whitlock, 2006; Whitlock et al., 2005). Approximately 10% of infants with Down syndrome will be diagnosed with TL; this form of leukemia usually disappears in the first three months of life. About 40% of those infants with Down syndrome who acquire TL will later acquire AMKL by their fourth year (Massey et al., 2006; Vyas & Roberts, 2006).

Solid Tumors

The incidence of solid tumors in individuals with Down syndrome is less than the general population (Dixon, Kishnani, & Zimmerman, 2006; Sullivan, Hussain, Glasson, & Bittles, 2007). However, there appears to be an increased risk of testicular germ cell tumors in males with Down syndrome (Dixon et al., 2006).

Growth and Obesity

Growth retardation is a prominent characteristic of individuals with Down syndrome. The growth rate of children with Down syndrome is not comparable to typically developing children. The velocity of growth is markedly different from typical children during the periods of infancy (6 months to 3 years of age) and adolescence (pubertal period) (Cronk et al., 1988; Meguid, El-Kotoury, Abdel-Salam, El-Ruby, & Afifi, 2004; Myrelid, Gustafsson, Ollars, & Anneréen, 2002). The height, weight, and head circumference measurements of infants with Down syndrome are less in comparison to infants without Down syndrome (Myrelid et al., 2002). Starting in late infancy, the issue of overweight is evident and persists throughout childhood and adulthood (Cronk et al., 1988; Myrelid et al., 2002). Puberty and final height occur earlier in youth with Down syndrome compared to typically developing youth. Final height is achieved at about 16 years of age (Myrelid et al., 2002).

Dermatologic Problems

Skin problems are common in Down syndrome and appear to increase with age. The most frequently occurring dermatologic problems are atopic dermatitis, cheilitis, fissured tongue, ichthyosis, premature graying, seborrheic dermatitis, and vitiligo (Daneshpazhooh, Nazemi, Bigdeloo, & Yoosefi, 2007).

Seizure Disorders

Seizures occur more frequently in children with Down syndrome, with estimates of incidence ranging from 5% to 10% (Cohen, 1999). Prevalence rates are increased during infancy and adulthood. Infantile spasms are the most common seizure type observed in infants (Chen, 2007). Forty percent of seizures occur during the first year of life (Roizen, 2007). Tonic-clonic seizures are the most frequently occurring type of seizure activity observed in adults. Besides infancy, the prevalence of seizures increases during this period of time. It is thought that seizure activity can be precipitated by other factors such as cardiac defects and infections (Cohen, 1999).

Sleep Problems

Obstructive sleep apnea is a potential problem to monitor for in children and adults with Down syndrome. The symptoms observed are restless sleep, difficulty awaking, daytime sleepiness, and behavioral changes (AAP, 2001; Chen, 2007). Parents may not recognize the problems associated with their child's sleep apnea; therefore, parental education is needed for proper identification and treatment implementation (Shott et al., 2006). For children who have cardiac problems, sleep apnea increases the workload of the heart because less oxygenation of the blood occurs, resulting in pulmonary hypertension and an enlarged right side of the heart. Other complications result due to the problems with oxygenation of the blood, such as recurrent pulmonary infections, gastroesophageal reflux disease, and decreased growth (Leshin, 2000). In adults with Down syndrome, the underlying causative mechanism of obstructive sleep apnea may not be due to obesity. The clinical features of Down syndrome of hypotonia and structural anomalies can be contributory (Smith, 2001).

MEDICAL MANAGEMENT OF SELECTED SECONDARY CONDITIONS

As discussed in the previous section, individuals with Down syndrome can manifest a range of associated problems that will affect their overall health status and level of functioning. The extent to which these associated conditions will have adverse effects will be mediated in part by the quality of interdisciplinary care and ongoing health surveillance provided. Specific conditions that warrant attention and monitoring across the life span are discussed in this section.

The immediate diagnostic priority for an infant born with Down syndrome is to determine if there are associated anomalies that require prompt medical attention. These anomalies are congenital heart disease, gastrointestinal anomalies, and cataracts (Crocker, 2006). Because infants with Down syndrome are at increased risk for congenital heart defects, a complete cardiac evaluation including an echocardiogram should be performed (AAP, 2001). Correction of the defect will be performed following diagnosis. Some experts have recommended that routine echocardiographic studies be performed during adolescence and early adulthood to detect the valve dysfunction problems of mitral valve prolapse, tricuspid valve prolapsed, and aortic valve regurgitation (Feingold & Geggel, 2001). If detected, corrective surgery will be necessary. Whatever the age, the individual with Down syndrome who has undergone surgical repair of their cardiac defect will require antibiotic prophylaxis prior to dental work to prevent subacute bacterial endocarditis (Chen, 2007). The early detection and treatment of cardiac problems have improved survival rates and life expectancy of individuals with Down syndrome (Roizen, 2007).

Clinical manifestations of GI anomalies mentioned previously will require immediate surgical intervention. The correction of GI problems requires ongoing monitoring for signs and symptoms of complications. For example, the child born with Hirschsprung disease will require ongoing care and monitoring through the two-stage surgical process for stomal complications of the temporary colostomy following the first stage of the surgical repair. Long-term management includes monitoring for incontinence, inadequate emptying, stenosis, and constrictions. Depending on the severity of the imperforate anus defect, the child may require ongoing management as well following surgical intervention (Betz & Sowden, 2008).

The ongoing screening guidelines for sensory problems are discussed in the section on the life-span approach to care and nursing role. However, it is known that ophthalmologic problems (e.g., keratoconus, cataracts, refractive errors) and hearing problems worsen with age and require ongoing monitoring and treatment. The deterioration of hearing and vision can create psychosocial problems if not treated properly. The inability to hear others correctly can lead to social isolation and depression (Smith, 2001). Problems with vision limit the ability of the individual to engage in recreational pursuits, social activities, and self-care activities; live independently; and move safely and comfortably within the community.

Atlantoaxial instability is monitored continuously for manifestation of signs and symptoms. The signs of atlantoaxial instability are spasticity, abnormal reflexes (presence of Babinski sign, deep tendon responses), clonus, changes in gait, neck pain, torticollis, and loss of upper or lower body strength (Cohen, 1999; Smith, 2001). Children should be screened for orthopedic problems whenever there are changes in gait, complaints of muscle pain, or fatigue. Radiographic studies may be necessary to assess the feasibility of sports participation and for diagnostic evaluation when clinical manifestations are apparent. A rare but serious complication of atlantoaxial instability is spinal decompression, which requires surgery to stabilize the spine (AAP, 2001; Chen, 2007; Smith, 2001).

Individuals who are overweight and obese need to be monitored for type 2 diabetes. Currently there are no available guidelines for monitoring serum glucose levels, although experts have provided recommendations for screening at least every 2 years (Smith, 2001). Hypothyroidism may be difficult to detect because its clinical manifestations are similar to behaviors of individuals with Down syndrome such as weakness, weight gain, constipation, and depression (Stoppler, 2006). The compromised immune systems of individuals with Down syndrome put them at risk for recurrent infections, especially during times of high communicability in schools, places of employment, and congregate living environments. Monitoring for illnesses and the institution of infection control precautions will be an important component of care.

If obstructive sleep apnea is suspected, an otolaryngological evaluation is needed. Sleep studies may be ordered to determine a diagnosis. Treatment approaches include removal of the adenoids and tonsils, and in severe cases, uvulopalatopharyngoplasty for children who have large and soft palates (Leshin, 2000). Continuous positive airway pressure devices may be used for individuals who can tolerate this treatment. Cor pulmonale is a serious complication of untreated sleep apnea in adults (Smith, 2001).

INTERDISCIPLINARY APPROACHES TO CARE

Individuals with Down syndrome will require interdisciplinary care throughout their lives. The demand for health care services will be based on each individual's unique health needs, as well as the particular stage of development. A child born with a cardiac defect will require prompt surgical intervention followed by a lifetime of surveillance. For others, routine screenings to monitor for later appearing cardiac problems, such as a prolapsed mitral value, will be needed.

Beginning in infancy, the child will require services and supports from interdisciplinary team members to foster the acquisition of developmental skills. Occupational and physical therapists will work with the child and family to implement a program of care to foster fine and gross motor development. The plan of care, whether provided in center-based or home settings by the occupational and/or physical therapist, will require strong family involvement to continue, reinforce, and practice newly learned skills and move on to acquire new ones. Children with feeding problems may require the combined services of the dietician, psychologist, social worker, developmental pediatrician, and occupational therapist to determine the needs for feeding and develop strategies to foster healthy growth. Nurses can provide the coordination needed to ensure services are provided in a timely, coordinated, and continuous manner and focus on ensuring well-child and special health needs are met.

Later in school, the child will benefit from the participation of the team of educational and related services personnel who can develop an individualized education program (IEP) that addresses the child's needs for services. The occupational and physical therapists may continue to provide consultation or services to foster gross and fine motor skills needed for physical activities. Recreational specialists or social workers associated with developmental disabilities agencies may be involved in programs to facilitate the development of recreational and social skills, such as learning how to play cooperatively with others or learning skills of social communication.

As adolescence approaches, the profile of interdisciplinary team members changes. As the youth prepares for adulthood, specialists in vocational rehabilitation and counseling, job training, housing, mobility training, and community living (e.g., budgeting, meal preparation) will become members of the youth's team of service providers, whether these services are provided in school, in a health care setting, or by a community agency, such as the developmental disabilities service agency. These supports will continue to varying degrees into adulthood.

As the individual ages, the composition of team members will be altered again. The emphasis will shift to supportive—and eventually for many, palliative care. Mental health changes may be evident in individuals for whom limited planning has occurred, which may result in a constriction of their social activities and network (Ailey, 2005). Alzheimer's disease is a major concern for adults with Down syndrome, as nearly 40% of individuals are affected (Crocker, 2006). For additional information on dual diagnosis, see Chapter 14.

Throughout the life span, nurses function in a variety of roles to facilitate the acquisition of the individual's needs for care and services. The nurse may act as the service coordinator, ensuring that the needs of the child and family are met by the interdisciplinary members of the team of care, as well as serving as the liaison on behalf of the team to the family. Another role of the nurse is as a direct service provider in a number of settings, including the hospital, a large or smaller congregate facility, and a community clinic or service program. As consultants, nurses provide input to interdisciplinary team members as to the nursing related needs and available services available to the child and family (Nehring et al., 2004).

LIFE-SPAN APPROACH TO CARE AND THE NURSING ROLE

In the following sections, the nursing role in the health care of persons with Down syndrome across various life stages will be discussed.

Infancy

The birth of an infant with Down syndrome will present the child's family with major challenges as the child's caregivers. Parents will be dealing with the reality of having an infant who has an intellectual disability and possibly a number of associated conditions that will require ongoing treatment and care. Parents may feel anxious about their own capabilities to safely and competently care for a child who has a variety of intellectual and physical needs. Feelings of inadequacy to care for the child may overwhelm the parents, which may affect their abilities to bond lovingly with their child. Other concerns may arise as to how this child will alter their lifestyle such as family routines, their spousal relationship, their relationships with their other children, and the effect on family finances. Nurses and other members of the child's specialized team can provide assurance, support, and instruction to allay parental concerns. Parents may need referrals to a social worker, mental health professional, and/or parent support group to provide ongoing support to cope with the stresses and adapt to their new caregiving demands (Van Cleve & Cohen, 2006).

In addition to these worries and concerns, parents need to be resilient to deal with the new caregiving demands while providing loving and developmentally appropriate care to their child. Parents need to be assured that they will be supported by the members of the child's specialized team to better understand the needs of their child, learn the knowledge and skills needed to provide care, and access the needed health care and community resources (Siklos & Kerns, 2006). Referrals to community resources will include the medical specialty clinics to treat the ongoing problems with associated conditions, early intervention programs, and parent support groups. Nurses will serve in a key role to instruct parents on home care management of their child's needs and to provide anticipatory guidance as to future needs.

Although infants diagnosed with Down syndrome present with clinical characteristics shared by all children with this diagnosis, the associated conditions and extent to which the child is intellectually disabled can vary significantly. Children with Down syndrome may present initially with other secondary conditions such as cardiac defects, respiratory problems, gastrointestinal anomalies, and hearing and vision deficits. These secondary conditions will require immediate and/or early treatment. Parents will need instruction to observe for and report changes in their child's physical status and/or behavior that may indicate the presence of an undetected secondary condition or complication (Van Cleve & Cohen, 2006).

Primary health care screenings are recommended every 2 months up to 12 months of age, followed by screenings at 15 and 18 months of age. Beginning at 2 years of age, the child should be seen by a pediatric primary care provider annually. These pediatric visits should include growth assessment, vision, hearing, and thyroid screenings and administration of immunizations according to the recommendations of the Advisory Committee on Immunization Practices, AAP, and the American Academy of Family Physicians (U.S. Department of Health and Human Services [USDHHS], Centers for Disease Control and Prevention [CDC], 2009a). The child's growth pattern should be noted during each clinic visit. The child's BMI, based on the height and weight, should be monitored closely.

If a visual screening during the visit is not possible, then seeking out options with another health care provider or the child's school nurse should be planned. If positive findings are found with the screening, then the child should be referred to a pediatric ophthalmologist. Ongoing dental care requires aggressive preventive care. Dental recommendations indicate that the child with Down syndrome should be seen by dentists with expertise in special needs dentistry on a quarterly basis (Tufts University School of Dentistry, 2008). Antibiotic prophylaxis will be needed for children who have undergone cardiac surgery (NIDCR, 2009).

All children diagnosed with Down syndrome should be referred to early intervention programs as mandated by Part C of the Individuals with Disabilities Education Improvement Act (IDEA) of 2004 (PL 108-446) (U.S. Department of Education, n.d.). The array of services available in the early intervention programs will assist to facilitate the child's development and family functioning. These services will be identified in the individualized family service plan (IFSP). For more information on early intervention programs and the IFSP, refer to Chapters 3 and 4.

Preschool and School Age

The child's fine and gross motor skills, speech and language, and psychosocial development will continue to be monitored by the array of service providers in health care, education, and community settings. Although the parents continue to be the child's primary advocates for services, the child is beginning to learn—through appropriate parental modeling and instruction, from caregivers, from typically developing peers and siblings, and from service providers—the developmentally appropriate skills to become as self-reliant as possible for this stage of development.

Pediatric health practitioners will provide primary health care based on the guidelines of care specific to the needs of children with Down syndrome. The surveillance visit begins with eliciting parental input about relevant changes in the child's level of functioning at home and school, emergence of behavioral problems, and problems related to sleep (e.g., interrupted sleep possibly due to sleep apnea) and elimination (e.g., constipation). Screening for growth using growth charts specific for children with Down syndrome, as well as vision, hearing, and thyroid functioning, will be conducted at each visit. Any positive findings should be referred to a specialist for additional testing and treatment.

During the preschool years, atlantoaxial instability or subluxation is assessed radiographically. Screening for celiac disease is done with immunoglobulin A (IgA) antiendomysium antibodies and total IgA between 2 and 3 years of age (AAP, 2001; Cohen, 1999). Immunizations are administered according to the recommendations of the Advisory Committee on Immunization Practices, AAP, and American Academy of Family Physicians (USDHHS, CDC, 2009a, 2009b). Additionally, it is important to assess the health literacy of parents as it pertains to understanding their child's condition and treatment approaches, as well as their ability to access needed services.

Parents may need assistance to fully understand their and their children's rights and protections pertaining to schooling as specified in Part B of IDEA. The process for developing an IEP as specified in IDEA is very different than the process for the IFSP. For additional information on the IEP process, refer to Chapters 3 and 4. Nurses in both the school and health care settings can assist parents to better understand the services and support provided by IDEA, as well as assure that the child's health-related needs that may adversely affect their learning performance are included in the IEP.

Adolescence

Annual primary care screenings for vision, hearing, and thyroid functioning continue. The youth's growth pattern related to height and weight on Down syndrome specific charts continues to be monitored. Quarterly visits to the dentist to monitor oral care needs continues with the use of antibiotic prophylaxis as needed prior to dental procedures for those who have had surgical repair of a cardiac defect or have mitral valve prolapse (NIDCR, 2009).

The physical changes associated with puberty can be assessed using the Tanner scale (Wheeler, 1991) because teens with Down syndrome undergo pubertal changes at the same progression as typically developing teens. The teen's health issues should be reviewed directly with the teen and also with the parent or guardian. It is important that time during the visit is allocated to discuss issues alone with the teen to foster their self-determination. Concerns related to pubertal changes, such as menstruation (e.g., dysmenorrheal), night ejaculations, acne, vaginal or penile discharge, and masturbation, are addressed. If teens are sexually active (or plan to be), then transmission of sexually transmitted diseases, contraception, and reproductive issues should be discussed. Also, a discussion of what constitutes unwelcomed sexual advances and means to deter them, as well as sexual abuse, should occur (Van Cleve, Cannon, & Cohen, 2006).

The American College of Obstetricians and Gynecologists (ACOG) recommends that adolescents have their first reproductive visit beginning between ages 13 and 15 (ACOG, 2003), whereas the Office of Women's Health suggests age 18 if sexually active or age 21 years if not (USDHHS, 2007). Also, the ACOG recommends that adolescents and young women from 9–13 years of age up to age 26 receive the quadrivalent human papillomavirus (HPV) vaccine (ACOG, 2006). HPV, which is transmitted sexually or by skin-to-skin contact, can cause genital warts, cervical changes, and cervical cancer.

Adolescence is a period of significant transitions in all areas of development for all teens. Youth with Down syndrome together with their parents will need to consider the future planning issues differently pertaining to high school completion. They will need to ensure that their transition IEP addresses these comprehensive needs. Many plans laying the groundwork for the future following completion of high school can be forged in the transition IEP, such as on-the-job training, learning the social skills needed to function independently in community and employment settings, and the learning of functional community skills, such as taking public transportation, cooking, and money management (Betz & Nehring, 2007).

Health care transition planning is an integral component for adulthood preparation. Several tasks should be accomplished to achieve the goals of health care transition planning (AAP, American Academy of Family Practice, & American College of Physicians American Society of Internal Medicine, 2002; Betz & Nehring, 2007):

1. Finding adult providers
2. Enrolling in adult health insurance plans
3. Learning or delegating responsibilities for ongoing self-care management
4. Obtaining referrals to community-based programs

Nurses as team consultants or coordinators can assist families by providing direct assistance or needed information to successfully navigate new service systems. For additional information on adolescent developmental concerns and transition planning, see Chapters 3 and 5.

Adulthood

Primary care is focused on the maintenance of health and prevention of secondary conditions and complications. Health screenings for individuals with disabilities correspond to those for adults without disabilities, except for condition-related issues. Adult screening guidelines that incorporate both typical and Down syndrome–related screenings are listed in Table 12.2. Adult immunizations are administered according to the guidelines of the American College of Physicians, Ad-

Table 12.2.   Screening guidelines for adults with Down syndrome

Test	Age range	Men	Women	Frequency
Body mass index measurement (height/weight)	20 years to 40 years	X	X	Every 1 to 2 years
	40 years and older	X	X	Annually
Vision screening	18 years and older	X	X	Every 2 years
Hearing screening	18 years and older	X	X	Every 2 years
Thyroid screening (sensitive thyroid-stimulating hormone)	18 years and older	X	X	Annually
Cholesterol	20 years and older with risk factors	X	X	Every 5 years
	35 years and older with no risk factors	X		Every 5 years
	45 years and older with no risk factors		X	Every 5 years
Blood pressure	20 years and older	X	X	Every 2 years
Colorectal cancer	50 years and older	X	X	Every 10 years if no nonmalignant polyps; if family history, then test more often
Serum glucose	No age parameters	X	X	When blood pressure or cholesterol level is elevated
Bone density test	Beginning at 65 years		X	Routinely
	Beginning at 60 years		X	If risk factors for osteoporosis fractures
Chlamydia and other sexually transmitted infections	Sexually active	X	X	
Human immunodeficiency virus (HIV)	Sexually active and meet criteria	X	X	If had unprotected sex with men or multiple partners, pregnant, used intravenous drugs, had sex with HIV-infected partner
Abdominal aortic aneurysm	Between 65 and 75 years	X		If history of smoking
Mental health screening	No age parameters	X	X	If reported feeling sad, withdrawn, changes in behavior and self-care for more than 2 weeks
Testicular examination	15 years and older	X		Routinely with primary care provider visit
Breast manual examination	20 years and older		X	Routinely with primary care provider visit
Mammogram	40 years and older		X	Every 1 to 2 years
Pap test	20 years and younger if sexually active		X	Every 1 to 3 years
	21 years to 61 years		X	Every 1 to 3 years; every 5 years if 3 consecutive negative findings
Monitor for symptoms of dementia, including Alzheimer's disease	18 years and older	X	X	

Sources: Agency for Healthcare Research and Quality (2007a, 2007b), American Academy of Pediatrics (2001), American College of Obstetricians and Gynecologists (2003, 2006), California Department of Developmental Services (2006), Chen (2007), Cohen (1999), Crocker (2006), Marshfield Clinic (n.d.), and Smith (2001).

visory Committee on Immunization Practices (2009). Ongoing monitoring of dental care needs continues on a quarterly basis. Antibiotic prophylaxis will be needed prior to dental procedures for those who have had surgical repair of a cardiac defect or have mitral valve prolapse (NIDCR, 2009).

Gynecologic care for women should include a pelvic examination and Pap test on an annual basis. Beginning at age 40, a mammogram should be conducted every 1 to 2 years. Testicular examinations should be done as part of the health screening visits. Beginning at age 50, men should have yearly prostate screening antigen tests to screen for prostate cancer (USDHHS, Office of Women's Health, 2007).

Of particular concern for individuals with Down syndrome is that the aging process is accelerated compared to typical adults. Evidence of this acceleration is demonstrated in the early signs of dementia and Alzheimer's disease such as memory loss, decline in self-care skills, job skills, and social skills, as well as changes in behavior (Cohen, 1999; Smith, 2001). Changes in behavior and/or the emergence of mental health problems are referred to a professional who has expertise in dual diagnosis. See Chapter 14 for more information on dual diagnosis.

Lifestyle choices pertaining to living arrangements, employment options, job training, community living, and recreational interests will be dependent on the individual's interests, needs, preferences, and level of functioning. The range of lifestyles will vary. One individual may live independently and work productively in a competitive employment setting, such as in a child care center or landscape company, whereas another individual might live in a congregate setting with several others with intellectual disabilities. For more information on adult developmental issues and systems of care, see Chapters 3 and 5.

Nurses function in a variety of roles and settings in working with adults with Down syndrome. Nurses may serve as nurse practitioners in community clinics providing primary care and health surveillance. Nurses are employed to work in large congregate facilities with organization structures similar to acute care settings but focused on rehabilitation and habilitation. In community settings, nurses may be employed as team consultants or coordinators in providing services to adults with Down syndrome in a variety of community settings wherein the individual lives independently, with family members, or in a supported housing arrangement. For additional information on adult developmental concerns, see Chapters 3 and 5.

CONCLUSION

Of the chromosomal disorders, most is known about Down syndrome or trisomy 21. However, much is still unknown about the etiology of this condition or the specific propensity for the numerous secondary conditions that are often comorbid. Further understanding of these factors, as well as the reasons for the premature aging that also characterizes this condition, are needed. In caring for a person with Down syndrome of any age, it is important to understand how each system can be affected and what the appropriate screening and treatment options are. Individuals with Down syndrome may lead full and happy lives. However, their lives are complicated and require health supervision that includes educational, social, residential, and recreational elements. The nurse is best prepared to offer the holistic care that is needed across the life span for these individuals and their family members.

REFERENCES

Agency for Healthcare Research and Quality. (2007a). *Men stay healthy at any age: Your checklist for health.* Retrieved on February 25, 2009, from http://www.ahrq.gov/ppip/healthymen.pdf.

Agency for Healthcare Research and Quality. (2007b). *Women stay healthy at any age: Your checklist for health.* Retrieved on February 25, 2009, from http://www.ahrq.gov/ppip/healthywom.htm.

Ailey, S. (2005). Behavior management and mental health. In W.M. Nehring (Ed.), *Core curriculum for specializing in intellectual and developmental disability: A resource for nurses and other health care professionals* (pp. 291–304). Boston: Jones & Bartlett.

Aitken, D.A., Crossley, J.A., & Spencer, K. (2006). Prenatal screening in neural tube defects and aneuploidy. In D.L. Rimoin, J.M. Connor, R.E. Pyeritz, & B.R. Korf (Eds.), *Emery and Rimoin's principles and practices of medical genetics* (5th ed, pp. 636–678.). New York: Churchill Livingstone.

Ali, F.E., Al-Busairi, W.A., & Al-Mulla, F.A. (1999). Treatment of hyperthyroidism in Down syndrome: Case report and review of literature. *Research in Developmental Disabilities, 20,* 297–300.

Alvarez, N. (2008). *Atlantoaxial instability in individuals with Down syndrome.* Retrieved on February 19, 2009, from http://emedicine.medscape.com/article/1180354-overview.

American Academy of Pediatrics, Committee on Genetics. (2001). Health supervision for children with Down syndrome. *Pediatrics, 107,* 442–449.

American Academy of Pediatrics, American Academy of Family Practice, & American College of Physicians-American Society of Internal Medicine. (2002). A consensus statement on health care transitions for young adults with special health care needs. *Pediatrics, 110,* 1304–1306.

American College of Physicians, Advisory Committee on Immunization Practices (2009). Recommended adult immunization schedule: United States, 2009. *Annuals of Internal Medicine, 140,* 40–44.

American College of Obstetricians and Gynecologists. (2003). *Primary and preventive health care for female adolescents.* Washington, DC: Author.

American College of Obstetricians and Gynecologists. (2006). *HPV vaccine: ACOG recommendations.* Retrieved on February 28, 2009, from http://www.acog.org/departments/dept_notice.cfm?recno=7&bulletin=3945.

Besser, L.M., Shin, M., Kucik, J.E., & Correa, A. (2007). Prevalence of Down syndrome among children and adolescents in metropolitan Atlanta. *Birth Defects Research A: Clinical and Molecular Teratology, 79,* 765–774.

Betz, C.L., & Nehring, W.M. (2007). *Promoting health care transition planning for adolescents with special health care needs and disabilities.* Baltimore: Paul H. Brookes Publishing Co.

Betz, C.L., & Sowden, L.A. (2008). *Mosby's pediatric nursing reference* (6th ed., pp. 256–263). St. Louis: Mosby Elsevier.

Bittles, A.H., Bower, C., Hussain, R., & Glasson, E.J. (2007). The four ages of Down syndrome. *European Journal of Public Health, 17,* 121–125.

California Department of Developmental Services. (2006). *Down syndrome.* Retrieved on February 17, 2009, from http://www.ddhealthinfo.org/.

Canfield, M.A., Honein, M.A., Yuskiv, N., Xing, J., Mai, C.T., Collins, J.S., et al. (2006). National estimates and race/ethnic-specific variation of selected birth defects in the United States, 1999–2001. *Birth Defects Research A: Clinical and Molecular Teratology, 76,* 747–756.

Capone, G., Goyal, P., Ares, W., & Lannigan, E. (2006). Neurobehavioral disorders in children, adolescents, and young adults with Down syndrome. *American Journal of Medical Genetics C (Seminars in Medical Genetics), 142,* 158–172.

Capone, G.T., Grados, M.A., Kaufmann, W.E., Bernad-Ripoll, S., & Jewell, A. (2005). Down syndrome and comorbid autism-spectrum disorder: Characterization using the Aberrant Behavior Checklist. *American Journal of Medical Genetics A, 134,* 373–380.

Capone, G.T., Roizen, N.J., & Rogers, P.T. (2008). Down syndrome. In P. J. Accardo

(Ed.). *Capute and Accardo's neurodevelopmental disabilities in infancy and childhood* (3rd ed., pp. 285–308). Baltimore: Paul H. Brookes Publishing Co.

Centers for Disease Control and Prevention. (2006). Improved national prevalence estimates for 18 selected major birth defects—United States, 1999–2001. *Morbidity and Mortality Weekly Report, 54,* 1301–1305.

Chen, H. (2007). *Down syndrome.* Retrieved on February 20, 2009, from http://emedi cine.medscape.com/article/943216-over view.

Cohen, W.I. (Ed.). (1999). *Health care guidelines for individuals with Down syndrome: 1999 revision.* Retrieved on February 27, 2009, from http://www.ndsccenter.org/resources/healthcare.pdf.

Concolino, D., Pasquzzi, A., Capalbo, G., Sinopoli, S., & Strisciuglio, P. (2006). Early detection of podiatric anomalies in children with Down syndrome. *Acta Paediatrics, 95,* 17–20.

Coppede, F., Colognato, R., Bonelli, A., Astrea, G., Bargagna, S., Siciliano, G. et al. (2007). Early detection of podiatric anomalies in children with Down syndrome. *American Journal of Medical Genetics A, 143A,* 2006–2015.

Crocker, A. (2006). Down syndrome. In I.L. Rubin & A.C. Crocker (Eds.), *Medical care for children & adults with developmental disabilities.* Baltimore: Paul H. Brookes Publishing Co.

Cronk, C., Crocker, A.C., Pueschel, S.M., Shea, A.M., Zackai, E., Pickens, G., et al. (1988). Growth charts for children with Down syndrome: 1 month to 18 years of age. *Pediatrics, 81,* 102–110.

Cushing, T., Chericuzio, C.L., Wilson, C.S., Taub, J.W., Ge, Y., Reichard, K.K., et al. (2006). Risk for leukemia in infants without Down syndrome who have transient myeloproliferative disorder. *Journal of Pediatrics, 148,* 687–689.

Daneshpazhooh, M., Nazemi, T.J.M., Bigdeloo, L., & Yoosefi, M. (2007). Mucocutaneous findings in 100 children with Down syndrome. *Pediatric Dermatology, 24,* 317–320.

Day, S.M., Strauss, D.J., Shavelle, R.M., & Reynolds, R.J. (2005). Mortality and causes of death in persons with Down syndrome in California. *Developmental Medicine & Child Neurology, 47,* 171–176.

Devlin, L., & Morrison, P.J. (2004). Accuracy of the clinical diagnosis of Down syndrome. *Ulster Medical Journal, 73,* 4–12.

Dinani, S., & Carpenter, S. (1990). Down's syndrome and thyroid disorder. *Journal of Mental Deficiency Research, 34,* 187–193.

Dixon, N., Kishnani, P.S., & Zimmerman, S. (2006). Clinical manifestations of hematologic and oncologic disorders in patients with Down syndrome. *American Journal of Medical Genetics C (Seminars in Medical Genetics), 142C,* 149–157.

Down Syndrome Center. (2007). Study of Down syndrome and congenital heart defects. Retrieved on February 22, 2009, from http://genetics.emory.edu/DSC/research/chd.cfm.

Durmowicz, A.G. (2001). Pulmonary edema in 6 children with Down syndrome during travel to moderate altitudes. *Pediatrics, 108,* 443–447.

Feingold, M., & Geggel, R.L. (2001). Letter to the editor. Health supervision for children with Down syndrome. *Pediatrics, 108,* 1384–1385.

Freeman, S.B., Taft, L.F., Dooley, K.J., Allran, K., Sherman, S.L., Hassold, M.J., et al. (1998). Population-based study of congenital heart defects in Down syndrome. *American Journal of Medical Genetics, 80,* 213–217.

Geggel, R.L., O'Brien, J.E., & Feingold, M. (1993). Development of valve dysfunction in adolescents and young adults with Down syndrome and no known congenital heart disease. *Journal of Pediatrics, 122,* 821–823.

Glasson, E.J., Sullivan, S.G., Hussain, R., Petterson, B.A., Montgomery, P.D., & Bittles, A.H. (2002). The changing survival profile of people with Down's syndrome: Implications for genetic counseling. *Clinical Genetics, 62,* 390–393.

Hattori, M., Fujiyama, A., Taylor, T.D., Newton, R., Robinson, Z.F., Bingley, P.J., et al. (2000). The DNA sequence of human chromosome 21: The chromosome 21 mapping and sequencing consortium. *Nature, 405,* 311–319.

Hecht, C.A., & Hook, E.B. (1996). Rates of Down syndrome at live birth at one-year maternal age intervals in studies with apparent close to complete ascertainment in populations of European origin: A proposed revised rate schedule for use in genetic and prenatal screening. *American Journal of Medical Genetics, 62,* 376–385.

Individuals with Disabilities Education Improvement Act (IDEA) of 2004, PL 108-446, 20 U.S.C. §§ 1400 *et seq.*

Jones, K.L. (2006). Down syndrome. In K. Jones (Ed.), *Smith's recognizable patterns of human malformation* (6th ed., p. 7–10). Philadelphia: Elsevier Saunders.

Khoshnood, B., Pryde, P., & Wall, S. (2000). Ethnic differences in the impact of advanced maternal age on birth prevalence of Down syndrome. *American Journal of Public Health, 90,* 1778–1781.

Lashley, F.R. (2005). *Clinical genetics in nursing practice* (3rd ed.). New York: Springer.

Lejeune, J., Gautier, M., & Turpin, R. (1959). Study of somatic chromosomes from 9 mongoloid children. *Comptes rendus hebdomadaires des séances de l'Acadmie des sciences, 248,* 1721–1722.

Leshin, L. (2000). *Obstructive sleep apnea and Down syndrome.* Retrieved on February 27, 2009, from http://www.talkabout sleep.com/sleep-disorders/archives/child rensdisorders_osadowns.htm.

Loureiro, A.C.A., Costa, F.O., & da Costa, J.E. (2007). The impact of periodontal disease on the quality of life of individuals with Down syndrome. *Down Syndrome Research and Practice, 12,* 50–54.

Malini, S.S., & Ramachandra, N.B. (2006). Influence of advanced age of maternal grandmothers on Down syndrome. *BMC Medical Genetics, 7,* 4.

March of Dimes. (2008). *Maternal screening for birth defects.* Retrieved on February 28, 2009, from http://www.marchofdimes .com/professionals/14332_1166.asp.

Marshfield Clinic. (n.d.). *Adult health screening guidelines.* Retrieved on February 25, 2009, from http://www.marshfieldclinic .org/patients/?page=wellness_adultScree ning.

Massey, G.V., Zipursky, A., Chang, M.N., Doyle, J.J., Nasim, S., Taub, J.W., et al. (2006). A prospective study of the natural history of transient leukemia (TL) in neonates with Down syndrome (DS): Children's Oncology Group (COG) study POG-9481. *Blood, 107,* 4606–4613.

Meguid, N.A., El-Kotoury, A.I.S., Abdel-Salam, G.M.H., El-Ruby, M.G., & Afifi, H.H. (2004). Growth charts of Egyptian children with Down syndrome (0–36 months). *Eastern Mediterranean Health Journal, 10,* 106–115.

Merrick, J. (2000). Incidence and mortality of Down syndrome. *Israel Medical Association Journal, 2,* 25–26.

Merrick, J., & Koslowe, K. (2001). Refractive errors and visual anomalies in Down syndrome. *Down Syndrome Research and Practice, 6,* 131–133.

Myrelid, A., Gustafsson, J., Ollars, B., & Anneren, G. (2002). Growth charts for Down's syndrome from birth to 18 years of age. *Archives of Diseases in Childhood, 87,* 97–103.

National Association for Down Syndrome. (n.d.). *Facts about Down syndrome.* Retrieved February 19, 2009, from http:// www.nads.org/pages_new/facts.html.

National Congress of Down Syndrome. (n.d.). *Frequently asked questions.* Retrieved on February 24, 2009, from http://www .ndsccenter.org/resources/faq.php.

National Dissemination Center for Children with Disabilities. (2004). *Disability fact sheet, No. 4, Down syndrome.* Washington, DC: Author.

National Institute of Dental and Craniofacial Research. (2009). *Practical oral care for people with Down syndrome.* Retrieved on February 25, 2009, from http://www .nidcr.nih.gov/OralHealth/Topics/Develop mentalDisabilities/PracticalOralCarePeople DownSyndrome.htm.

Nehring, W.M. (2004). Down syndrome. In P. Jackson Allen & J.A.Vessey (Eds.), *Primary care of the child with a chronic condition* (4th ed., pp. 446–468). St. Louis: Mosby Elsevier.

Nehring, W.M. (2008). Down syndrome. In C.L. Betz & L.A. Sowden (Eds.), *Mosby's pediatric nursing reference* (6th ed., pp. 149–161). St. Louis: Mosby Elsevier.

Nehring, W.M. (2010). Down syndrome. In P.L. Jackson Allen, J.A. Vessey, & N.A. Shapiro (Eds.), *Primary care of the child with a chronic condition* (5th ed., pp. 447–469). St. Louis: Mosby Elsevier.

Nehring, W.M., Roth, S.P., Natvig, D., Betz, C.L., Savage, T., & Krajicek, M. (2004). *Intellectual and developmental nursing: Scope and standards of practice*. Silver Spring, MD: American Nurses Association and Nursing Division of the American Association on Mental Retardation.

Newberger, D.S. (2000). Down syndrome: Prenatal risk assessment and diagnosis. *American Family Physician, 62,* 837–838.

Nicham, R., Weitzdorfer, R., Hauser, E., Friedl, M., Schubert, M., Wurst, E., et al. (2003). Spectrum of cognitive, behavioral and emotional problems in children with young adults with Down syndrome. *Journal of Neural Transmission, 67,* 173–191.

Olson, L.E., Richtsmeier, J.T., Leszl, J., & Reeves, R.H. (2004). A chromosome 21 critical region does not cause specific Down syndrome phenotypes. *Science, 306,* 687–690.

Pierpont, M.E., Basson, C.T., Benson, D.W., Gelb, B.D., Giglia, T.M., Goldmuntz, E., et al. (2007). Genetic basis for congenital heart defects: Current knowledge: A scientific statement from the American Heart Association Congenital Cardiac Defects Committee, Council on Cardiovascular Disease in the Young. *Circulation, 115,* 3015–3038.

Rasmussen, S.A., Wong, L.Y., Correa, A., Gambrell, D., & Friedman, J.M. (2006). Survival in infants with Down syndrome, metropolitan Atlanta, 1979–1998. *Journal of Pediatrics, 148,* 806–812.

Rex, A.P., & Preus, M. (1982). A diagnostic index for Down syndrome. *Journal of Pediatrics, 100,* 903–906.

Roizen, N.J. (2007). Down syndrome. In M.L. Batshaw, L. Pellegrino, & N.J. Roizen (Eds.), *Children with disabilities* (6th ed., pp. 263-273). Baltimore: Paul H. Brookes Publishing Co.

Roizen, N.J., & Patterson, D. (2003). Down's syndrome. *Lancet, 361,* 1281–1289.

Sherman, S.L., Allen, E.G., Bean, L.H., & Freeman, S.B. (2007). Epidemiology of Down syndrome. *Mental Retardation and Developmental Disabilities Research Reviews, 13,* 221–227.

Shott, S.R. (2006). Down syndrome: Common otolaryngologic manifestations. *American Journal of Medical Genetics, Part C (Seminars in Medical Genetics), 142C,* 131–140.

Shott, S.R., Amin, R., Chini, B., Heubi, C., Hotze, S., & Akers R. (2006). Obstructive sleep apnea: Should all children with Down syndrome be tested? *Archives of Otolaryngology Head & Neck Surgery, 132,* 432–436.

Siklos, S., & Kerns, K.A. (2006). Assessing need for social support in parents of children with autism and Down syndrome. *Journal of Autism and Developmental Disorders, 36,* 921–933.

Smith, D.S. (2001). Health care management of adults with Down syndrome. *American Family Physician, 64,* 1031–1038.

Snashall, S. (2002). *Hearing impairment & Down's syndrome.* Retrieved on February 20, 2009, from http://www.intellectual disability.info/complex_disability/hearing _ds.htm.

Staples, A.J., Sutherland, G.R., Haan, E.A., & Clisby, S. (1991). Epidemiology of Down syndrome in South Australia, 1960–1989. *American Journal of Human Genetics, 49,* 1014–1024.

Stephen, E., Dickson, J., Kindley, A.D., Scott, C.C., & Charleton, P.M. (2007). Surveillance of vision and ocular disorders in children with Down syndrome. *Developmental Medicine and Child Neurology, 49,* 513–515.

Stoppler, M. (2006). *Hypothyroidism symptoms.* Retrieved on February 27, 2009, from http://www.medicinenet.com/script/main/art.asp?articlekey=47277.

Sullivan, S.G., Hussain, R., Glasson, E.J., & Bittles, A.H. (2007). The profile and incidence of cancer in Down syndrome. *Journal of Intellectual Disabilities Research, 51,* 228–231.

Tolmie, J.L., & MacFadyen (2006). Clinical genetics of common autosomal trisomies. In D.L. Rimoin, J.M. Connor, R.E. Pyeritz, & B.R. Korf (Eds.), *Emery and Rimoin's principles and practices of medical genetics* (5th ed., pp. 1015–1037). New York: Churchill Livingstone.

Tomizawa, D., Tabuchi, K., Kinoshita, A., Hanada, R., Kigasawa, H., Tsukimoto, I., et al. (2007). Repetitive cycles of high-dose cytarabine are effective for childhood acute myeloid leukemia: Long-term outcome of the children with AML treated on two consecutive trials of Tokyo Children's Cancer Study Group. *Pediatric Blood and Cancer, 49,* 127–132.

Tufts University School of Dentistry. (2008). *Down syndrome: Dental manifestations, oral and dental considerations, management.* Retrieved on February 25, 2009, from http://ocw.tufts.edu/Content/56/learning units/669519.

Uibo, O., Teesalu, K., Metsküula, K., Reimand, T., Saat, R., Sillat, T., et al. (2006). Screening for celiac disease in Down's syndrome patients for revealed cases of subtotal villous atrophy without typical for celiac disease HLA-DQ and tissue transglutaminase antibodies. *World Journal of Gastronenterology, 12,* 1430–1434.

U.S. Department of Education. (n.d). *Building the legacy: IDEA 2004.* Retrieved on February 16, 2009, from http://idea.ed.gov/.

U.S. Department of Health and Human Services, Office of Women's Health. (2007). *Preventive screening tests and immunizations.* Retrieved on February 28, 2009, from http://www.womenshealth.gov/screening charts/general/part2.cfm.

U.S. Department of Health and Human Services, Centers for Disease Control and Prevention. (2009a). *The recommended immunization schedules for persons aged 0 through 6 years.* Retrieved on February 25, 2009, from http://www.cispimmunize.org/IZSchedule_Childhood.pdf.

U.S. Department of Health and Human Services, Centers for Disease Control and Prevention. (2009b). *The recommended immunization schedules for persons aged 7 through 18 years.* Retrieved on February 25, 2009, from http://www.cispimmunize.org/IZSchedule_Adolescent.pdf.

Van Cleve, S.N., Cannon, S., & Cohen, W.I. (2006). Part II: Clinical practice guidelines for adolescents and young adults with Down syndrome: 12 to 21 years. *Journal of Pediatric Health Care, 20,* 198–205.

Van Cleve, S.N., & Cohen, W.I. (2006). Part I: Clinical practice guidelines for children with Down syndrome from birth to 12 years. *Journal of Pediatric Health Care, 20,* 47–54.

Visootsak, J., & Sherman, S. (2007). Neuropsychiatric and behavioral aspects of trisomy 21. *Current Psychiatric Reports, 9,* 135–140.

Vyas, P., & Roberts, I. (2006). Down myeloid disorders: A paradigm for childhood preleukaemia and leukaemia and insights into normal megakaryopoiesis. *Early Human Development, 82,* 767–773.

Wheeler, M.D. (1991). Physical changes of puberty. *Endocrinology and Metabolism Clinics of North America, 20,* 1–14.

Whitlock, J.A. (2006). Down syndrome and acute lymphoblastic leukaemia. *British Journal of Haematology, 135,* 595–602.

Whitlock, J.A., Sather, H.N., Gaynon, P., Robison, L.L., Wells, R.J., Trigg, M. et al. (2005). Clinical characteristics and outcome of children with Down syndrome and acute lymphoblastic leukemia: A Children's Cancer Group study. *Blood, 106,* 4043–4049.

Winter, K., Baccaglini, L., & Tomar, S. (2008). A review of malocclusion among individuals with mental and physical disabilities. *Special Care Dentistry, 28,* 19–26.

Wouters, J., Weijerman, M.E., vanFurth, A.M., Schreurs, M.W.J., Crusius, J.B.A., von Blomber, B.M.E., et al. (2009). Prospective human leukocyte antigen, endomysium immunoglobulin A antibodies, and transglutaminase antibodies testing for celiac disease in children with Down syndrome. *The Journal of Pediatrics, 154,* 239–242.

Yang, Q., Rasmussen, S.A., & Friedman, J.M. (2002). Mortality associated with Down's syndrome in the USA from 1983 to 1997: A population-based study. *Lancet, 359,* 1019–1025.

Zigman, W.B., & Lott, I.T. (2007). Alzheimer's disease in Down syndrome: Neurobiology and risk. *Mental Retardation and Developmental Disabilities Research Reviews, 13,* 237–246.

CHAPTER 13

Cerebral Palsy

Martha Wilson Jones and Elaine Morgan

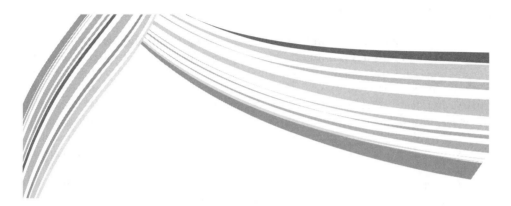

C erebral palsy (CP) is a neurodevelopmental condition identified in infancy or early childhood that continues to present challenges throughout the life of the affected individual. Individuals with CP may be encountered by nurses working in nearly every health care setting including inpatient, outpatient, primary or specialty care clinics, schools, residential care, and nursing homes.

This chapter provides information on the pathophysiology of CP, causes of CP, risk and causal factors, commonly associated secondary conditions, rates of incidence in the United States and worldwide, signs and symptoms, classifications, and the diagnostic testing process. This chapter also provides information on potential challenges and appropriate interventions presented in a review of systems format, which can be incorporated into the nursing process of care.

PATHOPHYSIOLOGY

CP, first described in 1843 by William Little, an English orthopedic surgeon, is a descriptive term describing a group of disorders caused by an insult to the developing fetal or infant brain (Little, 1843). The cerebral insult causes some degree of motor impairment due to abnormalities in movement and posture. Central nervous system (CNS) damage is nonprogressive; however, the resulting impairments have a neurodevelopmental presentation in which the full effects may not become apparent until months to years after diagnosis (Ashwal et al., 2004).

Epidemiology and advances in brain imagery have resulted in increased understanding of the neurobiology of brain injury. Inconsistency in definition and conceptualization of CP has complicated the determination of the incidence and prevalence of CP over time, as well as the validity and generalization of research studies. After an international workshop, the following definition incorporating associated disabilities and chronic health problems was proposed (Bax et al., 2005) and then published in 2007:

> Cerebral palsy describes a group of permanent disorders of the development of movement and posture, causing activity limitations that are attributed to nonprogressive

235

disturbances that occurred in the developing fetal or infant brain. The motor disorders of cerebral palsy are often accompanied by disturbances of sensation, perception, cognition, communication, and behavior: by epilepsy, and by secondary musculoskeletal problems. (Rosenbaum, Paneth, Levitron, Goldstein, & Bax, 2007, p. 9)

CAUSES OF CEREBRAL PALSY

Some of the causal etiologies in CP include interruption or failure in neuronal migration during brain development, failure of oligodendrocytes to deposit myelin on cell fibers causing inadequate transmission of nerve impulse, impaired function at brain cell synapse resulting in lack of or impaired transmission of nerve impulses, and death of gray matter cells. The specific area of the brain affected and the magnitude of CNS damage are directly related to the degree of impairment observed clinically, which then impacts attainment of function, management requirements, and life expectancy (Hemming, Hutton, & Pharoah, 2006; Hutton, Colver, & Mackie, 2000).

Research to determine causal and protective factors has been mixed. Barriers to long-term studies have been related to the technology in the neonatal world evolving so rapidly that it is difficult to conduct randomized controlled trials due the multitude of variables and the ethics of withholding a therapy in the interest of identifying long-term effects.

Fetal heart rate monitoring and surfactant replacement have positively impacted survival but have not reduced the risk for CP. Maternal antenatal treatment with magnesium sulfate was proposed to be protective against CP in cases of impending birth, but research thus far has been mixed without clear efficacy established (Doyle, Crowther, Middleton, & Merret, 2007). Infection of membranes has been associated with CP in both preterm and term infants, with treatment of bacterial vaginosis being the only preventative measure identified (Blair & Watson, 2006). There is strong evidence supporting the use of glucocorticoids given to mothers in preterm labor to decrease mortality and subsequent CP (O'Shea & Doyle, 2001).

Postnatal corticosteroids, administered prior to 96 hours of age to high-risk infants, decrease the incidence of chronic lung disease and early death; however, they increase the risk for CP (Doyle, Halliday, Ehrenkranz, Davis, & Sinclair, 2005). Hypothermia therapy following perinatal asphyxia has been associated with reduction in death and disability outcomes (Shankaran et al., 2005). Currently, there are no interventions that are able to repair existing brain damage.

RISK AND CAUSAL FACTORS IN CEREBRAL PALSY

CNS risk factors are associated with CP and may occur in the prenatal, perinatal, or postnatal time periods (see Table 13.1). Despite the many known risk factors, there are none identified in approximately 30% of cases (Rosenbaum, 2003). The most significant risk factors for CP are hypoxic-ischemic encephalopathy, intrauterine infections, multiple gestation, and low birth weight (Meberg & Broch, 2004; Odding, Roebroeck, & Stam, 2006).

Factors most likely to lead to CP in infants born prematurely include small for gestational age, prolonged rupture of membranes, patent ductus arteriosus, extended need for mechanical ventilation, periventricular leukomalacia, intraven-

Table 13.1.   Etiologies and risk factors associated with cerebral palsy

- Maternal abdominal trauma, iodine deficiency, or seizure disorder
- Antepartum co-fetal death, twin-to-twin transfusion, multiple gestation
- Perinatal exposure to toxins (e.g., methyl mercury ingestion) or teratogenic exposure
- Genetic disorders
- Malformation of brain structures
- Intrauterine infections (e.g., Rubella, cytomegalovirus, toxoplasmosis), chorioamnionitis
- Intrauterine growth restriction
- Preeclampsia, placental abruption, abnormal fetal presentation, cord prolapse, instrument delivery, prolonged rupture of membranes
- Premature birth
- Asphyxia, hypoxia, hypoxic ischemic encephalopathy
- Blood incompatibility, rhesus isoimmunization, hyperbilirubinemia, kernicterus
- Intraventricular hemorrhage, periventricular leukomalacia, cerebral infarction, hydrocephalus
- Head injury, shaken baby syndrome
- Meningitis, encephalitis, sepsis
- Metabolic or thrombophilic disorders
- Respiratory distress syndrome, chronic lung disease, postnatal steroids
- Result of early surgery to correct congenital heart defects (small percentage), patent ductus arteriosus
- Seizures within 48 hours of birth

Sources: Blair and Watson (2006); Cans et al. (2004); Drougia et al. (2007); Gibson, MacLennan, Goldwater, and Dekker (2003); Greenwood, Yudkin, Sellers, Impey, and Doyle (2005); Meberg and Broch (2004); Odding et al. (2006); Winter et al. (2002).

tricular hemorrhage, sepsis, and meningitis (Drougia et al., 2007). Periventricular white matter damage, intraventricular hemorrhage, and periventricular leukomalacia are highly predictive; up to 80% of infants with these conditions develop CP (Meberg & Broch, 2004).

SECONDARY CONDITIONS COMMONLY ASSOCIATED WITH CEREBRAL PALSY

In addition to causing some degree of motor impairment, CNS damage has a causal relationship in commonly occurring secondary conditions. These include disturbances of sensation (vision, hearing, and other sensory modalities), cognition, perception (incorporating and interpreting sensory and/or cognitive information), communication (expressive and/or receptive communication and/or social interaction skills), feeding and growth abnormalities, secondary musculoskeletal problems, behaviors and emotional disorders (e.g., features of autism, attention-deficit/hyperactivity disorder, mood disorders, anxiety disorders), and/or seizure disorders (Morris, 2007; Rosenbaum et al., 2007).

Severe visual disability is seen in approximately 11%–21% of individuals with CP, with up to 80% with some degree of visual impairment such as strabismus, nystagmus, and refractory errors (Cans, 2000; Ghasia, Brunstrom, Gordon, & Tychsen, 2008; Venkateswaran & Shevell, 2008). Sensorineural hearing loss occurs in approximately 30%–40% with intrauterine viral infections associated with high-frequency hearing loss (Cans, 2000; Morales, Azuara, Gallo, Gonzalez, & Rama, 2006). Sleep disorders occur in 23% of children with CP (compared to 5% in the general population) and may persist throughout the life span (Newman, O'Regan, & Hensey, 2006).

Impaired cognition, ranging from mild to some degree of intellectual and developmental disability, is seen in 30%–70% of individuals with CP, with higher levels of cognitive impairments associated with higher degrees of physical disability. Severe cognitive impairment is one of the most limiting comorbidities affecting long-term achievement and quality of life. Individuals with normal intelligence may have some degree of coexisting visual perceptual abnormalities and learning disabilities. The degree of overflow brain damage resulting from the initial insult may not be realized until the preschool or school-age period, when learning requires the use of higher brain functions (Cans, 2000; O'Shea, 2008).

Survival, quality of life, and life expectancy are associated with the severity and number of functional disabilities. Severe language and cognitive disability, tube feedings, severity of physical disability, and the presence and severity of seizures are most associated with increased rates of mortality (Blair, 2001; Hutton & Pharoah, 2002; Katz, 2003). The incidence of epilepsy in CP is as high as 38% and can be more refractive to treatment (Gururaj, Sztriha, Bener, Dawodu & Eapen, 2003).

RATES OF INCIDENCE IN THE UNITED STATES AND WORLDWIDE

The worldwide incidence of CP is approximately 2–2.5 per 1,000 live births, with approximately 90% of children with CP surviving to the age of 20 years (Rapp & Torres, 2000). The National United Cerebral Palsy Association reported that approximately 40% of individuals with CP are less than 20 years of age; however, a substantial number of individuals now live into their 50s and 60s—some even into their 70s and 80s. The precise number of adults with CP in the United States is not known, but has been estimated at around 400,000 (United Cerebral Palsy, 2001).

The prevalence of CP, worldwide and in the United States, has been fairly stable over the past 20 years, ranging from 1.5–2.5 cases per 1,000. However, the proportion of former premature infants now account for 40%–50% of all children with CP (Ashwal et al., 2004; Blair & Watson, 2006). Prevalence decreases significantly with increasing gestational age. The risk increases with increasing plurality due to tendency for shorter gestation, but this is also seen in term births of multiples due to antepartum co-fetal death, twin-to-twin transfusion, or intrapartum problems. Triplet births are associated with an 18-fold increased risk for CP (Blair & Watson, 2006).

SIGNS AND SYMPTOMS

CP is a clinical diagnosis determined from abnormal findings on the physical and neurological examination. It is made by either a physician or nurse practitioner working in a primary or speciality care setting. The first presenting symptom is typically a delay in gross motor milestones. Potential abnormal neurological signs include abnormal muscle tone, involuntary movements, brisk deep tendon reflexes, clonus, persistence of primitive reflexes and postural reactions, and side-to-side asymmetries in tone or functional abilities. Abnormal tone leads to abnormal posture and movement patterns (Roberts, Palfrey, & Bridgemohan, 2004). Loss of milestones is not typically seen in children with CP and may indicate a degenerative process. Ankle clonus is a reflex in which there is a spasmodic alteration of muscular relaxation and contraction elicited by quick dorsiflexion of the ankle followed by holding the ankle in flexion for approximately 3 seconds. Approximately 30% of infants with persisting ankle clonus will be diagnosed with CP (Futagi, Otani, & Goto, 1997). See Table 13.2 for warning signs associated with CP.

Table 13.2.   Warning signs of cerebral palsy

- Irritability, lethargy, problems with sleep
- Abnormal muscle tone
- Early rolling at 1–2 months of age using arching
- Opisthotonic posturing and extensor thrusting (extended/arched position)
- Weak suck, difficulty with swallowing, oral hypersensitivity, delayed feeding milestones
- Tonic bite, tongue thrust
- Poor weight gain/failure to thrive
- Adducted (cortical) thumbs, fisting of hands persisting past 5 months of age
- Declaring handedness prior to 18 months
- Not rolling by 6 months
- Head lag beyond 6 months of age
- Decreased rate of head growth in first 6 months of age
- Unable to sit with support by 8 months or sitting consistently in a *W* position
- Not walking by 15–18 months
- Poor trunk control and balance
- Discrepancies between intellectual and motor development
- Abnormal motor or gait patterns (e.g., toe walking, scissoring)
- Clonus persisting past 12 months and persistence of primitive reflexes
- Differences in functional ability of left and right extremities

Sources: Aneja (2004); Bennett (1999); Morgan and Aldag (1996); Roberts et al. (2004); Rosenbaum (2003); Venketaswaran and Shevell (2008); and Zafeiriou (2004).

Neuroimaging and laboratory analysis is not required for diagnosis; however, they may be used to explore for etiology and to rule out other possible disorders. Abnormal neuroradiological findings are found in up to 83% of individuals with CP, with white matter damage being the most common. Combined gray and white matter abnormalities are more commonly seen with hemiplegia, isolated white matter abnormalities with bilateral spasticity or athetosis, and isolated gray matter damage with ataxia. No abnormality is detectable by conventional magnetic resonance imaging or computed tomography in approximately 17% of children with CP (Korzeniewski, Birbeck, DeLano, Potchen, & Paneth, 2008). With hemiplegia, testing for coagulation disorders should be considered due to the high incidence of cerebral infarction. An electroencephalogram is not indicated unless there are features suggestive of epilepsy or specific epileptic syndrome. Metabolic and genetic studies are not routinely obtained, but may be considered if a brain malformation is identified or in the presence of dysmorphic features (Ashwal et al., 2004).

In infants and children, a complete developmental evaluation should include assessment of cognitive, speech, fine motor, gross motor, and adaptive skill levels. Screening for ophthalmologic and hearing impairments, oral-motor dysfunction, and sensory issues should additionally be included in the initial assessment. Therapies are most effective when started early (especially during the first 5 years of life) as developmental processes build on each other and form the foundation for future development.

CLASSIFICATION

Classification of CP has been inconsistent since it was first described (Little, 1843). This has presented difficulty in comparison of research studies and standardizing treatment options. In addition to working on a global definition of CP, an international workgroup proposed a new classification system (Bax et al., 2005; Rosenbaum et al., 2007). Because work is ongoing and research published to this point does not reflect the proposed system, both the proposed classification system and some of the older methods are described in this section.

The proposed classification system includes assessment of physical findings and motor impairments, but additionally includes the impact of CP on the individual, overall functioning, and associated conditions. There are four components (Rosenbaum et al., 2007):

1. Motor abnormalities

2. Accompanying impairments

3. Anatomical and neuroimaging findings

4. Causation and timing (if this is clearly identified)

Classification has previously been based on anatomical distribution of dysfunction, function, and type of neurological involvement. One method used is to describe the nature of the movement disorder (spastic, ataxic, dystonic, or athetotic) along with the topographic distribution or limb involvement affected by the motor abnormalities (monoplegia, diplegia, triplegia, hemiplegia or quadriplegia). A second method divides CP into two major physiological classifications—pyramidal (spastic) and extra pyramidal (nonspastic)—indicating the area of the brain that has been affected, as well as the resulting predominant motor disorder (Ashwal et al., 2004; Rosenbaum, 2003).

Spastic CP (pyramidal) accounts for approximately 70%–80% of all individuals with CP and is caused by damage to upper motor neurons in the motor tract fibers or corticospinal pathways. In the normal brain, inhibitory neural signals are delivered to the spinal cord, modulating reflex signals, and the muscle tone remains normal. CNS damage may lead to failure to generate signals or inadequate inhibitory signals sent, resulting in spasticity. Diplegia is caused by bilateral injury affecting primarily the lower extremities; hemiplegia is caused by unilateral damage and affects an upper and lower extremity on one side of the body. Quadriplegia is caused by a more severe CNS insult with a correspondingly higher level of disability affecting all extremities with truncal instability. Triplegia (three extremities) and monoplegia (one extremity) occur rarely and reflect focalized areas of injury along the motor tracts (Roberts et al., 2004; Venkateswaran & Shevell, 2008).

Dyskinetic CP (extrapyramidal) accounts for 10%–15% of all cases of CP and is caused by damage to nerve cells outside of the pyramidal tracts in the cerebellum or basal ganglia. The resulting disability is global and reflected by abnormal tone regulation, postural control, and coordination. Muscle tone may vary hour to hour and the characteristic movements observed are involuntary.

Dyskinetic CP is further divided into two subgroups: choreoathetotic CP and dystonic CP. Choreoathetotic CP is caused from damage to the deep motor neurons in the basal ganglia or thalamus. It is dominated by hyperkinesia and hypotonia, with tone predominately decreased but fluctuating. Rapid, random, involuntary, or jerky movements (choria) or slow, writhing, constantly changing, or contorted movements (athetosis) may be seen; when occurring together, they are referred to as *choreoathetosis*. Dystonic CP is dominated by abnormal rigid postures and hypertonia with tone fluctuation. Involuntary movements, distorted voluntary movements, and abnormal postures are due to sustained muscle contractions and fluctuate depending on body position, level of consciousness, tasks being attempted, and emotional state (Ashwal et al., 2004; Himmelmann, Hagberg, Wiklund, Eek, & Uvebrant, 2007).

Ataxic CP, accounting for approximately 5% of all cases CP, is caused by injury to the neurons in the cerebellum and affects overall coordination. Resulting clinical symptoms include problems with voluntary movement, balance, and depth perception, as well as tremors and poor head control. A wide-based gait (adaptation to abnormal balance) is observed, with rapid repetitive movements performed poorly with past pointing (over- or undershooting) of goal-directed movement (Sanger, 2003).

Hypotonic CP (central hypotonia) is included as a type of CP due to the resulting motor delays. Myopathy and neuropathy must be ruled out as potential causes prior to classifying as CP. Mixed CP is the terminology used when there is overlap in clinical symptoms reflecting more than one type of CP; the most dominant type should be used for classification (Ashwal et al., 2004; Sanger, 2003). See Figure 13.1 for an illustration of how different regions of the brain are affected in various forms of CP and Table 13.3 for impairments associated with the types of CP (Pellegrino, 2007).

Ambulation potential is dependent on the type and severity of CP; however, in all types, independent sitting by 2 years is a highly reliable predictive sign for eventual walking. Other predictors associated with independent ambulation include achievement of head balance before 9 months, the ability to put weight on the hands while prone and rolling from supine to prone by 18 months, and motor control of crawling by 30 months (Farmer, 2003; Fedrizzi et al., 2000). Other factors include active epilepsy and severe visual or hearing impairments; the presence of a severe intellectual impairment (IQ <50) is the most predictive variable in decreased potential for independent ambulation in all types of CP (Beckung, Hagberg, Uldall, & Cans, 2008; da Paz, Burnett, & Braga, 1994).

DIAGNOSTIC TESTING

Gross and fine motor functioning or impairments are important aspects in assessment in individuals with CP. The two streams of development can be at different levels and independent assessment of each is optimal (Carnahan, Arner, & Hagglund, 2007; Rosenbaum et al., 2002). The 2005 classification system supports the use of objective functional scales when assessing functional motor abilities (Rosenbaum et al., 2007). See Table 13.4 for some of the available standardized testing tools.

INTERDISCIPLINARY TREATMENT APPROACH

The team of professionals involved in the care of an individual with CP may vary greatly depending on the age of the individual, severity of impairments, and availability of specialists within a geographic area. General therapeutic interventions include physical therapy, occupational therapy, speech/language therapy, special education, surgical intervention, and medications. Ensuring that the individual client is receiving appropriate services as well as coordination of the interdisciplinary team may fall under the role of the nurse.

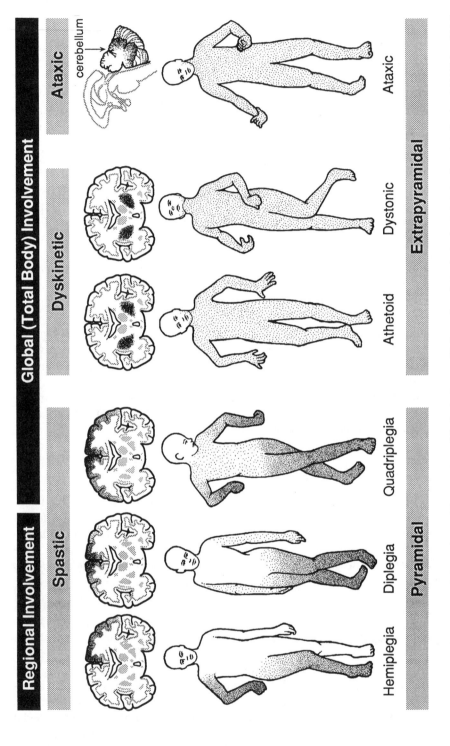

Figure 13.1. The effects of cerebral palsy on different regions of the brain. (From Pelligrino, L. [2007]. Cerebral palsy. In M.L. Batshaw, L. Pellegrino, & N.J. Roizen [Eds.], *Children with disabilities* [6th ed., p. 393]. Baltimore: Paul H. Brookes Publishing Co.; reprinted by permission.)

Table 13.3.   Types of cerebral palsy (CP) and associated secondary impairments

CP type	Details	Cognitive impairment	Functional motor ability	Vision/hearing/ epilepsy
Diplegia	30%–40% of spastic CP Preterm birth accounts for >50%	>70% with normal intelligence Learning disabilities, communication, and attention disorders common	Up to 80%–90% will walk with or without assistive devices	Risk for strabismus
Hemiplegia	20%–30% of spastic CP Associated with strokes, vascular malformation, and unilateral intraventricular hemorrhage or periventricular leukomalacia Middle cerebral artery vascular territory is the most commonly affected, with left side twice as common as right side	60% with normal intelligence Communication disorders common and unilateral sensory disorders possible	60% will walk with or without assistance by 36 months of age	Risk for strabismus and/or loss of portion of a visual field (hemianopsia) High rate of partial seizures
Quadriplegia	10%–15% of spastic CP Associated with severe asphyxia in preterm/ term infants, and severe bilateral intraventricular hemorrhage and periventricular leukomalacia in preterm infants	50% risk of intellectual disabilities Sensory impairments common, with up to 33% requiring assisted feedings	Up to 50% will eventually achieve some degree of assisted ambulation, 25% will need minimal assistance, and 25% will be severely impaired and nonambulatory	Up to 50% with severe hearing deficit or deafness, up to 80% with severe visual impairments, up to 50% with epilepsy
Dyskinetic		30%–78 % will have normal intelligence Speech problems (dysarthria and articulation) common	Up to 50% will achieve some degree of ambulation	Dyskinetic eye movements Associated with high incidence of sensorineural hearing loss, especially with kernicterus
Ataxic		Problems with voluntary movement, balance, depth perception, overall coordination Oral motor difficulties common (e.g., swallowing, drooling)	Wide-based, unsteady gait common	Nystagmus or involuntary oscillating eye movements may be present

Sources: da Paz, Burnett, and Braga (1994); Himmelmann et al. (2007); Himpens, Van den Broeck, Oostra, Calders, and Vanhaesebrouck (2008); Jan, Lyons, Heaven, and Matsuba (2001); Pueyo, Junque, and Vendrell (2003); Sanger (2003); Venkateswaran and Shevell (2008).

Table 13.4.   Assessment tools for assessing levels of functional ability of individuals with cerebral palsy (CP)

Tool	Description
Gross Motor Function Classification System (GMFCS)	• Assessment of gross motor function of children with CP based on severity of disability/functional limitations • Five levels of function and trajectories can can be used to predict gross motor development by plotting on a special chart (similar to curves on somatic growth charts) • Introduction and user instructions can be downloaded at http://canchild-mgm.icreate3.esolutionsgroup.ca/en/GMFCS/resources/GMFCS-ER.pdf • Palisano et al. (1997) and Rosenbaum et al. (2002)
Peabody Developmental Motor Scale 2	• Early child motor development program incorporating assessment and interventions for gross and fine motor skills from birth through 5 years of age • Darrah, Magill-Evans, Volden, Hodge, & Kembhavi (2007)
Manual Ability Classification System	• Corresponding classification of manual ability used with GMFCS in children 4–18 years of age • Eliasson et al. (2006)
Pediatric Evaluation of Disability Inventory	• Comprehensive clinical assessment and monitoring of key functional capabilities/skills including self care, mobility and social function • Used in children with disabilities ages 6 months to 7.5 years • Ketelaar and Vermeer (1998)
Pediatric Outcome Data Collection Instrument	• Functional health-related quality of life instrument for children and parents • Reflects child's participation in the community setting • Can be used to evaluate outcomes in relation to functioning, treatment planning, and goal setting, and to improve patient care • Gates, Otsuka, Saunders, and McGee-Brown (2008)

NURSING PROCESS OF CARE

The nursing process of care guides the nurse in all settings and throughout the life span of clients with CP in promotion of optimal health and wellness. In the assessment phase, the client may be an individual, family, group, or in some cases, a community. The role of the nurse will vary greatly depending on setting (acute, chronic, or rehabilitation), age of the client (pediatric to geriatric), and specific needs of the individual. There is a broad range of physical impairment associated with CP, with some individuals requiring minimal assistance to others requiring assistance with all activities of daily living, complex care coordination, and utilization of resources. Key aspects in nursing care for individuals with CP include coordination of professionals on the team, enrollment in services that will benefit the client, identification and treatment of associated conditions, prevention of secondary conditions, monitoring of therapies in place, promotion of the best adaptation in terms of physical impairments, management of spasticity, client/family education, support for stress relief, and positive coping (Ahlstrom, 2007; Camus, 2008; King, Teplicky, King, & Rosenbaum, 2004).

Assessment can be optimized by using a focused review of systems approach with both the history and physical examination. Awareness of potential challenges specific to individuals with CP can facilitate the assessment process and identify appropriate interventions. The identified challenges and strengths can then be used to identify an individual's problems and generate nursing diagnoses, a plan of care, implementation of the nursing plan, and evaluation of effectiveness. The basic principles of nursing care can be adapted to meet the needs of care regardless of severity of CP.

General Health

Assessment of accurate measurement of height and weight is important across the life span. Once children grow beyond the limits of the infant scale, scales with handlebars provide stability for ambulatory patients and scales with a wider platform can be used for the nonambulatory patient in a wheelchair. Measurement of height may be difficult; there is potential for inaccuracies when measuring individuals with hip or knee flexion contractures and/or scoliosis. Segmental measures to estimate stature can be used (Stevenson et al., 2006).

Children with moderate to severe CP have poor growth when compared to typical children, which is impacted by secondary health conditions (Stevenson et al., 2006). Growth charts for children with quadriplegia were developed by Krick, Murphy-Miller, Zeger, and Wright (1996) and are available from the Kennedy Krieger Institute (2008).

Assessment of head circumference in all infants up to the age of 2 years is important. Excessive growth is a warning sign for hydrocephalus, whereas a flat line on the curve may indicate that the brain is not growing, which is associated with a poor prognosis for cognition.

Ability for self-care in activities of daily living is impacted by the degree of physical impairment, cognition, and ability to communicate. These include eating (e.g., ability to self-feed, degree of assistance required), dressing (ability to change clothes), ambulation (need for cane, walker, gait trainer, ankle-foot orthotics, wheelchair), toileting (toilet independently, use of adaptive equipment, totally dependent), and hygiene (degree of independence with daily activities). Promoting independence yet ensuring safety is one of the most important aspects to address in all activities and across all settings.

Head, Eye, Ear, Nose, and Throat

Increased or decreased oral muscle tone may impact verbal communication due to inability to form words and may require alternative means of communication. Ear infections are especially common in children with CP; those with impaired communication at any age may not be able to communicate the pain or discomfort of an ear infection. Assessment for hearing impairments requires formal audiological evaluation, which is especially important if speech delays are identified in children. Hearing and vision ability may worsen with age and periodic reexamination is indicated.

There is a higher increased prevalence of dental caries in primary dentition in children with CP (Guare Rde & Ciamponi, 2003). Dental pain may be missed in those who are unable to verbally communicate. It is important to assess the oral cavity including state of dentition, inquire about access to dental care, promote dental hygiene, and ensure that the client is eating food rich in calcium and vitamin D. Refer to Chapter 17 for additional information on sensory impairment.

Sialorrhea (drooling) is common in moderate to severe CP due to hypersecretion of saliva, low oral muscle tone with poor lip closure, inadequate jaw control, postural problems, inability to recognize salivary spill, and dental malocclusion. This can lead to dehydration, dental enamel erosion, chapping of the skin around the mouth, odor, and social stigmatization (Hockstein, Samadi, Gendron, & Handler, 2004). Oral-motor therapy may be useful to teach techniques to close lips and swallow more effectively. Medications such as anticholinergics (e.g., glycopyrrolate, scopolamine patch) may be used but have the potential for undesirable side effects. Botulinum toxin injections also have been used and, in extreme cases, surgical options include removal of the salivary gland, salivary duct ligation, and duct rerouting (Yam, Yang, Abdullah, & Chan, 2005).

Medication side effects may lead to relaxed voluntary muscles causing delayed swallowing or suppression of protective reflexes, such as gag and cough. Muscles of the pharynx and larynx may be spastic or hypotonic depending on the type of CP. This raises the risk for aspiration with feedings, which may be further complicated by the presence of gastroesophageal reflux disease (GERD). The caregiver should assess for choking, coughing, gagging, or retching with feeding. However, it is important to keep in mind that aspiration may be subclinical or silent. Some signs that indicate further assessment are multiple episodes of pneumonia, a diagnosis of chronic bronchitis, and asthma (Edmunds, 2005). If there is suspicion of aspiration, this may be confirmed by a modified barium/video swallow test, with a speech or occupational therapist present to assess functional swallowing ability. It may also be necessary to thicken formula or alter food consistency to facilitate swallowing without aspiration. If the individual is cognitively capable of following instructions, maneuvers to facilitate effective swallowing (e.g., a chin tuck) can be learned.

Sleep apnea may occur due to airway obstruction secondary to enlarged tonsils or adenoids and/or from central apnea. The caregiver should assess for snoring, noisy breathing, apnea, or night awakenings due to any breathing problems. A tonsillectomy and/or adenoidectomy may improve airway space and improve sleep.

Cardiovascular

Thrombophlebitis is a potential risk for those who are sedentary or nonmobile. Standard assessment techniques and interventions are indicated. Hands and especially feet may be cool and slightly blue due to poor circulation in immobile patients.

Pulmonary

Frequent respiratory tract infections are common and may be secondary to an ineffective cough reflex, weak respiratory muscles, spasticity of the chest wall leading to restrictive breathing, or aspiration with feeding. The decline in functional ability in the second decade of life is often a result of respiratory issues, especially in those with decreased mobility (Katz, 2003).

Gastrointestinal

Maintaining adequate nutrition and hydration can be challenging for many individuals with CP due to abnormal oral motor tone leading to ineffective swallowing patterns. The degree of motor impairment can greatly affect independence in self-feeding skill abilities. Impairment in language skills and/or cognitive limitations may limit ability to indicate hunger or request food when hungry. GERD and dental issues are associated with pain during and after eating. Chronic constipation may lead to a diminished desire to eat. Sensory impairments and oral aversion are common; an occupational therapist experienced in this area may provide useful interventions. Brain growth may be affected by inadequate calories, which makes nutritional assessment especially important in infants and young children (Georgieff, 2007).

The type of CP may impact daily caloric needs, with more calories required in those with increased muscle movements due to spasticity or to the constant motor movements associated with athetoid CP. Comorbid medical conditions, such as chronic lung disease in preterm infants or patients with decreased intestinal absorption, may also require higher daily caloric intake. Additional calories can be provided if needed by concentration of formulas or by using higher caloric preparations. Continual assessment across the life span is essential. Some individuals with CP may take enough by mouth to thrive initially, but decline in the second decade and require a gastrostomy tube to augment oral intake (Katz, 2003).

There is also risk for intake beyond body requirements leading to obesity, which is not uncommon in those fed by gastrostomy tube. Immobility may also lead to a decrease in overall caloric needs. The obese child or adult with CP can be difficult to lift or move, making this a physical hardship for the parent or caregiver. Obesity can contribute to functional decline in the mobility of ambulatory adolescents and adults, thus negatively impacting overall health and quality of life.

An oral motor function assessment may identify issues with potential to affect oral feeding skills, such as a hyperactive gag reflex, persistent bite reflex, poor lip and tongue control, and difficulties with chewing or swallowing. Oral feeding is optimal but can be difficult and time consuming. Allow for sufficient time for the patient to eat. Small and frequent feedings may be helpful and potentially reduce stress during mealtimes.

It is important to remember that feeding skills occur in developmental sequence just as other skills. Therefore, the child or adult should be fed according to the individual's oral motor/swallowing ability and developmental age, not necessarily the chronological age. For example, a 3-year-old child with severe impairment may be at a 6-month-old level developmentally and may appropriately continue to be bottle fed. This may be the case even for an adult who does not progress beyond this developmental stage.

Fluid and fiber intake is often inadequate in individuals with low oral muscle tone, impaired oral motor coordination, and decreased gastric motility/motility, which may lead to constipation. Constipation in infants and toddlers may respond to dietary changes, such as changing formula to soy or 100% whey formula, adding sorbitol-containing juices (e.g., pear, prune, apple), or adding pureed vegetables and fruit (Loening-Baucke, 2005). Dietary fiber intake can be augmented by ingestion of foods high in fiber or supplements. With recurrent constipation or with patients not responsive to dietary interventions, the use of oxmotic agents such as Lactulose and MiraLax may be useful (Baker et al., 1999). Gastrointestinal motility problems such as slow gastric emptying can be treated with medications, such as erythromycin (Taketomo, Hodding, & Krauss, 2004). Ensuring regular bathroom times (e.g., 30 minutes after meals) may be helpful in establishing optimal stooling patterns.

Genitourinary

Bladder functioning may be impaired due to abnormal muscle tone and control, leading to difficulty in urinary continence. Voiding patterns and dysfunctional voiding should be included in the initial and ongoing assessment of the individual with CP. Some children and adults may never achieve continence and require on-going use of diapers, making ongoing assessment of skin integrity essential. Trips to the bathroom to void every 2 to 3 hours may help with continence.

Reproductive

For females, menarche history should be reviewed and Tanner stage should be assessed (Tanner, 1961). Individuals who are severely impaired intellectually or verbally may not communicate the discomfort associated with menstrual periods effectively. Often, there is a hygiene concern for the parent or caregiver.

Sexuality is an area not always addressed in clients with physical disability. However, secondary sex characteristics and puberty in individuals with CP develop within the typical age ranges. The parent may not be expecting the puberty changes and may benefit from anticipatory guidance. The physical ability to take care of the necessary aspects related to menstruation may be impaired and should be assessed and addressed appropriately. Review the options for contraception if the client is sexually active. Routine gynecologic care is indicated regardless of disability.

Endocrine

Growth problems frequently occur in children with CP. Children with hemiplegia will usually be smaller on the affected side. A bone-age wrist film can be done to make an initial assessment of failure of general growth, with further workup as indicated.

Skin

Assessment and maintenance of skin integrity is extremely important throughout the life span. In children, there is an increased risk for development of pressure sores or friction areas if they are wearing splints that become too tight following growth spurts. There are many different types of splints, including ankle/foot orthotics, wrist/hand orthotics, knee extension splints, and elbow extension splints; these should be removed to assess the integrity of the skin beneath. Children (and even adults with CP, depending on developmental level or level of function) may have thickened, dry, or hyperpigmented skin on the hands, elbows, or knees due to prolonged crawling (e.g., commando crawling, crawling quadruped, or crawling in a tall kneel position).

Individuals who self-propel their wheelchairs may have friction areas on their hands. If the client self-propels the wheelchair with hands on the rubber tires instead of on the wheel rim, sports gloves or neoprene gloves fitted by a therapist are helpful for skin protection. There is an increased risk for the development of decubiti in those unable to independently change position. Teaching aspects of self-care in skin hygiene is needed, as well as application of basic nursing interventions such as repositioning, keeping skin dry and clean, and use of special pressure relief mattress. Adolescents with CP may also be concerned with acne.

Neurological

Because seizures are more common with CP, assessment and promotion of safety is essential. Seizures may not be totally controlled by medications, so it is important to prevent injuries during seizures. Helmets may be used by individuals with frequent seizures. Older children can be taught awareness of an aura.

Pain assessment and management is important. Pain can occur due to muscle spasms and difficulty maintaining optimal posture. Other comorbid medical conditions also may cause pain, such as undiagnosed GERD or esophagitis, constipation, gallbladder disease, renal stones, occult fractures or hip dislocations, otitis media, sinusitis, pressure sores or skin breakdown, and dental decay (Breau, Camfield, McGrath, & Finley, 2004). Behavioral changes such as irritability, crying, or displaying self-injurious behaviors may be the only clue that pain exists. Finding the source of the pain can be challenging.

Musculoskeletal

Spasticity has the potential to impact the functional capacity of the individual with CP, resulting in impaired physical mobility. There may be safety issues associated with ambulation. Secondary effects impact other systems of the body such as cardiovascular, skin (decubiti), respiratory infections, bowel and bladder problems, and osteoporosis. With spasticity, there is an imbalance of the agonist and antagonist muscles, which commonly leads to contractures, scoliosis, and hip subluxation or dislocation. Management of spasticity is essential to promote function, decrease or prevent deformities (such as contractures), alleviate pain, and increase ease of care giving (see Table 13.5).

Continuous changes in muscle tone are required for walking, as well as the ability to maintain an upright posture. Even individuals with mild CP typically have impairments in gait. Toe walking and scissoring are the most common gait disturbances. There can be pain associated with stiff muscles and spasticity. Caregivers should be instructed to do daily passive range-of-motion and stretching exercises, with additional education about the need for frequent position changes throughout the day whether in a bed or wheelchair. To maintain good alignment, individuals can be assisted to obtain well-fitted equipment (e.g., wheelchair, bath chairs, adapted toilet, stander, splints) as indicated.

Scoliosis is common in children with CP (McCarthy, D'Andrea, Betz, & Clements, 2006) and occurs in 25%–64% of institutionalized adults (Majd, Muldowney, & Hold, 1997). Referral to orthopedics for treatment of scoliosis may reduce the risk of decreased mobility and other complications of severe scoliosis. Increased lumbar lordosis and thoracic kyphosis, spondylolysis, and pelvic obliquity may be seen along with the scoliosis (Morrell, Pearson, & Sauser, 2002).

Individuals with CP are at increased risk for hip disorders, especially if they are unable to achieve ambulation. Progressive hip adduction and flexion is common; it may lead to femoral anteversion, subluxation, deformities of the femoral head, and hip dislocation, which can progress to degeneration, sometimes with pain (Morrell, Pearson, & Sauser, 2002). Children who are walking by 3–4 years have less risk for dislocations. It is essential to recognize progressive deformity and provide treatment to prevent irreversible changes. Physical examination is not reliable in all cases and an anteroposterior x-ray of the pelvis is required for diagnosis (Flynn & Miller, 2002).

Table 13.5. Spasticity management

Intervention	Expected or potential effect
Physical therapy	Range of motion (ROM), stretching of muscles to prevent contractures
Casting and orthotics	Promotion of appropriate alignment of bone, adjustment of the ROM at joint, and to maintain stretch/position
Oral antispasticity medications (e.g., benzodiazepines, oral baclofen, dantrolene sodium)	Increases mobility by causing decreased resistance to passive ROM, decreased hyperreflexia, reduction in painful spasms and clonus Potential side effects include Benzodiazepines (e.g., diazepam, clonazepam, clorazepate dipotassium): sedation, weakness, hypotension, gastrointestinal symptoms, incoordination, depression, ataxia, and lethargy Dantrolene sodium: weakness (including respiratory muscles), drowsiness, diarrhea, nausea, lethargy, hepatotoxicity associated with maximum dose and long-term use Oral baclofen: weakness, sedation, hypotonia, ataxia, confusion, fatigue, nausea, dizziness, lower seizure threshold
Botulinum toxin (derived from claustridium botulinum)	Injection into the neuromuscular junction of a hypertonic or spastic muscle results in relaxation by blocking the release of acetylcholine Decreases focal muscle spasticity increasing mobility/motor function impeding activities of daily living without the systemic effects of oral muscle relaxants Effect is 4–6 months so repeated treatments are needed Physical therapy, serial casting, or use of splints may maximize the benefits
Nerve blocks	Phenol or alcohol blocks injected into the nerve supply of the spastic muscle to produce muscle relaxation
Baclofen pump	Intrathecal baclofen is delivered directly into the spinal cord via a pump implanted surgically to decrease lower limb spasticity and for general dystonia Less medication is needed, resulting in fewer side effects Increased risk for infection and mechanical failure with monthly appointments required to refill the pump Improves functional intelligibility of speech in some children
Neurosurgery	Selective dorsal rhizotomy involves the transaction of selected sensory nerves entering the lower spinal cord with decrease in spasticity of muscles associated with the severed nerves May lead to improved motor functioning In individuals without potential for ambulation, may facilitate ease of care and decrease the risk of contractures May have negative effect on bowel and bladder function Requires intense physical therapy for optimal functional effects on lower limb function
Orthopedic surgery	May be utilized to correct/prevent musculoskeletal deformities Heel cord lengthening may be required between 4 to 7 years

Sources: Gaebler-Spira and Revivo (2003); Leary et al. (2006); Murphy, Irwin, and Hoff (2002); Pennington, Goldbart, and Marshall (2004).

Osteoporosis is common in those individuals who cannot bear weight, which increases potential for fractures. Factors such as a decrease in light exposure, spasticity/immobility, and the metabolic conversion of the precursors of vitamin D to inactive metabolites by anticonvulsive medications may increase predisposition to fractures (Rapp & Torres, 2000).

Adaptive equipment may be used to optimize gait and mobility, with the goal to facilitate the highest level of independence possible. Although individuals who are severely affected may not achieve independent ambulation, others may do so with the help of walkers or various specially designed splints supporting their ankles and feet. Wheelchairs range from manual to those powered with a joystick, head switch, or sip/puff controls. Grab rails or bath chairs can facilitate bathing and toileting. A nonslip surface can be put on chairs to prevent slipping; night lights may promote safety in dimly lighted areas or during nighttime hours. An adapted chair or stander can be used to promote sitting and standing.

Functional deterioration occurs in approximately 35% of adults with CP, with a higher percentage seen in those with more involved movement disorders (Ando & Ueda, 2000). Deterioration of locomotion skills may occur and this is associated with advancing age, delayed debut of walking, and the severity of neurological impairments (Jahnsen, Villien, Egeland, Stanghelle, & Holm, 2004).

Developmental/Educational/Psychosocial

In children and adolescents with CP, the physical limitations associated with their disabilities can have a considerable impact on independence, communication, socialization, academics, emotions, self-esteem, and overall quality of life (Donkervoort, Roebroeck, Wiegerink, van der Heijen-Maessen, & Stam, 2007). See Chapters 4 and 5 for information regarding developmental issues associated with children and adolescents with disabilities.

Even with survival to adulthood, there is a diminished life expectancy in those with severe impairment. Immobility, incontinence, intellectual and developmental disabilities, inability to oral feed, and seizures are risk factors leading to death in the second decade of life (Hutton, Colver, & Mackie, 2000; Katz, 2003; Liptak, 2008). Approximately one third of adults with CP live at home; many of their parents are elderly and may not have the physical capability to care for the individual (Rapp & Torres, 2000).

Quality of life is typically related to the severity of impairments. Adults with CP tend to be less socially active than peers; impairments in communication skills and lack of social networks are the most important factors leading to depression or loneliness in up to 50% of adults with CP (Ballin & Balandin, 2007). Pain, joint deformities, and fatigue are the most common health problems in adults with CP. The strongest predictors of fatigue are pain, deterioration of functional skills, low life satisfaction, and limitations in emotional and physical role function (Jahnsen, Villien, Stanghelle, & Holm, 2003). Regardless of their disability, as many as 66% of adults with CP are regularly active; up to 84% will live independently, with or without ancillary services such as an attendant. Employment status is most affected by ambulation status, IQ, and speech ability (Anderson & Mattsson , 2001; Ballin & Balandin, 2007; Murphy, Molnar, & Lankasky, 2000). See Chapter 5 for further information regarding developmental issues of adulthood in individuals with disabilities.

COMPLEMENTARY AND ALTERNATIVE MEDICINE

Following diagnosis, many parents may explore the use of complementary and alternative medicine (CAM) such as massage and naturopathy. CAM therapy is used most frequently by parents of children with greater levels of CP severity. Most

CAM therapies do not change the level of disability. Some therapies sought are associated with significant out-of-pocket costs and are typically not covered by insurance (Samdup, Smith, & Song, 2006).

CONCLUSION

Children born with CP require lifelong care and management. The advances of science and technology and improvement in treatment approaches and supports for individuals with CP have resulted in increased life expectances. As this chapter has illustrated, nurses have an important role in assisting individuals with CP across their life span in the ongoing assessment of their comprehensive needs for services and supports and the coordination of an interdisciplinary plan of care.

REFERENCES

Ahlstrom, G. (2007). Experiences of loss and chronic sorrow in persons with severe chronic illness. *Journal of Clinical Nursing, 16*, 76–83.

Anderson, C., & Mattsson, E. (2001). Adults with cerebral palsy: A survey describing problems, needs, and resources with special emphasis on locomotion. *Developmental Medicine & Child Neurology, 43*, 76–82.

Ando, N., & Ueda, S. (2000). Functional deterioration in adults with cerebral palsy. *Clinical Rehabilitation, 14*, 300–306.

Aneja, S. (2004). Evaluation of a child with cerebral palsy. *Indian Journal of Pediatrics, 71*, 627–634.

Ashwal, S., Russman, B., Blasco, P., Miller, G., Sandler, A., & Shevell, M. Quality Standards Subcommittee of the American Academy of Neurology. (2004). Practice parameter: Diagnostic assessment of the child with cerebral palsy: Report of the Quality Standards Subcommittee of the American Academy of Neurology and the Practice Committee of the Child Neurology Society. *Neurology, 62*, 851–863.

Baker, S., Lipak, G., Colletti, B., Croffie, J., Di Lorenzo, C., Ector, W., et al. (1999). Constipation in infants and children: Evaluation and treatment. *Journal of Pediatric Gastroenterology and Nutrition, 29*, 612–626.

Ballin, L., & Balandin, S. (2007). An exploration of loneliness: Communication and the social networks of older people with cerebral palsy. *Journal of Intellectual & Developmental Disability, 32*, 315–326.

Bax, M., Goldstein, M., Rosenbaum, P., Levitron, A., Paneth, N., Dan, B., et al. (2005). Proposed definition and classification of cerebral palsy, April 2005. *Developmental Medicine & Child Neurology, 47*, 571–576.

Beckung, E., Hagberg, G., Uldall, P., & Cans, C. (2008). Probability of walking with cerebral palsy in Europe. *Pediatrics, 121*, 187–192.

Bennett, F. (1999). Diagnosing cerebral palsy—The earlier the better. *Contemporary Pediatrics, 16*, 208–216.

Blair, E. (2001). Life expectancy among people with cerebral palsy in Western Australia. *Developmental Medicine & Child Neurology, 43*, 508–515.

Blair, E., & Watson, L. (2006). Epidemiology of cerebral palsy. *Seminars in Fetal & Neonatal Medicine, 11*, 117–125.

Breau, L.M., Camfield, C.S., McGrath, P.J., & Finley, G.A. (2004). Risk factors for pain in children with severe cognitive impairments. *Developmental Medicine & Child Neurology, 46*, 364–371.

Camus, H. (2008). The way forward for learning disability nursing. *British Journal of Nursing, 17*, S18–S19.

Cans, C. (2000). Surveillance of cerebral palsy in Europe: A collaboration of cerebral palsy surveys and registers. *Developmental Medicine & Child Neurology, 42*, 816–824.

Cans, C., McManus, V., Crowley, M., Guillen. P., Platt, M., Johnson, A., et al. (2004). Cerebral palsy of post-neonatal origin: Characteristics and risk factors. *Paediatric and Perinatal Epidemiology, 18*, 214–220.

Carnahan, K., Arner, M., & Hagglund, G. (2007). Association between gross motor function (GMFCS) and manual ability (MACS) in children with cerebral palsy. A population-based study of 359 children. *BMC Musculoskeletal Disorders*. Retrieved on July 1, 2009, from http://www.biomedcentral.com/1471-2474/8/50.

da Paz, A.C., Burnett, S.M., & Braga, L.W. (1994). Walking prognosis in cerebral palsy: A 22-year retrospective analysis. *Developmental Medicine & Child Neurology, 36*, 130–134.

Darrah, J., Magill-Evans, J., Volden, J., Hodge, M., & Kembhavi, G. (2007). Scores of typically developing children on the Peabody Developmental Motor Scale: Infancy to preschool. *Physical and Occupational Therapy in Pediatrics, 27*, 5–19.

Donkervoort, M., Roebroeck, M., Wiegerink, D., van der Heijen-Maessen, H., & Stam, H. (2007). Determinants of functioning of adolescents and young adults with cerebral palsy. *Disability and Rehabilitation, 29*, 453–463.

Doyle, L., Crowther, C., Middleton, P., & Marret, S. (2007). Magnesium sulfate for women at risk of preterm birth for neuroprotection of the fetus. *Cochrane Database of Systematic Reviews, 3*. doi:10.1002/14651858.CD004661.pub2.

Doyle, L., Halliday, H., Ehrenkranz, R., Davis, P., & Sinclair, J. (2005). Impact of postnatal systemic corticosteroids on mortality and cerebral palsy in preterm infants: Effect modulation by risk for chronic lung disease. *Pediatrics, 115*, 655–661.

Drougia, A., Giapros, V., Krallis, N., Theocharis, P., Nikaki, A., Tzoufi, M., et al. (2007). Incidence and risk factors for cerebral palsy in infants with perinatal problems: A 15-year review. *Early Human Development, 83*, 541–547.

Edmunds, A. (2005). Gastroesophageal reflux disease in the pediatric patient. *Clinical Review, 15*, 74–82.

Eliasson, K.A., Krumlinde, S., Rosblad, B., Beckung, E., Arner, M., Ohrvall, A., et al. (2006). The Manual Ability Classification System (MACS) for children with cerebral palsy: Scale development and evidence of validity and reliability. *Developmental Medicine & Child Neurology, 48*, 459–554.

Farmer, S.E. (2003). Key factors in the development of lower limb co-ordination: Implications for the acquisition of walking in children with cerebral palsy. *Disability and Rehabilitation, 25*, 807–816.

Fedrizzi, E., Facchin, P., Marzaroli, M., Pagliano, E., Botteon, G., Percivalle, L., et al. (2000). Predictors of independent walking in children with spastic diplegia. *Journal of Child Neurology, 15*, 228–234.

Flynn, J., & Miller, F. (2002). Management of hip disorders in patients with cerebral palsy. *Journal of the American Academy of Orthopedic Surgeons, 10*, 198–209.

Futagi, Y., Otani, K., & Goto, M. (1997). Prognosis of infants with ankle clonus within the first year of life. *Brain Development, 19*, 50–54.

Gaebler-Spira, D., & Revivo, G. (2003). The use of botulinum toxin in pediatric disorders. *Physical Medicine and Rehabilitation Clinics of North America, 14*, 703–725.

Gates, P., Otsuka, N., Saunders, J., & McGee-Brown, J. (2008). Relationship between parental PODCI questionnaire and School Functional Assessment in performance in children with CP. *Developmental Medicine & Child Neurology, 50*, 690–695.

Georgieff, M. (2007). Nutrition and the developing brain: Nutritional priorities and measurement. *The American Journal of Clinical Nutrition, 85*, 6145–6205.

Ghasia, F., Brunstrom, J., Gordon, M., & Tychsen, L. (2008). Frequency and severity of visual, sensory and motor deficits in children with cerebral palsy: Gross Motor Function Classification Scale. *Investigative Ophthalmology & Visual Science, 49*, 572–580.

Gibson, C., MacLennan, A., Goldwater, P., & Dekker, G. (2003). Antenatal cause of cerebral palsy: Associations between inherited thrombophilias, viral and bacterial infection, and inherited susceptibility to infection. *Obstetrics Gynecology Survey, 58*, 209–220.

Greenwood, C., Yudkin, P., Sellers, S., Impey, L., & Doyle, P. (2005). Why is there a modifying effect of gestational age on risk factors for cerebral palsy? *Archives of Disease in Childhood, Fetal and Neonatal Edition, 90*, F141–F146.

Guare Rde, O., & Ciamponi, A. (2003). Dental caries prevalence in the primary dentition of cerebral-palsied children. *Journal of Clinical Pediatric Dentistry, 27*, 287–292.

Gururaj, A., Sztriha, L., Bener, A., Dawodu, A., & Eapen, V. (2003). Epilepsy in children with cerebral palsy. *Seizure, 12*, 110–114.

Hemming, K., Hutton, J., & Pharoah, P. (2006). Long-term survival for a cohort of adults with cerebral palsy. *Developmental Medicine and Child Neurology, 48*, 90–95.

Himmelmann, K., Hagberg, G., Wiklund, L., Eek, M., & Uvebrant, P. (2007). Dyskinetic cerebral palsy: A population-based study of children born between 1991–1998. *Developmental Medicine & Child Neurology, 49*, 246–251.

Himpens, E., Van den Broeck, C., Oostra, A., Calders, P., & Vanhaesebrouck, P. (2008). Prevalence, type, distribution, and severity of cerebral palsy in relation to gestational age: A meta-analytic review. *Developmental Medicine & Child Neurology, 50*, 334–340.

Hockstein, N., Samadi, D., Gendron, K., & Handler, S. (2004). Sialorrhea: A management challenge. *American Family Physician, 69*, 2628–2634.

Hutton, J., Colver, P., & Mackie, P. (2000). Effect of severity of disability on survival in north east England cerebral palsy cohort. *Archives of Disease in Childhood, 83,* 468–474.

Hutton, J., & Pharoah, P. (2002). Effects of cognitive, motor, and sensory disabilities on survival in cerebral palsy. *Archives of Diseases in Childhood, 86,* 84–89.

Jahnsen, R., Villien, L., Egeland, T., Stanghelle, J., & Holm, I. (2004). Locomotion skills in adults with cerebral palsy. *Clinical Rehabilitation, 18,* 309–316.

Jahnsen, R., Villien, L., Stanghelle, J., & Holm, I. (2003). Fatigue in adults with cerebral palsy in Norway compared with the general population. *Developmental Medicine & Child Neurology, 45,* 296–303.

Jan, J., Lyons, C., Heaven, R., & Matsuba, C. (2001). Visual impairment due to a dyskinetic eye movement disorder in children with dyskinetic cerebral palsy. *Developmental Medicine & Child Neurology, 43,* 108–112.

Katz, R. (2003). Life expectancy for children with cerebral palsy and mental retardation: Implications for life care planning. *NeuroRehabilitation, 18,* 261–270.

Kennedy Krieger Institute. (2008). *Growth charts for children with quadriplegic cerebral palsy.* Retrieved October 1, 2008, from http://www.kennedykrieger.org.

Ketelaar, M., & Vermeer, A. (1998). Functional motor abilities of children with cerebral palsy: A systematic literature review of assessment measures. *Clinical Rehabilitation, 2,* 369–380.

King, S., Teplicky, R., King, G., & Rosenbaum, P. (2004). Family-centered service for children with cerebral palsy and their families: A review of the literature. *Seminars in Pediatric Neurology, 11,* 78–86.

Korzeniewski, S., Birbeck, G., DeLano, M., Potchen, M., & Paneth, N. (2008). A systematic review of neuroimaging for cerebral palsy. *Journal of Child Neurology, 23,* 216–227.

Krick, J., Murphy-Miller, P., Zeger, S., & Wright, E. (1996). Pattern of growth in children with cerebral palsy. *Journal of the American Dietetic Association, 96,* 680–685.

Leary, S.M., Gilpin, P., Lockley, L., Rodriguez, L., Jarrett, L., & Stevenson, V.L. (2006). Intrathecal baclofen therapy improves functional intelligibility of speech in cerebral palsy. *Clinical Rehabilitation, 20,* 228–231.

Liptak, G.S. (2008). Health and well being of adults with cerebral palsy. *Current Opinion in Neurology, 21,* 136–142.

Little, W.J. (1843). Lectures on the deformity of the human frame. *Lancet, 1,* 318–320.

Loening-Baucke, V. (2005). Prevalence, symptoms, and outcomes of constipation in infants and toddlers. *The Journal of Pediatrics, 146,* 359–363.

Majd, M., Muldowney, D., & Holt, R. (1997). Natural history of scoliosis in the institutionalized adult cerebral palsy population. *Spine, 22,* 1461–1466.

McCarthy, J., D'Andrea, L., Betz, R., & Clements, D. (2006). Scoliosis in the child with cerebral palsy. *Journal of the Academy of Orthopedic Surgeons, 14,* 367–375.

McDonagh, M., Morgan, D., Carson, S., & Russman, B. (2007). Systematic review of hyperbaric oxygen therapy for cerebral palsy: The state of the evidence. *Developmental Medicine & Child Neurology, 49,* 942–947.

Meberg, A., & Broch, H. (2004). Etiology of cerebral palsy. *Journal of Perinatal Medicine, 32,* 434–439.

Morales, A.C., Azuara, B.N., Gallo, T.J., Gonzalez, A.A, & Rama, Q.J. (2006). Sensorineural hearing loss in cerebral palsy patients. *Acta Otorrinolaringol Espanola, 57,* 300–302.

Morgan, A.M., & Aldag, J.C. (1996). Early identification of cerebral palsy using a profile of abnormal motor patterns. *Pediatrics, 98,* 642–649.

Morrell, D., Pearson, J., & Sauser, D. (2002). Progressive bone and joint abnormalities of the spine and lower extremities in cerebral palsy. *Radiographics, 22,* 257–268.

Morris, C. (2007). Definition and classification of cerebral palsy: A historical perspective. *Developmental Medicine & Child Neurology Supplement, 109,* 3–7.

Murphy, K., Molnar, G., & Lankasky, K. (2000). Employment and social issues in adults with cerebral palsy. *Archives of Physical Medicine and Rehabilitation, 81,* 807–811.

Murphy, N., Irwin, M., & Hoff, C. (2002). Intrathecal baclofen therapy in children with cerebral palsy: Efficacy and complications. *Archives of Physical Medicine and Rehabilitation, 83,* 1721–1725.

Newman, C.J., O'Regan, M., & Hensey, O. (2006). Sleep disorders in children with cerebral palsy. *Developmental Medicine & Child Neurology, 48,* 564–568.

O'Shea, M. (2008). Cerebral palsy. *Seminars in Perinatology, 32,* 35–41.

O'Shea, T., & Doyle, L. (2001). Perinatal glucocorticoid therapy and neurological outcome in epidemiologic perspective. *Seminars in Neonatology, 6,* 293–207.

Odding, E., Roebroeck, M., & Stam, H. (2006). The epidemiology of cerebral palsy: Incidence, impairments, and risk factors. *Disability and Rehabilitation, 28,* 183–191.

Palisano, R., Rosenbaum, P., Walter, S., Russell, D., Wood, E., & Galuppi, B. (1997). Development and reliability of a system to classify gross motor function in children with cerebral palsy. *Developmental Medicine & Child Neurology, 39,* 214–223.

Pellegrino, L. (2007). Cerebral palsy. In M.L. Batshaw, L. Pellegrino, & N.J. Roizen (Eds.), *Children with disabilities* (6th ed., p. 387–408). Baltimore: Paul H. Brookes Publishing Co.

Pennington L., Goldbart J., & Marshall J. (2004). Interaction training for conversational partners of children with cerebral palsy: A systematic review. *International Journal of Language & Communication Disorders. 39,* 151–170.

Pueyo, R., Junque, C., & Vendrell, P. (2003). Neuropsychologic differences between bilateral dyskinetic and spastic cerebral palsy. *Journal of Child Neurology, 18,* 845–850.

Rapp, C., & Torres, M. (2000). The adult with cerebral palsy. *Archives of Family Medicine, 9,* 466–472.

Roberts, G., Palfrey, J., & Bridgemohan, C. (2004). A rational approach to the medical evaluation of a child with developmental delay. *Contemporary Pediatrics, 21,* 76.

Rosenbaum, P. (2003). Cerebral palsy: What parents and doctors want to know. *British Medical Journal, 326,* 970–974.

Rosenbaum, P., Paneth, N., Leviton, A., Goldstein, M., & Bax, M. (2007). A report: The definition and classification of cerebral palsy, April 2006. *Developmental Medicine & Child Neurology Supplement, 109,* 8–14.

Rosenbaum, P., Walter, S., Hanna, S., Palisano, R., Russell, D., & Raina, P., et al. (2002). Prognosis for gross motor function in cerebral palsy: Creation of motor development curves. *JAMA, 288,* 1357–1363.

Samdup, D., Smith, R.I., & Song, S. (2006). The use of complementary and alternative medicine in children with chronic conditions. *American Journal of Physical Medicine & Rehabilitation, 85,* 842–846.

Sanger, T. (2003). Pathophysiology of pediatric movement disorders. *Journal of Child Neurology, 18,* S9–S24.

Shankaran, S., Laptook, A., Ehrenkranz, R., Tyson, J., McDonald, S., & Donavan, E., et al. (2005). Whole-body hypothermia for neonates with hypoxic-ischemic encephalopathy. *New England Journal of Medicine, 353,* 1574–1584.

Stevenson, R., Conaway, M., Chumlea, W., Rosenbaum, P., Fung, E., Henderson, R., et al. (2006). Growth and health in children with moderate-to-severe cerebral palsy. *Pediatrics, 118,* 1010–1018.

Taketomo, C., Hodding, J., & Kraus, D. (2004). *Lexi-Comp's pediatric dosage handbook* (11th ed.). Hudson, OH: Lexi-Comp.

Tanner, J.M. (1961). *Growth at adolescence* (2nd ed.). Oxford: Blackwell.

United Cerebral Palsy. (2001). *Cerebral palsy: Facts and figures.* Retrieved May 1, 2008, from http://www.ucp.org/ucp_generaldoc.cfm/1/9/37/37-37/447.

Venkateswaran, S., & Shevell, M. (2008). Comorbidities and clinical determinants of outcome in children with spastic quadriplegic cerebral palsy. *Developmental Medicine & Child Neurology, 50,* 216–222.

Winter, S., Autry, A., Boyle, C., & Yearsin-Allsopp, M. (2002). Trends in the prevalence of cerebral palsy in a population-based study. *Pediatrics, 110,* 1220–1225.

Yam, W.K., Yang, H.L., Abdullah,, B., & Chan, C. (2005). Management of drooling for children with neurological problems in Hong Kong. *Brain Development, 28,* 24–29.

Zafeiriou, D.I. (2004). Primitive reflexes and postural reactions in the neurodevelopmental examination. *Pediatric Neurology, 31,* 1–8.

CHAPTER 14

Mental and Behavioral Health Disorders in Individuals with Intellectual and Developmental Disabilities

Sarah H. Ailey and Tanya Melich-Munyan

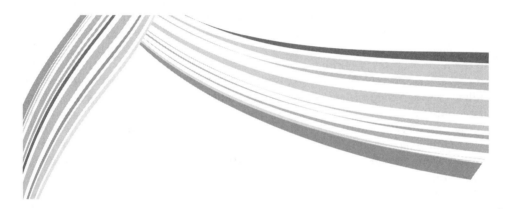

Mental health disorders are often underrecognized and undertreated in individuals with intellectual and developmental disabilities (IDD). Individuals with IDD experience all of the mental health disorders that individuals without IDD experience, including affective disorders, anxiety disorders, schizophrenia, panic disorders, posttraumatic stress disorder (PTSD), and others (Brown & Marshall, 2006). Behavior disorders are a significant concern among individuals with IDD and are the most common reason for mental health referrals. Terms for psychiatric conditions and behavior disorders are often used interchangeably in literature for individuals with IDD, although individuals with IDD manifest challenging behaviors, such as aggression or destructive tendencies, without underlying psychopathology (Allen & Davies, 2007). Prevalence studies of mental health disorders among individuals with IDD use different assessment methods, definitions of mental health, and diagnostic criteria. Based on a review of the literature, most studies report rates for individuals with IDD much higher than the general population. The point prevalence (including behavior disorders) of mental health disorders is likely to be between 30% and 50% (Smiley, 2005).

Mental health and behavior disorders have major consequences in working and living situations. Numerous studies indicate that particularly the challenging behaviors of being destructive, disruptive, and hurtful to self and others are a major concern for individuals with IDD (Whittington & Burns, 2005). A recent Swedish study found that 31% of caregivers working in group homes with individuals with IDD experienced violent behavior from residents within a year (Lundstrom, Saveman, Eisemann, & Astrom, 2007). Aggressive and self-injurious behavior result in greater public and individual health care costs (Harris, 2006). Furthermore, with the high prevalence of behavior disorders, individuals whose behavior is not challenging may not receive needed treatment for mental health disorders.

Despite the prevalence of mental health disorders, individuals with a dual diagnosis of IDD and mental illness are often underserved. Historical literature indicates that until the mid 1980s, it was common for clinicians to doubt that individuals with IDD could have a dual diagnosis with other disorders, such as depression (Sovner & Pary, 1993). The mental health care system continues to remain ill-equipped to manage their care (Palmer, Llanos, Tobias, & Bella, 2006), and a lack of qualified providers limits access to care (Moseley, 2004).

A past and current aspect of inadequacies in care for individuals with IDD is that both physical and mental health symptoms have been attributed to the IDD by health care professionals. Attributing mental health disorders to IDD has been called *diagnostic overshadowing.* Reiss, Levitan, and Szysko conducted a classic study on the phenomenon published in 1982. Professional psychologists were given the same case descriptions for individuals identified to have average intelligence and individuals identified to have intellectual disabilities. Psychopathology was identified more often for the individuals with average intelligence than for the individuals with intellectual disabilities. The phenomenon was not different for psychologists with experience in working with individuals with intellectual disabilities (Reiss & Szyszko, 1983). Mason and Scior (2004) also found that diagnostic overshadowing appears to occur more commonly among psychiatrists than psychologists while evaluating an individual with IDD.

Individuals with IDD who have mental health disorders often require medical and social services as well. Collaborative interdisciplinary practice for people with multiple physical and psychological disorders has been identified as the exemplary model of care, and benchmarks for models of interdisciplinary practice and care are needed (Braden, 2006). Individuals with IDD are also disadvantaged by the current state of mental health research. Scientific studies often specifically exclude this population (National Institute of Neurological Disorders and Stroke, 2001), making it difficult to assess their true service deficiencies and needs.

GENERAL NURSING PROCESS FOR INDIVIDUALS WITH IDD

Nursing care of individuals with IDD who also have mental health disorders is often complex. Ecological models of mental health care systematically assess the individual in relation to social and environmental conditions that affect mental health (Ailey & Miller, 2004). Thorough assessment that includes a detailed physical evaluation and history is critical. A conscientious nursing assessment should address history of current complaints, presence of particular syndromes or diagnoses, psychosocial history, family history, medication history, and functional health patterns. Other health care providers, family, and residential staff serve as valuable resources in compiling a comprehensive assessment. Recognizing and understanding the interrelationship and the differences between IDD, mental health disorders, and physical disorders is essential. Assessing social and environmental conditions is important in evaluating mental health and in the development of treatment plans for individuals with IDD.

Planning also involves a life-span approach. From birth to the process of dying and death, care should be integrated to support each phase of life. A life-span approach includes primary prevention and early intervention during infancy and supports the transitions to adolescence, adulthood, and later years (Drew & Hardman, 2007; Harris, 2006). It affords support for the client in coping with sexuality, grief, and other aspects of living that are often quieted or ignored (Ailey, Marks, Crisp, & Hahn, 2003; Ailey, O'Rourke, Breakwell, & Murphy, 2008). Biological, cognitive, psychological, and social dimensions are given equal consideration as the wellness and mental health of clients with IDD are addressed. Embracing this approach considers, for example, the challenges of an individual with Down syndrome and a significant visual impairment who may be experiencing depression. Individuals with Down syndrome age more rapidly and may face the additional burden of Alzheimer's-like dementia. A life-span approach incorporates principles of case management to coordinate care between the individual, health professionals, family, and staff (Brown, 2005). This approach is comprehensive and is well suited as an overarching framework for the development, implementation, and evaluation of interdisciplinary treatment plans.

Evaluation involves setting individualized goals and objectives and measuring progress toward achievement of these goals. Goals should be dynamic, should reflect real-time progress, and should be periodically reevaluated throughout the course of care.

HISTORY AND PHYSICAL ASSESSMENT

The gathering of data pertaining to history and physical health is important for a mental/behavioral health assessment. History of current complaints, family history, illness, and medication history should be obtained. Other issues, including genetic and other biological issues, social and environmental considerations, and life changes, should also be considered when gathering a history and physical assessment.

Physical health problems and complaints, such as sleep disorders, hypo- or hyperthyroidism, nutritional problems, unrecognized pain, and anemia may mimic or complicate mental health disorders for individuals with IDD or may be misattributed to the IDD. Symptoms of sleep disorders include behavior changes, mood swings, depression, and appetite changes; these are symptoms that may be mistaken for depression, intermittent explosive disorders, or anxiety (Benson & Ivins, 1992). Symptoms of hypothyroidism include weight gain, sleep changes, and depression, whereas symptoms of hyperthyroidism include nervousness, sleep changes, behavior changes, and fatigue (Heuther, 2004). Symptoms of both disorders might be mistaken for mental health disorders. Individuals with IDD may have difficulties with communication that affect their own and others' awareness of a change in physical or mental health status (Atherton, 2006). This underlines the significance of a thorough, effective, person-centered nursing assessment. A comprehensive description of the symptomatology of major psychiatric disorders can be found in the Diagnostic Manual–Intellectual Disabilities (Fletcher, Laschen, Stavrakaki, & First, 2007).

Genetic and Other Biological Issues

Information on the presence or absence of particular syndromes is important in the mental/behavioral health assessment. Specific mental health and behavioral disorders are associated with specific syndromes and genetic disorders. Knowledge of the presence of particular syndromes can help to guide the nursing assessment. See Table 14.1 for descriptions of health issues associated with specific syndromes or conditions, including autism spectrum disorder, fragile X syndrome, and Prader-Willi syndrome. The list is not all inclusive; literature can be searched regarding mental health and behavior disorders often associated with other syndromes and conditions.

Social and Environmental Considerations

Social and environmental concerns are also risk factors for mental health disorders. For an individual with IDD, the educational, work, or family setting may contribute to the development of or exacerbate a mental health disorder. Interpersonal risk factors for mental health disorders include a history of physical, sexual, or psychological abuse; social isolation; stigmatization; family stress; substance abuse; and involvement with the correctional system. These risk factors are important to assess.

Life Changes

Major life changes may include death of a parent, other family member, or an individual important in one's life. Developing programs to support individuals with IDD in grieving is an important issue because grief may be a risk factor for depression (Ailey et al., 2008). Hollins and Esterhuyzen (1997) found that 26% of individuals who had lost a parent within 2 years could be characterized as depressed. However, it is important to do a thorough assessment and not to interpret behavioral manifestations of grief as troublesome behavior or psychopathology (MacHale & Carvey, 2002). Other major life changes include moving, changing schools or jobs, and the loss of a pet, housemate, or important staff member.

Other Potential Issues

Individuals with IDD may be socially isolated, may be at risk for abuse, or may be abusing substances. Individuals with IDD may also have PTSD or cognitive features of other mental health disorders. These potential factors should also be considered when assessing a person with IDD.

Social Isolation   Individuals with IDD may be socially isolated. Job and social opportunities may be limited because of a lack of social skills in interacting with colleagues in work environments and with others at school or in the community. In addition, individuals with mild or moderate IDD may understand that they are stigmatized. A phenomenological study in the United Kingdom (Jahoda & Markova, 2004) found that individuals with IDD transitioning from a family home or care facility to a more independent community setting were aware of the stigma related to IDD and believed they were stigmatized. Social isolation and stigmatization can lead to increased difficulty with mental health disorders.

Table 14.1. Issues associated with specific syndromes and disorders

Syndrome	Etiology	Associated health problems	Associated mental health disorders	Nursing interventions
Autism spectrum disorders	Multiple causation, suspected genetic, environmental, immunologic[a]	Decreased nociception, chronic diarrhea, *Candida*	Anxiety, depression, mood swings, repetitive behavior, obsessive-compulsive disorder[a,b]	Sensory integration Structured environment Nutritional management Social skills instruction[a]
Down syndrome	Chromosome 21 trisomy[a]	Congenital heart defects, weight gain, diabetes, hypothyroidism, skeletal disorders, gastrointestinal disorders[a]	Depression, autism, early onset Alzheimer's, attention deficits, obsessive-compulsive tendencies[a,b]	Depression screening Nutritional assessment Weight management Promote physical activity Maintain routines[a]
Fetal alcohol spectrum disorder	Exposure to alcohol during gestation[c]	Hearing loss[c], congenital heart defects, cerebral palsy	Panic disorder, depression, impulsive behavior, attention-deficit hyperactivity disorder[e]	Early intervention and referral for inter-disciplinary services (mother and infant) Teach impulse control Structured environment[d]
Fragile X syndrome	Mutation of FMR-1 gene[a]	Mitral valve prolapse, fragile skin, poor coordination, seizures, hernias[a]	Autistic behaviors, pervasive speech, self-injurious behaviors, progressive dementia, anxiety[a,e]	Sensory integration Sensorimotor therapy Maintain safety Low stress environment[a]
Prader-Willi	Loss of gene activation on chromosome 15[e]	Weight gain, diabetes, dental caries, scoliosis, strabismus, osteoporosis, decreased nociception[f]	Depression, anxiety, obsessive-compulsive tendencies, self-injurious behavior, extreme anger[e]	Minimize change Nutritional management Promote physical activity Assess skin integrity Reinforce appropriate display of emotions[f]
Williams syndrome	Deletion at 7q11.23[f]	Supraventricular aortic stenosis, hyperacusis, hypercalcemia, rectal prolapse, kidney abnormalities[g]	Anxiety, attention deficits, hypersociability[e,g]	Promote adequate fluid intake Monitor bowel/bladder function Reinforce appropriate socialization Promote motor skills development[h]

[a]McKinney, James, Murray, and Ashwill (2005); [b]Blacher and McIntyre (2006); [c]Cohen-Kerem, Bar-Oz, Nulman, Papaioannou, and Koren (2007); [d]Caley, Shipkey, Winkleman, Dunlap, and Rivera (2006); [e]Sadock and Sadock (2003); [f]Bellon-Harn (2005); [g]Holin and Udwin (2006); [h]Tsai, Wu, Liou, and Shu (2008).

Risk for Abuse   Abuse is a risk for mental health disorders. A case-controlled study in the United Kingdom found a significant association between sexual abuse and psychiatric disorders in individuals with IDD (Sequeira, Howlin, & Hollins, 2003). As mandated reporters, nurses should be particularly alert for signs of abuse including changes in eating habits, hygiene, or activity level. Individuals with IDD may be at greater risk than the general population for abuse, including incest, rape and assault, abuse by caregivers and individuals in authority, abuse by family members and other individuals with IDD, victimization, and exploitation (American Academy of Pediatrics, 2001; Nettlebeck & Wilson, 2002).

Most of the research establishing risk for abuse was conducted in the 1990s. In a study in the United Kingdom, McCarthy and Thompson (1997) found 61% of women and 25% of men with IDD experienced sexual abuse, while a study in the United States found 79% of women with IDD were likely to have experienced sexual abuse (Stromsness, 1993). Victims usually know the abusers, who are often family members, staff, and other individuals with IDD (Furey, 1994). Aspects of the lives of individuals with IDD, such as different caretakers, the need for assistance with personal care, being used to obeying and complying, and lack of skills to defend and speak up for themselves put them at further risk for abuse and exploitation (Aylott, 1999).

Substance Abuse   As individuals with IDD live longer and more independently, some individuals may engage in more substance-related health risk behaviors. Individuals with IDD may be at less risk of substance use than the general population, but are more likely to abuse than their peers without disabilities. Among individuals with IDD who use alcohol, approximately 50% misuse it (McGillicuddy & Blane, 1999). Internationally, smoking rates among individuals with IDD have been reported from 6.2% to 36% (Taylor, Standen, Cutajar, Fox & Wilson, 2004; Tracy & Hosken, 1997). Research on education, prevention, and treatment with individuals with intellectual disabilities has not been done (McGillicuddy, 2006). For individuals with IDD living in residential placements, state-mandated policies protecting all residents and all employees from environmental tobacco smoke were almost nonexistent until the mid 1990s when policies mandating the restrictions in state-run facilities went into effect (Minihan, 1999, 2003).

Posttraumatic Stress Disorder   Individuals with IDD develop PTSD at a rate comparable to that of the general population when exposed to trauma (Ryan, 1994). As with other mental health alterations, individuals with IDD may perceive and react to traumatic events in a different manner, and it is often expressed through challenging behaviors (Doyle & Mitchell, 2003). Turk, Robbins, and Woodhead (2005) have expressed concern that clinicians fail to properly diagnose PTSD among individuals with IDD. Individuals with IDD experiencing PTSD may exhibit regression from their current developmental stage or new expressions of aggression or other challenging behavior (Turk et al., 2005). If nurses detect any history of abuse or other trauma, assessment for PTSD should be considered.

Cognitive Features of Other Mental Health Disorders   Individuals with mild or moderate IDD may manifest cognitive features of mental health disorders. Unwarranted or inappropriate anxiety or changes in language patterns may become evident. Individuals with IDD report suicidal ideation, lack of desire to participate in personal hygiene, social withdrawal, poor self-esteem, self-hatred, and lack of self-confidence (Ailey, 2009; Ailey, Miller, Heller, & Smith, 2006). Depression is also associated with frequency of automatic negative thoughts, feelings of hopelessness, rates of self-reinforcement, amount of negative social support (Nezu, Nezu, Rothenberg, DelliCarpini, & Groag, 1995), and social comparison (Dagnan & Sandhu, 1999). Conversely, the absence of depression in adolescents with IDD is associated with global self-worth and positive self-image (Zigler, Bennet-Gates, & Hodapp, 1999).

DIAGNOSTIC PROCESS

Mental health disorders in individuals with IDD often go undetected and are associated with poor outcomes. Screening is an active process aimed at detecting disease, illness, or deficit and is useful in identifying and referring for follow-up individuals who may have previously unrecognized mental health disorders. Nurses working with individuals with IDD in school, employment, residential, and community settings should screen for mental health disorders as part of providing routine, optimal care.

In the following sections, screening instruments and tools, clinical interviews, behavioral observations, and functional analysis are discussed as options of the diagnostic process. Regardless of the diagnostic tools and methods used, best practice assessment should follow a biopsychosocial model. This model draws from multiple sources of information including family, medical, developmental, and psychiatric history. It also includes informant interviews, direct observation, and a clinical interview with the individual with IDD (Fletcher, 2008). A comprehensive diagnosis informs the planning, implementation, and evaluation of the plan of care.

Screening Instruments and Tools

A variety of screening instruments for psychopathology are available, including tools used in the general population, tools developed specifically for individuals with IDD, and tools that are specifically informant rated about individuals with IDD. This section will specifically discuss the *Diagnostic and Statistical Manual of Mental Disorders (DSM)*, the *International Classification of Diseases (ICD)*, and *Diagnostic Criteria for Psychiatric Disorders for Use with Adults with Learning Disabilities/Mental Retardation (DC-LD)*. See also Table 14.2 for a description of screening measures specifically developed for use with individuals with IDD.

Diagnostic and Statistical Manual of Mental Disorders   The *DSM*, now in its fourth edition, text revision (*DSM-IV-TR;* American Psychiatric Association, 2000), is the principal system for psychiatric diagnosis in the United States. The *DSM* evolved in the early 1900s from a need to collect uniform statistics in psychiatric hospitals (Clark, Watson, & Reynolds, 1995). The *DSM-IV-TR* uses criteria based on specific symptoms to determine a diagnosis and to differentiate one diagnosis from another. The *DSM* attempts to disengage itself from behavioral theory with regard to etiology and the developmental nature of the various psychiatric disorders (Clark et al., 1995). Symptoms are generally given equal weight within a diagnosis and a certain number of criteria must be met to make a diag-

Table 14.2.   Screening measures developed for individuals with intellectual and developmental disabilities (IDD)

Measure	Description
Glasgow Depression Scale for People with a Learning Disability	Self-report tool for clients with mild/moderate IDD
	20 items scored on 3-point Likert scale
	Items derived from Diagnostic Criteria for Psychiatric Disorders for use with Adults with Learning Disabilities/ Mental Retardation (DC-LD)[a]
	Higher score indicates greater depression
Psychopathology Instrument for Mentally Retarded Adults	Two-part interview: others and self-report
	Among the most widely used for individuals with IDD[b]
	Criteria similar to *DSM-IV*
	Scores (1 or 0) indicate presence or absence of symptoms
	Scores are summed to provide a disorder subscale and total[c]
Reiss Screen for Maladaptive Behaviors	Informant rated behavior scale for individuals with mild to severe IDD
	38 items scored on 3-point scale: *1* = no problem to *3* = major problem
	Items address symptom category or psychiatric concept
	Based on *DSM-III-R* disorders[d]
Reiss Scale for Children's Dual Diagnosis	Comparable to Reiss Screen for Maladaptive Behavior, for use with clients up to age 21
	60-item instrument
	Valid for identifying presence of psychopathology, but not specific diagnosis[e]
Self-Report Depression Questionnaire	Self report measure for clients with mild IDD
	32 items scored as *almost, sometimes,* or *most* for occurrence of symptoms during the past 2 weeks[f]
Strohmer-Prout Behavior Rating Scale	Informant rated behavior and emotion measure for individuals with borderline/mild IDD
	135-item scale, 2 global factors and 12 clinical subscales[g]
	Considered to be one of the more superior informant scales[b]

Key: DSM, Diagnostic and Statistical Manual of Mental Disorders; [a]Cuthill, Espie, and Cooper (2003); [b]Kazdin, Matson, and Senatore (1983); [c]Nezu, Ronan, Meadows, and McClure (2000); [d]Reiss (1988); [e]Reiss and Valenti-Hein (1990); [f]Esbensen, Seltzer, and Greenberg (2005); [g]Strohmer and Prout (1998).

nosis. Diagnoses based on the *DSM-IV-TR* facilitate clinical practice and communication and are used to determine access to treatment, therapies, and third-party payment.

The *Diagnostic Manual–Intellectual Disability* (*DSM-ID;* Fletcher, Loschen, Stavrakaki, & First, 2007) covers all *DSM-IV-TR* diagnoses. For the majority of diagnoses, no adaptations in criteria were made. The manual presents considerable information on the application of diagnostic criteria to people with IDD including etiology, genetic considerations, and manifestations (e.g., Charlot et al., 2007; Cooray, Gabriel, & Gaus, 2007; Lee & Friedlander, 2007). It includes a critique of the application of *DSM-IV-TR* criteria for specific disorders. In field testing, preliminary assessment of the data indicates that clinicians were better able to make diagnoses using the *DSM-ID* as a supplement to the *DSM-IV-TR* than with the *DSM-IV-TR* alone (Fletcher et al., 2007).

International Classification of Diseases   The *International Classification of Diseases 10* (*ICD-10;* World Health Organization, 2007) is another classification system used in mental health. The *ICD-10* is an international standard for diagnostic and treatment categorization. It provides a structure to track prevalence, morbidity, and mortality of mental health disorders. Like the *DSM-IV-TR*, the *ICD-10* uses criteria based on specific symptoms to determine a diagnosis and to differentiate one diagnosis from another. Diagnoses in both systems are broadly comparable.

Diagnostic Criteria for Psychiatric Disorders for Use with Adults with Learning Disabilities/Mental Retardation   In 2001, the Royal College of Psychiatrists published the *DC-LD* (2001). This textbook provides guidelines for diagnostic criteria based on *ICD-10,* focusing primarily on adults with moderate to profound disabilities. Its criteria form the basis for the development of screening tools including the Glasgow Depression Scale for People with a Learning Disability (Cuthill, Espie, & Cooper, 2003).

Clinical Interviews

A medical diagnosis of a mental health disorder is made by a nurse practitioner, physician, psychologist, or psychiatrist using a variety of tools. A clinical diagnostic interview, commonly used to diagnose psychopathology in the general population, may also be conducted with a client with IDD. In addition to client history, physical examination, and laboratory studies, the interview is used to determine the cause of and formulate a prognosis for the mental health disorder.

Individuals with severe or profound intellectual disabilities may experience greater difficulty in expressing their thoughts and feelings (Myrbakk & von Tetzchner, 2008) and screening may have to rely on reports of informants. As intellectual levels vary with degree of disability, the interviewer must adjust the language and tempo of interview to elicit the most accurate response. Treating an adult individual with IDD like their mental age is not productive or therapeutic and may elicit anger and other justifiably uncooperative behavior in response (Sadock & Sadock, 2003). Age-appropriate communication affords dignity and demonstrates respect.

Psychiatric Assessment Schedule for Adults with Developmental Disabilities   The Psychiatric Assessment Schedule for Adults with Developmental Disabilities 10 (PAS-ADD 10; Moss, Goldberg, Patel, Prosser, & Ibbotson, 1996) is a semistructured clinical diagnostic interview specifically designed to assist in clinical interviews for individuals with all levels of IDD. The 145-item instrument is both client and informant reported. A diagnosis derived from client interview may differ from a diagnosis derived from informant interview.

In the normative research, agreement between diagnoses derived from the interviews with the individuals with IDD and diagnoses derived from interviews with informants was 40.7%. In addition, 35.2% of diagnoses would have been missed if the interview with the individuals with IDD was not used (Moss, Prosser, Ibbotson, & Goldberg, 1996). With depression, the diagnosis of depression was derived from an informant interview for only 30.8% of the cases, in which a diagnosis of depression was derived from interviews with individuals with IDD (Ailey, 2009). The findings indicate that it is important that the interviewer speak directly with the individual with IDD whenever possible or practical. In some cases, it may be necessary to see the client with IDD while a family member or residential staff is present.

Behavioral Observations

Diagnosis of a mental health alteration should also rely on behavioral observations (American Academy of Child and Adolescent Psychiatry, 1999) and descriptions of behavior from informants including family, staff, and other supporting individuals. An individual with IDD exhibiting an episode of uncharacterized aggression may be experiencing a medication side effect or displaying irritability secondary to undiagnosed depression or other mood disorder. The clinician must gather all the relevant data and use diagnostic judgment to affect a definitive diagnosis.

Functional Analysis

A functional analysis approach or method may also be used to diagnose behavior disorders among individuals with IDD. The analysis focuses on the individual client and the identification of environmental and personal variables that influence or predispose challenging behaviors in the individual. Functional analysis methods include direct observation and measurement of challenging behavior. To be complete, these methods generally involve manipulation of an environmental variable under controlled conditions in an attempt to show a relationship between the environmental variable and the challenging behavior. If aggression was the challenging behavior, antecedents would be identified. It is also important to note the communicative intent, if any, of the behavior. This allows a positive behavior to be substituted in reaction to the antecedent. Behavioral management of disorders is improved with plans based on the hypotheses on the functions of behaviors.

Controversy exists among clinicians and researchers between the *DSM* and functional analysis methods. Behaviorists argue that the diagnostic concepts of the *DSM* system are more stigmatizing, less efficient, and more mechanistic than functional analysis (Andersson & Ghaderi, 2006). Combining *DSM-IV-TR* or *ICD-10* diagnosis with the contextual understanding of the individual's issues provided by functional analysis might lead to a more thorough understanding of the individual's disorder, resulting in better outcomes and a higher quality of life (Andersson & Ghaderi, 2006). However, Medicare/Medicaid and private insurance does not always reimburse for functional analysis.

PLANNING AND IMPLEMENTATION PROCESS

Planning and implementing the nursing and interdisciplinary treatment plan for mental health care of an individual with IDD requires understanding the client as a whole and the client in relation to their social and environmental conditions. Prioritizing nursing diagnoses, creating goals and objectives, managing medication, researching nonpharmacologic measures and alternative approaches, and using interdisciplinary approaches are all useful steps in the planning and implementation process.

Creating a Nursing Diagnosis

A nursing diagnosis uses patterns of client responses to a health alteration to identify a nurse-treatable cause and characterize related symptoms. When the alteration requires additional attention from another health care professional, the diagnosis becomes collaborative. Nursing diagnoses allow the practitioner to formulate an individualized plan of care. As with clients in the general population, nursing diagnoses also inform interdisciplinary treatment plans for individuals with IDD. Because these diagnoses are not medical, they help ensure the person-centeredness of mental health care for a client with IDD.

For an individual with autism spectrum disorder, a nursing diagnosis might reveal a risk for self-mutilation related to feelings of depression and psychogenic polypharmacy as evidenced by healing scratches and bite marks on arms. When an individual with IDD is hospitalized, the nursing diagnosis might note ineffective coping related to vulnerability secondary to developmental age and separation from familiar surroundings, as evidenced by uncharacteristic aggression and change in usual communication patterns.

Creating Goals and Objectives

Goals and objectives must be client-centered and measurable with both process and outcome measures. Goals guide the choice of intervention. For example, if the goal is related to reducing aggression or other challenging behaviors, the interventions might include ruling out physical problems that might contribute to aggression, exploring trigger points for anger, role playing to practice positive adaptive responses to anger, or medication review to determine if the behavior is a side effect of a particular drug.

Managing Medication

Another role for nurses in assessment, planning, and implementation of care is the assessment and monitoring of medications. As with the general population, mental health treatment for individuals with IDD may include pharmacological and/or psychosocial interventions. A combination of these interventions may be better than either alone.

A further aspect of the nursing assessment and treatment is to assess the rationale for psychoactive drugs. Individuals with IDD may be one of the most over-medicated populations (Holden & Gitlesen, 2004). A statewide survey conducted for the year 2000 found that 35.4% of individuals with IDD served in Oklahoma system received at least one psychoactive medication (Spreat, Conroy, & Fullerton, 2004), and Norwegian researchers found that 37% of individuals with IDD were prescribed psychoactive medications (Holden & Gitlesen, 2004). The Oklahoma study attributed the dramatic rise in the use of antidepressants to an increased use of selective serotonin reuptake inhibitors between 1994 and 2000. Spreat, Conroy, and Fullerton (2004) also found that when individuals with IDD were moved from an institutional to a community setting, they used more antipsychotics.

Behavior disorders are a common reason for prescribing psychotropic drugs. This marks an important difference from the prescribing practices for individuals without IDD. Despite changes to legislation and practice guidelines, a large portion of individuals with IDD and challenging behaviors remain subject to medication restraint (McGillivrary & McCabe, 2004). As with the general population, psychotropic drugs should only be prescribed to treat definite clinical symptoms and diagnoses (Matson et al., 2000; McGillivrary & McCabe, 2004). The use of psychotropic medication in the absence of sound clinical evidence is contrary to good clinical practice and amounts to chemical restraint (Matson et al., 2000). Key classes of psychotropic medications used with individuals with IDD include antipsychotics, anxiolytics, antidepressants, and mood stabilizers.

Antipsychotic Medications   In the general population, psychotropic medications are usually used to treat symptoms of schizophrenia. However, in individuals with IDD, psychotropics are frequently used to treat both psychotic disorders and nonpsychotic disorders, including behavior disorders. The use of psychoactive drugs to treat behavior disorders is controversial. Psychotropic therapies should not be employed for convenience of caregivers, but rather to improve quality of life for individuals with IDD (Tanaka, Aita, & Hirano, 2006).

A Cochrane systematic review of randomized clinical trials regarding the use of antipsychotic medications for behavior disorders of individuals with IDD found the results to be inconclusive (Brylewski & Duggan, 2004). Of the nine randomized controlled trials evaluated, no study demonstrated that antipsychotic medications clearly helped or harmed adults with intellectual disabilities and behavior issues. Tyer et al. (2008) demonstrated that risperidone and haloperidol were less effective than a placebo in curtailing challenging or aggressive behavior. This study recommended that antipsychotics should no longer be used as standard treatment for behavior disorders for individuals with IDD. Experts suggest that psychotropics may be helpful in managing acute behavior disorders, but adaptive behaviors and overall activity may also be reduced (Matson et al., 2000).

As severe and permanent side effects are associated with long-term use of psychotropics, a cautious approach is indicated. Individuals with IDD may be particularly sensitive to developing side effects such as tardive dyskinesia (Friedlander, Lazar, & Klancnik, 2001). In addition to frequent reevaluation of the appropriateness of psychotropic drug therapy nurses should routinely screening for movement disorders.

Antidepressant Medications   In the general population, antidepressants are used to treat depression and anxiety disorders and for smoking cessation. Antidepressives include selective serotonin reuptake inhibitors, tricyclic antidepressives, and monoamine oxidase inhibitors. Methodological problems exist with the research on use of antidepressants for individuals with IDD; thus, the results of existing studies warrant further investigation (Deb & Unwin, 2007).

Mood Stabilization Medications   Treatment of symptoms of bipolar disorders is the common usage of mood stabilizers. The classic drug of choice is lithium. Anticonvulsants such as carbamazepine, topiramate, and divalproex sodium have also been shown to have a mood-stabilizing effect in the general population (Stoner, Lea, Wolf, & Berges, 2005; Yerevanian, Koek, & Mintz, 2003). Again, challenging behaviors are a frequent reason for the use of mood-stabilizing drugs for individuals with IDD. Research on the use of mood stabilizers to manage challenging behaviors is limited and has methodological problems (Deb & Unwin, 2007).

Risks versus benefits should be considered with all medications. Efficacy, side effects, the potential of interaction with other drugs, and potential long-term effects of the drugs must continually be evaluated. The benefits and risks of particular drugs with specific syndromes should also be assessed. Medication errors remain an important concern (van de Bernt, Robertz, de Jong, van Roon, & Leufkens, 2007). Continual evaluation of medication management is part of planning overall care for individuals with IDD and mental health disorders.

Using Nonpharmacologic Approaches

For individuals with IDD, nonpharmacological treatments may be a useful adjunct or alternative when appropriate. These types of interventions assist in addressing behaviors, cognitive manifestations, and interpersonal factors in mental health disorders. Environmental management is an important first-line consideration. Interventions and treatment modalities should include the least restrictive setting for care. Creating a therapeutic atmosphere for an individual with IDD includes continuity of care. A known health care provider adds to a sense of comfort for that individual and affords a safe, stable environment for treatment. Continuity of care also affords the clinician the opportunity for thoughtful assessment to help identify and understand the root cause of a client's behavior.

Cognitive Behavioral Therapies
Cognitive behavioral therapies—in which changing or modifying thoughts, feelings, and attitudes are addressed—may offer benefits for individuals with mild and moderate IDD. Studies indicate that cognitive behavioral therapies are an effective anger management therapy for individuals with IDD (Taylor, Novaco, Gillmer, & Thorne, 2002). Using the stop-think-relax technique (Chapman, Sheclack, & France, 2006), a clinician may work with clients in an individual or group setting. This strategy teaches individuals with IDD and anger management or anxiety issues to identify the trigger or disquieting emotion (i.e., stop), consider alternatives to displaying anger (think), and engage in activities such as deep breathing or self-talk (relax).

Complementary and Alternative Treatments
In the general population, alternative therapies for mental health disorders such as meditation and exercise have shown potential benefits. Nutritional assessment and dietary considerations are part of good nursing care, but no methodologically sound studies support a specific nutritional intervention for mental and behavioral health disorders. Mindfulness training includes focused breathing, concentration on a single thought, and other meditative techniques. It has been used to help individuals with mild IDD control aggression (Singh et al., 2007). A study conducted in Israel found that physical activities including exercise improved the sense of well-being among older adults with mild IDD (Carmeli, Zinger-Vankin, Morad, & Merrick, 2004).

Case Management and Interdisciplinary Approaches

Nursing care for individuals with IDD requires work and coordination with the client, family members and significant others, various specialists, and community agency personnel. Similar to clients in the general population, individuals with IDD may have a number of physical and mental health complaints. The body–mind connection mandates that nursing interventions and treatment modalities address both somatic and psychological complaints. In that context, case management of individuals with IDD and mental health disorders involves working with other health-related disciplines, including primary care providers, neurologists, endocrinologists, sleep disorder specialists, nutritionists, psychologists, and psychiatrists along with families and community center or residential staff. The nurse may need to become the catalyst for the creation of an interdisciplinary team. Cutting across professional boundaries and establishing interdisciplinary affiliations affords the client with IDD the highest standard of care.

EVALUATION PROCESS

Evaluation is a standard in all practice settings. As with any other individual, when creating a plan for mental health care for individuals with IDD, properly defining measurable, expected outcomes are important. Evaluation involves describing and measuring the effect of the nursing intervention on the expected outcomes. For example, an individual might have depressive symptoms including change in appetite, decreased interest levels for usual activities, and sadness along with new behavior disorders. With successful nursing intervention and interdisciplinary treatment, expected outcomes might include reduction in depressive symptoms, a renewed interest in usual activities, and display of positive adaptive behaviors. If the depressive symptoms were intensified by physical health symptoms such as chronic pain, the care plan and treatment should focus on those symptoms too.

Some general issues should be kept in mind when evaluating care for individuals with IDD. Mental health disorders often negatively impact the ability of an individual with IDD to function as part of society. A commonly expected outcome would be to promote maximum functioning of the client. Evaluation of that outcome may include examination of school or work performance or social/family unit function to determine if it has improved or been enhanced. The outcome and evaluation measure should correlate with the life-span approach to treatment and care.

Other overall questions include whether the data collected were adequate and included feedback from other interdisciplinary team members, family, and community or residential staff; if the concerns of the individual and his/her family and staff were addressed; and whether the planning and implementation were mutual. Answering these questions speaks to a suggestion that nursing care and evaluation of service delivery for individuals with IDD should address that person's social presence, individual choice, meaningful characteristics and behaviors, positive image, and participatory abilities (Gilbert, Todd, & Jackson, 1998). In addition, providing culturally competent nursing care for individuals with IDD may be even more critical than for the general population. Cultural insensitivity in mainstream health care practice in conjunction with the stigma of IDD may add to the burden many families and care providers experience when caring for an individual with IDD (Nehring, 2007; O'Hara, 2003).

CONCLUSION

Nurses frequently serve as client advocates. This role may be crucial to ensure that individuals with IDD who also have mental health disorders receive adequate, comprehensive care. As agencies that provide services for individuals with IDD also begin to offer a social model of service delivery, nurses become "agents of social inclusion" (Gates, 2006, p. x) and positively affect access to care.

Nurses may also advocate for improved intervention and treatment models and a life-span approach to care. As a member of an interdisciplinary team that includes the client, family, staff, and other professionals, nurses are responsible for coordination of care, and in that leadership role can advocate for thorough evaluation, appropriate medication use, and appropriate psychosocial interventions for their clients.

REFERENCES

Ailey, S.H. (2009). Evaluating the sensitivity and specificity of depression screening tools among individuals with intellectual and developmental disabilities. *Journal of Mental Health Research in Intellectual Disability, 2*, 45–64.

Ailey, S.H., Marks, B.A., Crisp, C., & Hahn, J.E. (2003). Promoting sexuality across the lifespan for individuals with intellectual and developmental disabilities. *The Nursing Clinics of North America, 38*, 229–252.

Ailey, S.H., & Miller, A.M. (2004). Psychosocial theories of depression for individuals with intellectual and developmental disabilities: A historicist perspective. *Research and Theory in Nursing Practice, 18*, 131–148.

Ailey, S.H., Miller, A.M., Heller, T., & Smith, E.V., Jr. (2006). Evaluating an interpersonal model of depression with adults with Down syndrome. *Research and Theory in Nursing Practice, 20*, 229–246.

Ailey, S.H., O'Rourke, M., Breakwell, S., & Murphy, A. (2008). Supporting a community of individuals with intellectual and developmental disabilities in grieving. *Journal of Hospice & Palliative Nursing, 10*, 285–292.

Allen, D., & Davies, D. (2007). Challenging behavior and psychiatric disorder in intellectual disability. *Current Opinions in Psychiatry, 20*, 450–455.

American Academy of Child and Adolescent Psychiatry. (1999). Practice parameters for the assessment and treatment of children, adolescents, and adults with mental retardation and comorbid mental disorders. *Journal of the American Academy of Child and Adolescent Psychiatry, 38*, 5S–31S.

American Academy of Pediatrics. (2001). Assessment of maltreatment of children with disabilities. *Pediatrics, 108*, 508–512.

American Psychiatric Association. (2000). *Diagnostic and Statistical Manual of Mental Disorders IV Text Revision.* Washington, DC: American Psychiatric Association.

Andersson, A., & Ghaderi, A. (2006). Overview and analysis of the behaviourist criticism of the Diagnostic and Statistical Manual of Mental Disorders (DSM). *Clinical Psychologist, 10*, 67–77.

Atherton, H. (2006). Care planning for good health in intellectual disabilities. In B. Gates (Ed.). *Care planning and delivery in intellectual disability nursing* (pp. 257–276). Oxford, UK: Blackwell Publishing.

Aylott, J. (1999). Preventing rape and sexual assault of people with learning disabilities. *British Journal of Nursing, 8*, 871–874.

Bellon-Harn, M.L. (2005). Clinical management of a child with Prader-Willi syndrome form maternal uniparental disomy (UPD) genetic inheritance. *Journal of Communication Disorders, 38*, 459–472.

Benson, B.A., & Ivins, J. (1992). Anger, depression and self-concept in adults with mental retardation. *Journal of Intellectual Disability Research, 36*, 169–175.

Blacher, J., & McIntyre, L.L. (2006). Syndrome specificity and family impact. *Journal of Intellectual Disability Research, 50*, 184–198.

Braden, K. (2006). *Appendix D: Health disparities and mental retardation: Programs and creative strategies to close the gap.* Retrieved November 26, 2008, from http://www.nichd.nih.gov/publications/pubs/closingthegap/sub18.cfm.

Brown, M. (2005). Promoting health, supporting inclusion: Developments in the nursing and midwifery contributions to improving the health of people with intellectual disabilities in Scotland. *International Journal of Nursing in Intellectual and Developmental Disabilities, 2*, 3.

Brown, M., & Marshall, K. (2006). Cognitive behaviour therapy and people with learning disabilities: Implications for developing nursing practice. *Journal of Psychiatric and Mental Health Nursing, 13*, 234–241.

Brylewski, J., & Duggan, L. (2004). Antipsychotic medication for challenging behaviour in people with learning disability. *The Cochrane Database of Systematic Reviews, 3*, CD000377.

Caley, L.M., Shipkey, N., Winkleman, T., Dunlap, C., & Rivera, S. (2006). Evidence-based review of nursing interventions to prevent secondary disabilities in fetal alcohol spectrum disorder. *Pediatric Nursing, 32*, 155–162.

Carmeli, E., Zinger-Vankin, T., Morad, M., & Merrick, J. (2004). Can physical training have an effect on well-being in adults with mild intellectual disability? *Mechanisms of Aging and Development, 126,* 299–304.

Chapman, R.A., Sheclack, K.J., & France, J. (2006). Stop-Think-Relax: An adapted self-control training strategy for individuals with mental retardation and coexisting psychiatric illness. *Cognitive and Behavioral Practice, 13,* 205–214.

Charlot, L., Fox, S., Silka, V.R., Hurley, A., Lowry, M., & Pary, R. (2007). Mood disorders. In R. Fletcher, E. Laschen, C. Stavrakaki, & M. First (Eds.), *Diagnostic Manual-Intellectual Disability: A textbook of mental disorders in persons with intellectual disability* (pp. 271–316). Kingston, NY: NADD Press.

Clark, L.A., Watson, D., & Reynolds, S. (1995). Diagnosis and classification of psychopathology: Challenges to the current system and future direction. *Annual Review of Psychology, 46,* 121–153.

Cohen-Kerem, R., Bar-Oz, B., Nulman, I., Papaioannou, V.A., & Koren, G. (2007). Hearing in children with fetal alcohol spectrum disorder (FASD). *Canadian Journal of Clinical Pharmacology, 14,* e307–e312.

Cooray, S., Gabriel, S. & Gaus, V. (2007). Anxiety disorders. In R. Fletcher, E. Laschen, C. Stavrakaki, & M. First (Eds.), *Diagnostic Manual-Intellectual Disability: A textbook of mental disorders in persons with intellectual disability* (pp. 317–348). Kingston, NY: NADD Press.

Cuthill, F.M., Espie, C.A., & Cooper, S.A. (2003). Development and psychometric properties of the Glasgow Depression Scale for people with a learning disability: Individual and carer supplement versions. *British Journal of Psychiatry, 182,* 347–353.

Dagnan, D., & Sandhu, S. (1999). Social comparison, self-esteem and depression in people with intellectual disability. *Journal of Intellectual Disability Research, 43,* 372–379.

Deb, S., & Unwin, G.L. (2007). Psychotropic medication for behaviour problems in people with intellectual disability: A review of the current literature. *Current Opinion in Psychiatry, 20,* 461–466.

Drew, C.J., & Hardman, M.L. (2007). *Intellectual disabilities across the lifespan* (9th ed.). Upper Saddle River, NJ: Prentice Hall.

Doyle, C., & Mitchell, D. (2003). Post-traumatic stress disorder and people with learning disabilities: A literature based discussion. *Journal of Intellectual Disabilities, 7,* 23–33.

Esbensen, A.J., Seltzer, M.M., & Greenberg, J.S. (2005). Psychometric evaluation of a self-report measure of depression for individuals with mental retardation. *American Journal on Mental Retardation, 110,* 469–481.

Fletcher, R. (2008). *Dual diagnosis: Serving consumers with intellectual disability and mental illness.* Retrieved on July 2, 2009 from http://thenationalcouncil.net/Handouts08/handouts/E02-Milius-Fletcher-1.pdf.

Fletcher, R., Loschen, E., Stavrakaki, C., & First, M. (Eds.). (2007). *Diagnostic manual–intellectual disability (DM-ID): A textbook of diagnosis of mental disorders in persons with intellectual disability.* Kingston, NY: NADD Press.

Friedlander, R., Lazar, S., & Klancnik, J. (2001). Atypical antipsychotic use in treating adolescents and young adults with developmental disabilities. *Canadian Journal of Psychiatry, 46,* 741–745.

Furey, E. (1994). Sexual abuse of adults with mental retardation: Who and where. *Mental Retardation, 32,* 173–180.

Gates, B. (2006). Preface. In B. Gates (Ed.), *Care planning and delivery in intellectual disability nursing* (p. x). Oxford, UK: Blackwell Publishing.

Gilbert, T., Todd, M., & Jackson, N. (1998). People with learning disabilities who also have mental health problems: Practice issues and directions for learning disability nursing. *Journal of Advanced Nursing, 20,* 1151–1157.

Harris, J.C. (2006). Family, psychoeducational, behavioral, interpersonal and pharmacologic interventions. In J.C. Harris (Ed.), *Intellectual disability: Understanding its causes, classification, evaluation, and treatment* (pp. 289–332). New York: Oxford University Press.

Heuther, S. (2004). Alterations of hormone regulation. In S. Heuther & K.L. McCance

(Eds.), *Understanding pathophysiology* (3rd ed., pp. 481–484). St. Louis: Mosby.

Holden, B., & Gitlesen, J.P. (2004). Psychotropic medication in adults with mental retardation: Prevalence and prescription practices. *Research in Developmental Disabilities, 25,* 509–521.

Holin, P., & Udwin, O. (2006). Outcome in adult life for people with Williams syndrome—results from a survey of 239 families. *Journal of Intellectual Disability Research, 50,* 151–160.

Hollins, S., & Esterhuyzen, A. (1997). Bereavement and grief in adults with learning disabilities. *British Journal of Psychiatry, 170,* 497–501.

Jahoda, A., & Markova, I. (2004). Coping and social stigma: People with intellectual disabilities moving from institutions and family home. *Journal of Intellectual Disability Research, 48,* 719–729.

Kazdin, A.E., Matson, J.L., & Senatore, V. (1983). Assessment of depression in mentally retarded adults. *American Journal of Psychiatry, 140,* 1040–1043.

Lee, P., & Friedlander, R. (2007). Attention-deficit and disruptive behavior disorders. In R. Fletcher, E. Laschen, C. Stavrakaki, & M. First (Eds.), *Diagnostic Manual–Intellectual Disability: A textbook of mental disorders in persons with intellectual disability* (pp. 127–144). Kingston, NY: NADD Press.

Lundstrom, M., Saveman, B.I., Eisemann, M., & Astrom, S. (2007). Prevalence of violence and its relation to caregivers' demographics and emotional reactions: An explorative study of caregivers working in group homes for persons with learning disabilities. *Scandinavian Journal of Caring Sciences, 21,* 84–90.

MacHale, R., & Carvey, S. (2002). An investigation of the effects of bereavement on the mental health and challenging behaviour in adults with learning disability. *British Journal of Learning Disabilities, 30,* 113–117.

Mason, J., & Scior, K. (2004). "Diagnostic overshadowing" amongst clinicians working with people with intellectual disabilities in the UK. *Journal of Applied Research in Intellectual Disabilities, 17,* 85–90.

Matson, J.L., Bamburg, J.W., Matville, E.A., Pinkston, J., Bielecki, J., Kuhn, D., et al.,

(2000). Psychopharmacology and mental retardation: A 10 year review (1990–1999). *Research in Developmental Disabilities, 21,* 263–296.

McCarthy, M., & Thompson, D. (1997). A prevalence study of sexual abuse of adults with intellectual disabilities referred for sex education. *Journal of Applied Research in Intellectual Disabilities, 10,* 105–124.

McGillicuddy, N.B. (2006). A review of substance use research among those with mental retardation. *Mental Retardation and Developmental Disabilities Research Reviews, 12,* 41–47.

McGillicuddy, N.B., & Blane, H.T. (1999). Substance use in individuals with mental retardation. *Addictive Behaviors, 24,* 869–878.

McGillivrary, J.A., & McCabe, M.P. (2004). Pharmacological management of challenging behavior of individuals with intellectual disability. *Research in Developmental Disabilities, 25,* 523–537.

McKinney, E.S., James, S.R., Murray, S.S., & Ashwill, J.W. (2005). The child with a cognitive impairment. In E.S. McKinney, S.R. James, S.S. Murray, & J.W. Ashwill (Eds.), *Maternal child nursing* (2nd ed., pp. 1561–1579). St. Louis: Elsevier Science.

Minihan, P.M. (1999). Smoking policies and practices in a state-supported residential system for people with mental retardation. *American Journal of Mental Retardation, 104,* 131–142.

Minihan, P.M. (2003). *Compliance is not enough: Smoking policies in state mental retardation and developmental disabilities agencies.* Unpublished doctoral dissertation, Brandeis University.

Moseley, C. (2004). *NASDDDS Technical Report: Survey on state strategies for supporting individuals with co-existing conditions.* Retrieved September 23, 2007, from http://www.nasddds.org/pdf/NTRCoexistingConditions.pdf.

Moss, S., Goldberg, D., Patel, P., Prosser, H., & Ibbotson, S. (1996). *The psychiatric assessment schedule for adults with a developmental disability (PAS-ADD 10): Manual.* Manchester, UK: Hester Adrian Research Centre and the Institute of Psychiatry.

Moss, S., Prosser, H., Ibbotson, B., & Goldberg, D. (1996). Respondent and informant accounts of psychiatric symptoms in a sample of patients with learning disability. *Journal of Intellectual Disability Research, 40,* 457–465.

Myrbakk, E., & von Tetzchner, S. (2008). Screening individuals with intellectual disability for psychiatric disorders: Comparison of four measures. *American Journal on Mental Retardation, 113,* 54–70.

National Institute of Neurological Disorders and Stroke. (2001). *Emotional and behavioral health in persons with mental retardation/developmental disabilities: Research challenges and opportunities.* Retrieved September 23, 2007, from http://www.ninds .nih.gov/news_and_events/proceedings/ Emotional_Behavioral_Health_2001.htm.

Nehring, W. (2007). Cultural considerations for children with intellectual and developmental disabilities. *Journal of Pediatric Nursing, 22,* 93–102.

Nettlebeck, T., & Wilson, C. (2002). Personal vulnerability to victimization of people with mental retardation. *Trauma, Violence & Abuse, 3,* 289–306.

Nezu, A., Ronan, G.F., Meadows, F.A., & McClure, K.S. (Eds.). (2000). *Practitioner's guide to empirically-based measures of depression.* New York: Kluwer Academic/Plenum Publishers.

Nezu, C.M., Nezu, A.M., Rothenberg, J.L., DelliCarpini, L., & Groag, I. (1995). Depression in adults with mild mental retardation: Are cognitive variables involved? *Cognitive Therapy and Research, 19,* 227–239.

O'Hara, J. (2003). Learning disabilities and ethnicity: Achieving cultural competence. *Advances in Psychiatric Treatment, 9,* 166–174.

Palmer, L., Llanos, K., Tobias, C., & Bella, M. (2006). *Integrated care program: Performance measures recommendations.* Retrieved September 23, 2007, from http://www.chcs .org/publications3960/publications_show .htm?doc_id=379026.

Reiss, S. (1988). *Reiss Screen for maladaptive behaviors: Test manual* (2nd ed.). Worthington, OH: IDS Publishing.

Reiss, S., Levitan, G.W., & Szyszko, J. (1982). Emotional disturbance and mental retardation: Diagnostic overshadowing. *American Journal of Mental Deficiency, 86,* 567–574.

Reiss, S., & Szyszko, J. (1983). Diagnostic overshadowing and professional experience with mentally retarded persons. *American Journal of Mental Deficiency, 87,* 396–402.

Reiss, S., & Valenti-Hein, D. (1990). Development of a psychopathology rating scale for children with mental retardation. *Journal of Consulting and Clinical Psychology, 62,* 28–33.

Royal College of Psychiatrists. (2001). *Diagnostic criteria for psychiatric disorders for use with adults with learning disabilities/mental retardation (DC/LD).* London: Gaskell.

Ryan, R. (1994). Post-traumatic stress disorder in persons with developmental disabilities. *Community Mental Health Journal, 30,* 45–53.

Sadock, B.J., & Sadock, V.A. (2003). Mental retardation. In B.J. Sadock & V.A. Sadock (Eds.), *Synopsis of psychiatry: Behavioral sciences/clinical psychiatry* (9th ed., pp. 1161–1179). Philadelphia: Lippincott Williams & Wilkins.

Sequeira, H., Howlin, P., & Hollins, S. (2003). Clinical effects of sexual abuse on people with learning disability. *The British Journal of Psychiatry, 182,* 13–19.

Singh, N.N., Lancioni, G.E., Winton, A.S.W., Adkins, A.D., Singh, J., & Singh, A.N. (2007). Mindfulness training assists individuals with moderate mental retardation to maintain their community placements. *Behavior Modification, 31,* 800–814.

Smiley, E. (2005). Epidemiology of mental health problems in adults with learning disability: An update. *Advances in Psychiatric Treatment, 11,* 214–222.

Sovner, R., & Pary, R.J. (1993). Affective disorders in developmentally disabled persons. In J.L. Matson & R.P. Barrett (Eds.), *Psychopathology in the mentally retarded* (pp. 87–147). Needham Heights, MA: Allyn & Bacon.

Spreat, S., Conroy, J.W., & Fullerton, A. (2004). Statewide longitudinal survey of psychotropic medication use for persons with mental retardation: 1994 to 2000. *American Journal on Mental Retardation, 109,* 322–331.

Stoner, S.C., Lea, J.W., Wolf, A.L.,& Berges, A.A.(2005). Levetiracetam for mood stabilization and maintenance of seizure control following multiple treatment failures. *Annals of Pharmacotherapy, 39,* 1928–1931.

Strohmer, D.C., & Prout, H.T. (1998). *Strohmer-Prout Behavior Rating Scale.* Schenectady, NY: Genium Publishing.

Stromsness, M. (1993). Sexually abused women with mental retardation: Hidden victims, absent resources. *Women and Therapy, 14,* 139–152.

Tanaka, K., Aita, C., & Hirano, M. (2006). Clinical characteristics and pharmacotherapy of extremely disruptive behavior disorders in people with mental retardation. *No To Hattatsu, 38,* 19–24.

Taylor, J.L., Novaco, R.W., Gillmer, B., & Thorne, I. (2002). Cognitive-behavioural treatment of anger intensity among offenders with intellectual disabilities. *Journal of Applied Research in Intellectual Disabilities, 15,* 151–165.

Taylor, N.S., Standen, P.J., Cutajar, P., Fox, D., & Wilson, D.N. (2004). Smoking prevalence and knowledge of associated risks in adult attenders at day care centers for people with learning disabilities. *Journal of Intellectual Disability Research, 48,* 239–244.

Tracy, J., & Hosken, R. (1997). The importance of smoking education and preventative health strategies for people with intellectual disability. *Journal of Intellectual Disability Research, 41,* 416–421.

Tsai, S.W., Wu, S.K., Liou, Y.M., & Shu, S.G. (2008). Early development in Williams syndrome. *Pediatrics International: Official Journal of the Japan Pediatrics Society, 59,* 221–224.

Turk, J., Robbins, I., & Woodhead, M.

(2005). Post-traumatic stress disorder in young people with intellectual disability. *Journal of Intellectual Disability Research, 49,* 872–875.

Tyer, P., Oliver-Africano, P.C., Ahmed, Z., Bouras, N., Cooray, S., & Deb, S., et al. (2008). Risperidone, haloperidol, and placebo in the treatment of aggressive challenging behaviours in patients with intellectual disability: A randomized controlled trial. *The Lancet, 371,* 57–63.

van de Bernt, P.M.L.A., Robertz, R., de Jong, A.L., van Roon, E.N., & Leufkens, H.G.M. (2007). Drug administration errors in an institution for individuals with intellectual disability: An observational study. *Journal of Intellectual Disability Research, 51,* 528–536.

Whittington, A., & Burns, J. (2005). The dilemmas of residential care staff working with the challenging behaviour of people with learning disabilities. *British Journal of Clinical Psychology, 44,* 59–76.

World Health Organization. (2007). *The ICD-10 classification of mental health and behavioral disorders: Clinical descriptions and diagnostic guidelines.* Geneva: Author.

Yerevanian B.I., Koek, R.J. & Mintz, J. (2003). Lithium, anticonvulsants and suicidal behavior in bipolar disorder. *Journal of Affective Disorders, 73,* 223-228.

Zigler, E., Bennett-Gates, D., & Hodapp, R.M. (1999). Assessing personality traits of individuals with mental retardation. In E. Zigler & D. Bennett-Gates (Eds.), *Personality development in individuals with mental retardation.* (pp. 206–225). New York: Cambridge University Press.

CHAPTER *15*

Autism

Jean E. Beatson

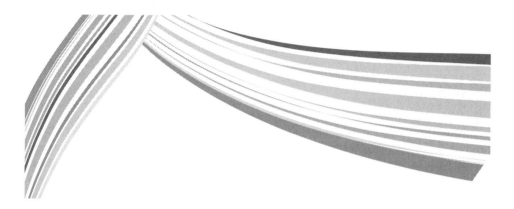

The term *autism spectrum disorders* (ASDs) refers to a group of developmental disabilities for which there is no known etiology or cure to date (Association of University Centers on Disabilities [AUCD], 2008). ASDs cross all cultural, ethnic, and socioeconomic groups, occurring in boys four times more than in girls (Centers for Disease Control and Prevention [CDC], 2009). The onset is usually before 3 years of age and lasts throughout the life span.

Since first being described in the 1940s, the conceptualization of autism has changed over time and is now considered to be a spectrum of disorders (Prelock & Contompasis, 2006). Although trends in diagnosis, assessment, and intervention in autism continue to evolve, the core impairments first described by Kanner (1943) remain relevant. Individuals with ASDs demonstrate impairment in some or all of the following areas: communication, social interaction, play, and behavior (Whalen & Schreibman, 2003). Although understood as a behavior disorder that is diagnosed clinically, research is uncovering a genetic and neurological basis for ASDs (Fombonne, 2008; Prelock & Contompasis, 2006).

There is marked variance in the expression of symptoms, making diagnosis, assessment, and intervention very challenging (Prelock & Contompasis, 2006). Individuals affected by ASDs can range from being extremely gifted to severely impaired (AUCD, 2008). Because of the complexities in etiology, screening, diagnosis, symptomology, assessment, and intervention, an interdisciplinary and collaborative teaming approach is the best model for providing care to individuals with complex needs, such as those with ASDs (Prelock & Vargas, 2004). Experts agree that early identification and intervention is critical to enhancing outcomes for individuals with ASDs (AUCD, 2008).

This chapter provides information on the definitions, incidence, prevalence, and impact of ASDs. The current thinking in the pathophysiology of ASDs is presented, followed by interdisciplinary approaches to care across the life span. The chapter concludes with a discussion of the importance and relevance for nursing in caring for individuals affected by ASDs and their families.

DEFINITIONS

ASDs are currently defined as a group of related disorders, including classic autism or autistic disorder, pervasive developmental disorder-not otherwise specified (PDD-NOS), and Asperger syndrome (CDC, 2009; Prelock & Contompasis, 2006). Along with Rett syndrome and childhood disintegrative disorder (CDD), these disorders are included in the broad category of pervasive developmental disabilities. Although the disorders share many features, they differ in onset, expression, and severity. Each is more fully described below.

Classic Autism

Classic autism, or autistic disorder, is characterized as a marked impairment in communication, as well as an impairment in the ability to develop peer relationships, share enjoyment or interests with others, initiate social interactions, and participate in imaginative play (American Psychiatric Association [APA], 2000). Individuals with classic autism may also demonstrate stereotypical behaviors that are repetitive, such as hand flapping or spinning. There are delays in social communication and interaction before 3 years of age, and Rett syndrome or CDD have been ruled out.

Pervasive Developmental Disorder-Not Otherwise Specified

A diagnosis of PDD-NOS is used when the criteria cannot be met for a specific pervasive developmental disorder, schizophrenia, schizotypal personality disorder, or avoidant personality disorder (APA, 2000). There is a severe and pervasive impairment in the development of reciprocal social interaction and communication skills or the presence of stereotyped behavior, interests, and activities. This category includes atypical autism. This diagnosis is used when the criteria cannot be met for autistic disorder because of late age at onset, atypical symptomology, or subthreshold symptomology, or all of these.

Asperger Syndrome

Asperger syndrome is characterized by a qualitative impairment in social interaction and restrictive or repetitive behaviors (APA, 2000). There are also significant impairments in occupational or social functioning. Unique to Asperger syndrome, however, is that there is no clinically significant language delay or cognitive impairment. Individuals with Asperger syndrome develop typical self-help skills and curiosity.

Rett Syndrome

The characteristics of Rett syndrome differ from autism disorder and others on the autism spectrum. The child develops typically up to 5 months of age, at which time there is a decrease in head circumference and psychomotor development (APA, 2000). Between 5 and 30 months there is a loss of hand skills, with noted hand wringing. Other symptoms include severe impairments in communication and interest in social interaction.

Childhood Disintegrative Disorder

Children diagnosed with CDD demonstrate typical development for at least the first 2 years of age, having a later onset than Rett syndrome or autistic disorder (APA, 2000). There is a clinically significant loss of skills manifested before age 10 in at least two of the following areas: language, play, bowel or bladder control, social skills or motor skills. There are also qualitative impairments in two of the three areas: social interaction, communication, and repetitive and stereotypical patterns of behavior including motor patterns. CDD is rare and associated with a poor prognosis (Prelock & Contompasis, 2006).

INCIDENCE AND PREVALENCE

The Autism and Developmental Disabilities Monitoring Network is a set of programs funded through the CDC for the purpose of monitoring the prevalence of (i.e., the percentage of the population with) ASDs in the United States (CDC, 2009). Prevalence reports are issued periodically. The first two prevalence reports were issued in 2007 and reported on data gathered in 2000 and 2002. Prevalence for ASDs was estimated at 6.6 and 6.7 per 1,000 in 2000 and 2002, respectively (More recently, the CDC reported a prevalence rate of approximately 1 in 150 children)—a significantly higher number than previously cited (CDC, 2009). The publication of the report sparked media uproar, focusing the public spotlight on the incidence and impact of ASDs (Autism Society of America [ASA], 2008).

It is commonly accepted that the prevalence of ASDs has increased over the years, from British studies in 1970s that estimated a prevalence of 0.2% to recent estimates of 0.7% (Fombonne, 2008). However, there is much discussion within the media and the research community about whether the incidence (i.e., the number of individuals with ASDs) is rising within the population. Known explanations regarding the increase in prevalence in ASDs includes more accurate diagnostic tools, medical professionals who are better trained at diagnosis, broader definitions of ASDs, and inclusion of comorbidities, such as intellectual and developmental disabilities (Fombonne, 2008; Prelock & Contompasis, 2006). The debate over whether there is an increase in incidence remains unanswered, pointing to the need for further research (Fombonne, 2008). Current research is looking at genetic and environmental impacts. To date, the role of environmental toxins related to incidence is unknown.

Worldwide population-based studies estimate the prevalence of ASDs to be 2–6 per 1,000 children (American Academy of Pediatrics [AAP], 2004; Fombonne, 2003; Yeargin-Allsopp et al., 2003). Although there are variations from place to place, it appears as if the prevalence of ASDs is similar in the United States and worldwide.

IMPACT

Regardless of the incidence debate, the impact of the rising prevalence of ASDs is felt by systems of care, providers, and most importantly, individuals affected by ASDs and their families. Currently, the ASA estimates that the lifetime cost of caring for a child with autism ranges from $3.5 million to $5 million, and that the United States is facing almost $90 billion annually in costs for autism. This figure includes research, insurance costs and noncovered expenses, Medicaid waivers for autism, educational spending, housing, transportation, employment, therapeutic services, and caregiver costs (ASA, 2008).

The impact on providers is broad, from pediatricians being presented with children with atypical development to school-based providers designing and implementing programs for children with ASDs. Physicians are often presented with a complex set of issues and symptoms from which they are to make a differential diagnosis (Prelock & Vargas, 2004). In addition, the AAP, American Academy of Family Physicians, and others issued a joint statement on the intent for all primary care practices to provide a medical home for their patients and families (AAP, 2008). Medical home principles include care that is culturally competent, family-centered, and coordinated across complex systems of care for patients and families throughout the life span. These added competencies, skills, and services that primary health care providers need to learn and institutionalize in their practices create challenges in implementation of a medical home primary care practice (Contompasis & Prelock, 2006). For more information on medical home principles, refer to Chapter 2.

The pressure is intense for early intervention to provide comprehensive interdisciplinary programs to address the complex needs of children with ASDs and their families (Smith & Dillenbeck, 2006). In addition, most preservice programs focus on discipline-specific knowledge and skills, with less emphasis on family-centered care, collaborative teaming, or cultural competence (Beatson, 2006). Health care providers should keep current with training in assessment and intervention in ASDs, despite increasing case loads and limited resources (Beatson, 2008; Beatson & Prelock, 2002).

The impact of ASDs on families is all encompassing. Families often feel disengaged and disempowered from the systems with which they need to interact (Beatson & Prelock, 2002). At times, they feel socially isolated because the behavior of their child with ASD prevents them from enjoying their usual activities or traveling. Families of children with ASDs must focus their resources on helping their children, at times to the exclusion of other priorities or family activities (ASA, 2008). Every member of the family is affected.

For individuals with ASDs, the world is a chaotic and confusing place. Sean Baron, an individual with ASD, described it this way: "I've spent nearly 10 years sharing with numerous audiences my experiences from the inside, specifically many of my struggles to merely make sense of a chaotic world, let alone fit into it" (Prelock, 2006, p. xvi). Also, many adults on the autism spectrum are fully able to work but often do not get the opportunity to do so (Jarbrink, McCrone, Fombonne, Zanden, & Knapp, 2007). Unemployment creates social isolation, as well as costs to the individual and society. There is a need for more supported employment programs to help individuals with ASDs and employers fill this gap.

PATHOPHSYIOLOGY

Much is still being learned about the pathophysiology of ASDs. Questions regarding the rate of autism in the population, the role of genetics, the genetic–environmental link, specific areas of brain involvement, and etiology are driving research related to the pathophysiology of ASDs (Szpir, 2006). Still more is unknown about assessment and intervention than the brain abnormalities, genetics, and etiology

(Prelock & Contompasis, 2006). It is an exciting and dynamic research era for those impacted by ASDs. This section presents current information on brain abnormalities in ASDs, genetics, and etiology.

Brain Abnormalities

Early brain studies in those with ASDs showed a general increase in brain size, with a smaller corpus callosum (Prelock & Contompasis, 2006). Research is revealing brain abnormalities and genetic links in those with autism (Szpir, 2006).The neuropathology indicates prenatal abnormal brain development, perhaps occurring at or shortly after conception (Fombonne, 2008). Earlier brain studies failed to report consistent neurological findings. However, with improved brain imaging techniques, including positron emission tomography, single photon emission tomography (SPECT), and functional magnetic resonance imaging (MRI), specific links between brain and behavior are being suggested (Zilbovicius, Meresse, & Boddaert, 2006). Temporal lobe abnormalities are being shown in children with autism, with decreased grey matter in the superior temporal sulcus. Initial studies suggest a correlation between severity of autistic syndromes and cerebral blood flow (Zilbovicius et al., 2006). Temporal regions abnormalities are thought to impact perception, cognition, and emotion, which are relevant domains of ASDs. The temporal lobe is considered to be central to sensory processing as well, another area of impairment to ASDs. These areas all impact the way in which a person decodes experiences and makes meaning of the world.

The first SPECT study suggests abnormal cortical activation in the left temporal cortex resulting in differences in recognizing and responding to auditory input (Zilbovicius et al., 2006). In their review of the literature, Zilbovicius et al. (2006) found that early studies using functional MRI suggested abnormal brain responses in face and voice perception. It appears that many of the significant impairments in ASDs can be linked to brain abnormalities and/or differences in activation of specific brain centers.

Genetics

There is increasing evidence for a strong genetic basis in ASDs (Fombonne, 2008). Twin studies have been particularly compelling. If one identical twin has ASD, it is very likely the other one will also have ASD, or at least some autistic symptoms (Volkmar & Wiesner, 2004). The rate of autism is clearly increased in siblings as well. Multiple genes seem to be involved as well as several chromosomes (Volkmar & Wiesner, 2004). It is hoped that in the next few years, a genetic cause for autism can be found.

Etiology

The precise cause(s) of autism are still unknown (Prelock & Contompasis, 2006; Volkmar & Wiesner, 2004). As discussed, brain abnormalities and genetic links have been clearly demonstrated; however, to date, they do not fully explain the etiology of ASDs. There is some thought that a genetic predisposition can be unlocked by environmental toxins or early birth difficulties, yet that evidence is still not established. To complicate matters more, different types of ASDs may have different etiologies, with perhaps the most being known about autism (Volkmar & Wiesner, 2004).

Immunizations

The public perception of the measles, mumps, and rubella (MMR) vaccine causing an expression of autism led to a series of studies trying to establish a causal relationship (Doja & Roberts, 2006; Volkmar & Wiesner, 2004). Also, there was concern that thimerosal, a mercury additive in vaccines, was responsible for the potential link between immunizations and onset of autism. In both incidences, no link was established between immunizations and autism (Doja & Roberts, 2006; Fitzpatrick, 2007). However, because of the general toxic nature of mercury, thimerosal has been eliminated in the MMR and other vaccines. Since thimerosal was discontinued in vaccines, the autism prevalence still continued to rise, thereby lending more credence to the evidence that it did not cause an increase in autism (Fitzpatrick, 2007; Rutter, 2005; Silverman, 2009).

Comorbidities

Various medical disorders are associated with, but not known to cause, autism. These include seizure disorder, intellectual disability, fragile X syndrome, disruptions of metabolism, tuberous sclerosis, and congenital rubella (Volkmar & Wiesner, 2004). Many of these disorders can result in moderate to severe intellectual disabilities; therefore, children may be diagnosed as having autism when they have autistic characteristics perhaps related to their cognitive disability. There is variance among clinicians when diagnosing autism, with some taking a broad view of the criteria and others rather a strict one.

The CDC's Centers for Autism and Developmental Disabilities Surveillance and Epidemiology are collaborating on a research study called the "Study to Explore Early Development." Its purpose is to enhance our understanding of risk factors, causes, and hopefully, prevention of autism (CDC, 2009).

SYMPTOMOLOGY AND CLINICAL MANIFESTATIONS

ASDs are characterized by impairments in social interaction, communication, narrow or unusual interests, and stereotypical motor patterns and sensory differences (Prelock & Contompasis, 2006). There is great variance in the preponderance of these impairments depending on which ASD the individual has and also among individuals in each category. This more fully discussed in the section on diagnosis.

Up to 70% of individuals on the autism spectrum have cognitive limitations (Volkmar & Wiesner, 2004). They may also have *scatter skills,* meaning they can be competent at one skill, such as puzzles, but very limited in others. The presence of scatter skills differentiates individuals on the autism spectrum from those with a primary diagnosis of intellectual disability.

Social Interaction

Children and individuals on the autism spectrum experience difficulties in perceiving the social and emotional responses of others (Prelock, 2006). This can be manifested by indifference to others or socially inappropriate responses to a situation, such as laughing at a funeral. They seem to prefer to be alone and not have similar needs for socialization as neurotypical individuals. The social world is mysterious and confusing to individuals on the autism spectrum. Interventions that focus on social interaction and exploration of emotions are critical.

Communication

Communication difficulties are a central impairment in ASDs (Volkmar & Wiesner, 2004). The *Diagnostic and Statistical Manual of Mental Disorders, Fourth Edition, Text Revision* (*DSM-IV-IR*; APA, 2000) describes the communication impairment as a delay or lack of verbal language, impairment in the ability to initiate or maintain communication, repetitive or idiosyncratic use of language (echolalia), and lack of pretend play. Individuals on the autism spectrum can range from being nonverbal to being highly verbal but coupled with the inability to read another person's body language or facial cues. Speech patterns are also different (Volkmar & Wiesner, 2004) and may sound more robotic and echolalic. Communication intervention may initially focus on establishing verbal language skills. If verbal language does not develop, alternative modes of communication will need to be targeted.

Narrow or Unusual Interests

Individuals on the autism spectrum have very focused interests (e.g., dinosaurs, trains) and will not be motivated to share another's interests or participate in group activities on a different topic (Prelock, 2006). They tend to exhibit a lack of flexibility, preferring strict routines. This impairment is problematic for children with ASDs when they are learning to play with other children. Play development is crucial to teaching communication and social interaction skills.

Motor Patterns and Sensory Differences

Usually, there are marked differences in the sensory and motor expression of individuals with ASDs. Stereotypical motor patterns may include hand flapping, hand wringing, swinging, or spinning (Dennis, Edelman, & Prelock, 2006). There may be balance or coordination difficulties. Motor planning may be affected; for example, a child may not know what to do first when putting on a pair of pants. There may be marked differences in regulating sensory input in any of the senses: smell, hearing, taste, visual, touch, pain reaction, and/or sight. Individuals may be hypo- or hypersensitive. Interventions often need to include sensory accommodations so that affected individuals can manage the daily sensory input and function across environments.

INTERDISICPLINARY APPROACHES TO CARE

It is commonly accepted that an interdisciplinary approach to care for individuals and families affected by developmental disabilities, including ASDs, is best practice (O'Rourke & Dennis, 2004). The array of clinical manifestations of ASDs requires a team approach to ensure that the complexities are addressed appropriately (Prelock, 2006). This section will address the theoretical frameworks of family-centered care, cultural competence, collaborative teaming, and the nursing process. Information on assessment and diagnosis will be presented, followed by intervention and care through the life span.

Theoretical Frameworks

Integrating the theoretical frameworks of family-centered care, cultural competence, and interdisciplinary collaborative teaming within clinical practice prepares service providers to address the complexities of caring for individuals and families affected by neurodevelopmental disabilities, including ASDs (Prelock & Vargas, 2004). The nursing process of care lends itself well to these frameworks, providing the lens through which nurses can become vital team members (Wright & Leahey, 2005). Family-centered care, cultural competence, interdisciplinary collaboration, and the nursing process are the theoretical frameworks embedded in the discussion on assessment, diagnosis, intervention, and care of individuals with ASDs and their families across the life span. Each framework is discussed below.

Family-Centered Care
Family-centered care is at the core of service provision, recognizing that families are consistent in an individual's life, while service providers come and go (Shelton & Stepanek, 1995). Family-centered care has as its focus respect and honor for the family's values and choices (Dunst, Trivette, & Hamby, 2007; Wright & Leahey, 2005). The ability to form trusting family/professional partnerships is crucial to being a family-centered nurse. Other key elements of family-centered care include unbiased information sharing, being flexible and accessible, and honoring cultural differences (Shelton & Stepanek, 1995). When families receive family-centered services they feel empowered and function as active and important members of the team (Beatson & Prelock, 2002). Providers who practice family-centered care feel authentically connected to families and better situated to collaboratively create meaningful care plans (Beatson, 2008). Closely related to family-centered care is cultural competence.

Cultural Competence
Before discussing cultural competence, one must understand the pervasive nature of culture. Every human being is raised and lives within a cultural framework, of which they may or may not be aware (Vargas & Beatson, 2004). It is a worldview shaped through the interplay of religion, ethnicity, race, environment, language, beliefs, customs, and habits. Culture is dynamic and ever changing. It influences roles people assume, as well as how they define family, daily habits, childrearing, family decision making, and health care practices.

Cultural competence is the journey of learning how to work effectively with individuals with a cultural worldview different from one's own (Vargas & Beatson, 2004). It has been shown that when health care providers do not practice cultural and linguistic competence, devastating health outcomes may result (Fadiman, 1997). *Linguistic competence* refers to ensuring that appropriate language interpretation and written translation is used for those with limited English proficiency or low literacy levels.

Health care professions also have a culture unique to their discipline (Kalyanpur & Harry, 1999; Vargas & Beatson, 2004). Many of the disciplines have within their origins some roots in the Western medical model. Certainly this is true for nursing, although current nursing assessment models embrace a strengths-based, holistic approach to care (Wright & Leahey, 2005).

Self-awareness is critical in the journey of becoming culturally competent. It is imperative that nurses understand themselves before they engage with families: "When we recognize the values behind our own practice, we become more open and responsive to the values of the families whom we serve" (Kalyanpur & Harry, 1999, p. xix). Systems of care among diverse cultural groups differ greatly, and nurses need to be prepared to meet the needs of an increasingly diverse society.

Interdisciplinary Collaborative Teaming
Because individuals with complex developmental disabilities, such as ASDs, require the services of many disciplines, the need for coordinated and integrated care is paramount (O'Rourke & Dennis, 2004). Interdisciplinary collaborative teaming provides such care. It is important to understand the difference between interdisciplinary and multidisciplinary approaches. A multidisciplinary approach involves many disciplines, but they do not necessarily collaborate with one another. This approach can lead to frustrations as recommendations may conflict with one another (O'Rourke & Dennis, 2004).

Interdisciplinary collaboration is key to creating meaningful recommendations and services (O'Rourke & Dennis, 2004). Consider the common issue of toilet training a 5-year-old child with ASD who has no verbal language, hates loud noises, and has some hypotonia and decreased motor skills. Imagine the efficiency of a collaborative team with the primary health care provider, family, occupational therapist (OT), physical therapist (PT), speech and language pathologist (SLP), special educator, and school nurse thinking about the issue in the same room at the same time. All the issues impacting this child can be addressed as everyone considers the best way to toilet train him. The primary care provider can monitor the medications, and the family can bring important history and the home environment into the plan. The OT can think about the sensory issues, and the PT can plan for posture on the toilet. The SLP can support communication and language in the toileting plan, and the special educator can work the toileting plan into the child's educational goals, and the nurse can provide the care coordination needed to link the care between home, school, and primary care to prevent discontinuities in the implementation of the toileting plan. Contrast this model with a multidisciplinary approach where the family, and perhaps the primary care provider, may obtain several different reports: one from the OT, one from the PT, and one from the SLP. There is no group thinking, sharing of ideas, and no synthesis of the information or coordination of services and care. They are left with trying to put it all together.

Nursing Framework of Care
The Calgary Family Assessment Model provides a holistic, strengths-based framework for working collaboratively with families (Wright & Leahey, 2005). It embraces the concepts of family-centered care, cultural competence, and interdisciplinary collaboration. During the nursing assessment, the structure, developmental phase and function of a family is described. Genograms and ecomaps are pictorial representations of the structure of a family. A genogram is the graphic depiction of the family tree. It allows the nurse to see health and illness patterns within multiple family generations. An ecomap is a drawing of the community surrounding a family, including professional and personal supports.

Understanding where a family and/or individual are within a developmental life cycle framework is essential to providing appropriate care. Wright and Leahey (2005) provided examples of diverse developmental life cycles representing different types of families, such as married heterosexual couples, homosexual couples, and divorced families, among others. The functional aspect of assessment has to do with how a family behaves in day-to-day life. This includes routines such as eating, sleeping, working, and playing. Also included are tasks related to caring for ill or family members with special needs or disabilities. Function also has to do with the ways in which a family communicates, ascribes roles, solves problems, shares power and beliefs, and forms alliances within the family (Wright & Leahey, 2005).

Once the assessment is completed with (not for) the family or a member of the family, then together with them, strengths and problems are identified. Decisions are made collaboratively about where to focus the care or intervention (Wright & Leahey, 2005). Priorities need to be set and the developmental phase of the individual or family needs to be considered. For example, the nurse discovers the 5-year-old child who needs a toileting program also is not sleeping at night, frequently walking through the house. The family is going through a divorce, and the children are spending time in different households. Together with the mother, the nurse decides that implementing a toileting plan right now would be too much for the child given the emotional turmoil and multiple environments involved. However, the sleep issue is more pressing not only because of the impact of sleep deprivation on the child's school day, but also because of the safety issues at home. The nurse can contact the school team to enlist their help in developing a collaborative plan to address the sleep problem (O'Rourke & Dennis, 2004).

Periodically checking in with the family to see which interventions are useful (and which are not) is a method of dynamic evaluation that allows refinement of the overall plan as the work continues (Wright & Leahey, 2005). It also allows problem solving and resource finding to continue as needed.

ASSESSMENT AND DIAGNOSIS

It is essential that the diagnosis of ASDs be made as early as possible to ensure the child's enrollment in an early intervention program. Participation in early intervention programs is associated with better outcomes for most children on the spectrum (AUCD, 2008; Volkmar & Wiesner, 2004). Two levels of assessment are recommended for screening and diagnosis (Filipek et al., 2000). The first level of assessment requires developmental surveillance done by anyone that has regular contact with young children, such as nurses in pediatric and family practice offices. This screening should include lead screening; hearing testing; screening using a developmental checklist; language development; sibling's social, communication, and play skills; and, a formal autism screening tool.

If the initial screening reveals delays and/or problems, then additional testing is needed. The second level of assessment requires diagnosis by an experienced and licensed physician or psychologist, and should include detailed family history, physical examination (e.g., head circumference), and patterns of regression in cognition and language (Filipek et al., 2000). At this level, observations need to be done of verbal and nonverbal communication, and sensory and motor challenges. Necessary testing may be include genetic, metabolic, and sleep electroencephalogram. Also, assessment of intellectual level, particularly nonverbal IQ by an experienced psychologist, is important (Volkmar & Wiesner, 2004). Ideally, this comprehensive assessment and diagnostic protocol is done in collaboration with families and practitioners from several disciplines (Prelock & Contompasis, 2006). Although the diagnosis needs to be made by a licensed physician or psychologist, the participation of the interdisciplinary team composed of SLP, OT, PT, and other professionals as needed and family can contribute a tremendous amount of vital assessment information.

A wide range of screening and assessment tools can be used for diagnosis and ongoing assessment of ASDs (Prelock, 2006). The Early Indicators or Red Flags of ASD Checklist is a screening tool that can be used to detect early indicators of autism (Prelock, 2006). This tool can be administered in primary care offices and during other health care or preschool screenings. Early warning signs of ASDs include failure to orient to name, failure to look at others, and language delay, among others (see Figure 15.1).

When making a referral for an autism diagnosis, it is most efficient to provide some information to the physician (Prelock & Contompasis, 2006). This information should include a videotape of the child in various contexts, such as play, structured and unstructured activities, and interaction with family. Completion of one of the autism screening tools is also indicated; selecting which tool to use is dependent upon the child's age and other factors related to clinical manifestations. It is helpful to review the *DSM-IV-TR* (APA, 2000) criteria for autism, providing comments on each answer. Disciplines involved may include a nurse, psychologist, speech pathologist, OT, PT, nutrition, special educator, or early interventionist (see Table 15.1).

The diagnostic criteria for ASDs are well described in the *DSM-IV-TR*, the diagnostic tool used by physicians and psychologists (APA, 2000). It clearly differentiates between autism, Asperger syndrome, CDD, PDD-NOS, and Rett syndrome. Further differential diagnosis needs to be made with disorders not considered part of the spectrum but that may have some similar clinical manifestations (Prelock & Contompasis, 2006), including specific language impairment, learning disabilities, intellectual disabilities, obsessive-compulsive disorder (OCD), attention-deficit/hyperactivity disorder, personality disorders, and schizophrenia. These disorders are described in the *DSM-IV-TR* and need to be considered carefully when making a diagnosis (APA, 2000). The complexity of accurately diagnosing ASDs makes a compelling case for accessing an experienced physician who will employ a diagnostic protocol that includes supporting evidence from the team and family (Prelock & Contompasis, 2006).

INTERVENTION AND CARE

ASDs are lifelong conditions that require lifelong intervention and care (Volkmar & Wiesner, 2004). Intervention and care are provided primarily through the health care and educational systems until a child graduates high school and transitions to adult services. Adult services vary from state to state and mostly originate through the state's vocational rehabilitation office and the state's health and human services agency, including mental health and developmental disabilities. An Internet search should produce results for what services are available in a specific state for children and adults with disabilities. Additional information pertaining to transition and adult services can be found in Chapters 3 and 5.

Child's Name: _____   Date: ____ / ____ / ____

Date of Birth: ____ / ____ / ____   Person(s) completing checklist: _____

Indicator	Yes	No	Uncertain/Comments
1. Demonstrates poor nonsocial visual orientation/attention (Adrien et al., 1992; Baranek, 1999)			
2. Fails to point to express interest**/**** (pointing usually develops by 8-10 mos.; may be delayed or never develop in ASD) (Baron-Cohen et al., 1992; Lord, 1995; Osterling & Dawson, 1994; Wetherby & Woods, 2003)			
3. Uses hand leading or another's body as a tool** (sees 'hand' as a tool, often replacing pointing) (Lord, 1995)			
4. Mouths objects excessively (Baranek, 1999)			
5. Stops talking after 3 or more meaningful words (Lord, 2000)			
6. Uses fewer than 5 meaningful words on a daily basis at age 2; lack of vocalizations with consonants**** (Lord, 2000; Wetherby & Woods, 2003)			
7. Fails to look at others***; abnormal eye contact or inappropriate eye gaze (Adrien et al., 1992; Osterling & Dawson, 1994; Wetherby & Woods, 2003)			
8. Fails to show interest in other children; ignores people; prefers to be alone (Adrien et al., 1992)			
9. Fails to orient to name***; shows delayed response to name, or lacks attention to voice* (especially neutral voice) (Baranek, 1999; Lord, 1995; Osterling & Dawson, 1994; Wetherby & Woods, 2003)			
10. Lacks symbolic play (e.g., pretending to make a meal, talk on the telephone, etc.); lacks playing with a variety of toys conventionally*** (Baron-Cohen et al., 1992; Wetherby & Woods, 2003)			
11. Exhibits unusual hand & finger mannerisms;** exhibits repetitive movements or posturing of body, arms, hands or fingers*** (Lord, 1995; Wetherby & Woods, 2003)			

Item			
12. Displays aversions to social touch (Baranek, 1999)			
13. Lacks coordination of gaze, facial expression, gesture & sound*** (Wetherby & Woods, 2003)			
14. Lacks expressive postures & gestures or exhibits unusual postures (Adrien et al., 1992)			
15. Fails to share enjoyment or interest**/*** (Lord, 1995; Wetherby & Woods, 2003)			
16. Fails to show objects***, show an interest in or joint attention to games for pleasure or connection with another; fails to spontaneously direct another's attention* (Baron-Cohen et al., 1992; Lord, 1995; Osterling & Dawson, 1994; Wetherby & Woods, 2003)			
17. Fails to show warm, joyful expressions with gaze***; lacks emotional facial expression & social smile (Adrien et al., 1992; Wetherby & Woods, 2003)			
18. Makes repetitive movements with objects*** (Wetherby & Woods, 2003)			
19. Unusual prosody*** (Wetherby & Woods, 2003)			
20. Fails to respond to contextual cues**** (Wetherby & Woods, 2003)			

*clearest discriminators at age 2 (Lord, 1995)

**clearest discriminators at age 3 (Lord, 1995)

***distinguishes children with ASD from children with developmental delays & those who are typically developing (Wetherby & Woods, 2003)

****distinguishes children with ASD from children who are typically developing but not children with developmental delays (Wetherby & Woods, 2003)

Note: Identification of the presence (a "Yes" response) of at least two of these red flags may indicate the need for further assessment

Figure 15.1. Early Indicators/Red Flags of ASD Checklist. (From Autism and related disorders: Trends in diagnosis and neurobiologic considerations, by P. A. Prelock and S.H. Contompasis, 2006, *Autism spectrum disorders: Issues in assessment and intervention* [pp. 23–24], P.A. Prelock [Ed.], Austin, TX: PRO-ED. Copyright 2006 by PRO-ED); reprinted with permission.)

Table 15.1. Summary of screening and diagnostic tools for autism spectrum disorders

Assessment tool	Age	Type of tool	Mode of assessment	Area(s) of assessment	Reliability & validity
TITLE: Asperger Syndrome Diagnostic Scale AUTHORS: Myles, B.S., Bock, S.J., & Simpson, R.L. YEAR: 2001 PUBLISHER: Austin, TX: PRO-ED	5 to 18 years	Diagnostic	Organizational tool used by those having sustained contact with the individual being assessed for at least 2 weeks	Probe areas: • Language • Social • Maladaptive • Cognitive • Sensorimotor	Internal consistency => Strong with an alpha of .83 for the Asperger Syndrome Quotient (ASQ) Interrater reliability => Strong correlation coefficient of .93 for the ASQ Content-description validity => acceptable coefficients (.47–.67) Criterion-prediction validity => accurate in discriminating individuals with & without Asperger syndrome Construct-identification validity => all items significantly related to the ASQ, making strong contributions to the measured construct
TITLE: Autism Spectrum Screening Questionnaire (ASSQ) RELATED REFERENCE: Ehlers, S., Gillberg, C., & Wing, L. (1999). A screening questionnaire for Asperger syndrome and other high-functioning autism spectrum disorders in school age children. *Journal of Autism and Developmental Disorders, 29*, 129–141.	6 to 17 year olds	Screening	A 27-item checklist completed by parents and/or teachers	Assesses symptoms of ASD in children and adolescents with strong or only mildly impaired cognitive skills Uses a 3-point scoring scale: 0 => normality 1 => some abnormality 2 => definite abnormality	Test-retest reliability => r = .94 for teacher sample & .96 for parent sample Inter-rater reliability => for parent & teacher @ time 1, r = .66 Divergent validity => r = .75 & .77 with Rutter Scale & .58 & .70 with Conners' Scale for parents & teachers, respectively Concurrent validity => ASSQ differentiated children with ASD from children with attention deficit & behavioral disorders while the Rutter & Conners' Scales did not differentiate ASD

TITLE / Reference	Population	Purpose	Format	Probe areas	Psychometrics
TITLE: Australian Scale for Asperger's Syndrome RELATED REFERENCE: Garnett, M.S., & Attwood, A.J. (1998). The Australian Scale for Asperger's Syndrome. In T. Attwood (Ed.), *Asperger's syndrome: A guide for parents and professionals* (pp. 17–19). Philadelphia, PA: Jessica Kingsley Publishers.	School-age children with high cognitive skills	Screening	Rating scale for teachers or parents	Probe areas: • Social/Emotional • Communication Skills • Cognitive Skills • Specific Interests • Movement Skills • Behavior	Not reported
TITLE: Autism Behavior Checklist (ABC), Subtest of the Autism Screening Instrument for Educational Planning (2nd ed.). AUTHORS: Krug, D.A., Arick, J.R., & Almond, P.J. YEAR: 1993 PUBLISHER: Austin, TX: PRO-ED	All ages	Screening	Structured checklist completed teacher & parent	Probe areas: Checklist of 57 non-adaptive behaviors, comparing an individual to his or her peers in 5 areas: • Sensory • Relating • Body & object use • Language • Social interaction & self-help	Standardized norms available for the teacher checklist only Inter-rater reliability = 95%; intra-rater reliability (based on split-half reliability test) yielded .87 correlation Content validity => 55 of 57 descriptors significant predictors of ASD Criterion-related validity => 86% of individuals with autism had ABC scores within 1 standard deviation of the mean ABC profile Poor convergent validity with other tools

(continued)

Table 15.1. (continued)

Assessment tool	Age	Type of tool	Mode of assessment	Area(s) of assessment	Reliability & validity
TITLE: Autism Diagnostic Interview–Revised (ADI-R) RELATED REFERENCES: LeCouteur, A., Rutter, M., Lord, C., Rios, P., Robertson, S., Holdgrafer, M., & McLennan, J. (1989). Autism Diagnostic Interview: A standardized investigator-based instrument. *Journal of Autism & Developmental Disorders, 19,* 363–387. Lord, C., Pickles, A., McLennan, J., Rutter, M., Bregman, J., Folstein, S., et al. (1997). Diagnosing autism: Analyses of data from the Autism Diagnostic Interview. *Journal of Autism and Developmental Disorders, 27,* 501–517. Lord, C., Rutter, M., LeCouteur, A. (1994). Autism Diagnostic Interview–Revised: A revised version of a diagnostic interview for caregivers of individuals with possible pervasive developmental disorders. *Journal of Autism & Developmental Disorders, 24,* 659–685. Lord, C., Storoschuk, S., Rutter, M., & Pickles, A. (1993). Using the ADI-R to diagnose autism in preschool children. *Infant Mental Health Journal, 14,* 234–252.	18 months to adulthood	Diagnostic	Structured parent interview	Probe areas: • Reciprocal social interaction • Communication and language • Restricted repetitive behaviors & interests	Internal consistency => alpha of .95 for social area; .84 for communication area; & .69 for behavior area Test-retest reliability => exceeding 83% Validity => individual items were strong discriminators of children with ASD & children with mental retardation or specific language impairment

| TITLE: Autism Diagnostic Observation Schedule–Generic (ADOS-G)

AUTHORS: Lord, C., Rutter, M., DiLavore, P., & Risi, S.

YEAR: 1999

PUBLISHER: Los Angeles, CA: Western Psychological Services

RELATED REFERENCES:

Lord, C., Risi, S., Lambrecht, L., Cook, E.H., Leventhal, B.L., DiLavore, P.C., Pickles, A., & Rutter, M. (2000). The Autism Diagnostic Observation Schedule–Generic: A standard measure of social and communication deficits associated with the spectrum of autism. *Journal of Autism and Developmental Disorders, 30,* 205–223. | 2 years through adult | Diagnostic | Semi-structured & standardized observational tool using 4 modules determined by expressive language level

Combination of the Autistic Diagnostic Observation (5–12 years) and the Pre-Linguistic Autistic Diagnostic Observation (2–5 years) with 2 new modules added | Probe areas:
• Communication
• Social interaction
• Play | Inter-rater reliability of individual items => kappas exceeded .60 for Module 1 with mean agreement of 91.5%; kappas ranged from .40 to over .60 for Module 2 with mean agreement of 89%; kappas ranged from .47 to .65 for Module 3 with mean agreement of 88.2%; kappas ranged from .41 to .66 with mean agreement 88.25%

Inter-rater agreement in diagnostic classification (Autism vs. nonspectrum) => 100% for Modules 1 & 3; 91% for Module 2; & 90% for Module 4

Test-retest reliability => excellent stability for social, communication & total; good stability for Behavior

Internal consistency => alphas of .86–.91 (social); .74–.84 (communication); .47–.65 (behavior) across the 4 modules |

(continued)

Table 15.1. *(continued)*

Assessment tool	Age	Type of tool	Mode of assessment	Area(s) of assessment	Reliability & validity
TITLE: Autism Screening Questionnaire (ASQ) RELATED REFERENCE: Berument, S.K., Rutter, M., Lord, C., Pickles, A., & Bailey, A. (1999). Autism Screening Questionnaire: Diagnostic validity. *British Journal of Psychiatry, 175,* 444–451.	Version 1: under 6 years Version 2: over 6 years	Screening	Rating scale indicating presence (scored as 1) or absence (scored as 0) of abnormal behavior completed by primary caregiver	Probe areas: • Social interaction • Language/communication • Repetition/stereotyped behavior	Good discriminative validity between individuals with ASD & those without ASD Sensitivity => 0.85 Specificity => 0.75 Predictive value => 0.93
TITLE: Checklist for Autism in Toddlers (CHAT) RELATED REFERENCES: Baron-Cohen, S., Allen, J., & Gillberg, C. (1992). Can autism be detected at 18 months? The needle, the haystack and the CHAT. *British Journal of Psychiatry, 161,* 839–843. Baron-Cohen, S., Cox, A., Baird, G., Swettenham, J., Nightingale, N., Morgan, K., Drew, A., & Charman, T. (1996). Psychological markers in the detection of autism in infancy in a large population. *British Journal of Psychiatry, 168,* 158–163.	18 month olds	Screening	Interview questions asked of parents Observation by practitioners	Probe areas: • Pretend play • Taking an interest in other children • Pointing • Gaze monitoring	Re-administration of CHAT found children failing the criterion items to receive a diagnosis of autism at 20 & 42 months Less sensitive to milder symptoms of ASD Sensitivity => 0.20–0.38 Specificity => 0.98

| TITLE: Childhood Autism Rating Scale (CARS)
AUTHORS: Schloper, E., Reichler, R.J., & Rochen-Renner, B.
YEAR: 1988
PUBLISHER: Los Angeles, CA: Western Psychological Services
RELATED REFERENCE:
Schloper, E., Reichler, R., DeVellis, R., & Daly, K. (1980). Toward objective classification of childhood autism: Childhood Autism Rating Scale (CARS). *Journal of Autism & Developmental Disorders, 10,* 91–103. | 24 months and older | Diagnostic | Structured interview & observation | Probe areas:
• Relating to people
• Imitation
• Emotional response
• Body use
• Object use
• Adaptation to change
• Visual response
• Listening response
• Taste, smell, & touch response & use
• Fear of nervousness
• Verbal communication
• Nonverbal communication
• Activity level
• Level & consistency of intellectual functioning
• General impressions | Discriminates child with autism from children without autism but other mental handicaps
Convergence with Autistic Diagnostic Interview good for children with autism
Internal consistency => Alpha = .94
Inter-rater reliability => 71%
Test-retest reliability => correlation of .88 & kappa of .64
Criterion-related validity => Correlation of .84 |

(continued)

Table 15.1. *(continued)*

Assessment tool	Age	Type of tool	Mode of assessment	Area(s) of assessment	Reliability & validity
TITLE: Gilliam Asperger's Disorder Scale AUTHOR: Gilliam, J.E. YEAR: 2001 PUBLISHER: Austin, TX: PRO-ED	3 to 22 years	Diagnostic	Behavioral rating scale used by parents, teachers & practitioners with sustained contact with individual for at least 2 weeks	Probe areas: • Social interaction • Restricted patterns of behavior • Cognitive patterns • Pragmatic skills • Early Development (optional subscale)	Internal consistency => Moderate to strong alphas for Asperger's Disorder Quotient (ADQ) (.87–.95) Test-retest reliability => Correlation coefficient for ADQ was .93 Inter-rater reliability => Correlation coefficient for ADQ was .89 Content-description validity => acceptable item discrimination coefficients Criterion prediction validity => strong degree of accuracy in discriminating between Asperger disorder vs. non-Asperger disorder group Construct-identification validity => significant correlations for the subscales indicating items across subscales measure same construct, i.e., behavioral characteristics of Asperger disorder
TITLE: Gilliam Autism Rating Scale (GARS) AUTHOR: Gilliam, J.E. YEAR: 1995 PUBLISHER: Austin, TX: PRO-ED	3 to 22 years	Diagnostic	Checklist used by parents, teachers & practitioners to identify symptoms of autism & indicate severity	Probe areas: • Stereotyped behaviors • Communication • Social Interaction • Developmental Disturbances	Internal consistency => Alpha of .96 for total test Test-retest reliability => correlations ranged from .81 to .86 Inter-rater reliability => correlations ranged from .72 to .95 Content validity => items coefficients of .61 to .69 Criterion related validity => correlated with the ABC

TITLE: Krug Asperger's Disorder Index (KADI) AUTHOR: Krug, D.A., & Arick, J.R. PUBLISHER: Western Psychological Services	6–22 years	Diagnostic	Index completed by a parent, caregiver or teacher at home or school	Probe areas: 32 items that help differentiate Asperger disorder from other forms of high-functioning autism	Standardized on 486 individuals with & without autism across 30 states and 10 countries
TITLE: Modified Checklist for Autism in Toddlers (M-CHAT) RELATED REFERENCES: Robins, D.L. Fein, D., Barton, M.L., & Green, J.A. (2001). The Modified Checklist for Autism in Toddlers: An initial study investigating the early detection of autism and pervasive developmental disorders. *Journal of Autism & Developmental Disorders, 31*, 131–144. Charman, T., Baron-Cohen, S., Baird, G., Cox, A., Wheelwright, S. Swettenham, J., & Drew, A. (2001). Commentary: The Modified Checklist for Autism in Toddlers. *Journal of Autism & Developmental Disorders, 31*, 145–148. Robins, D.L., Fein, D., Barton, M.L., & Green, J.A. (2001). Reply to Charman et al.'s Commentary on the Modified Checklist for Autism in Toddlers. *Journal of Autism & Developmental Disorders, 31*, 149–151.	18 months	Screening	Checklist completed by parents at pediatric visit	Probe areas: • Pretend play • Social relatedness • Communication • Sensory • Motor	Internal consistency => alpha of .85 Sensitivity => 0.87 Specificity => 0.99 Positive predictive power => 0.80 Negative predictive power => 0.99

(continued)

Table 15.1. (continued)

Assessment tool	Age	Type of tool	Mode of assessment	Area(s) of assessment	Reliability & validity
TITLE: Parent Interview for Autism (PIA) RELATED REFERENCE: Stone, W.L., & Hogan, K.L. (1993). A structured parent interview for identifying young children with autism. *Journal of Autism & Developmental Disorders, 23,* 639–652.	Preschool & younger	Diagnostic	Structured interview with parents: • Questions about observable behaviors • Ratings of frequency of occurrence	Probe areas: • Social relating • Affective responses • Motor imitation • Peer interactions • Object play • Imaginative play • Language understanding • Nonverbal communication • Motoric behaviors • Sensory responses • Need for sameness	Internal consistency & test-retest reliability for total PIA => .90 Construct validity => successfully differentiated children with ASD from children with mental retardation Concurrent validity with Diagnostic and Statistical Manual of Mental Disorders-IV & CARS
TITLE: Screening Tool for Autism in Two-Year Olds (STAT) RELATED REFERENCE: Stone, W.L., Coonrod, E.E., & Ousley, O.Y. (2004). Brief report: Screening tool for autism in two-year-olds (STAT): Development & preliminary data. *Journal of Autism & Developmental Disorders, 30,* 607–612.	24–35 month olds	Screening	20 minute play interaction with child	Probe areas: • Play (pretend & reciprocal social play) • Motor imitation • Nonverbal communicative development (requesting & directing attention)	Strong sensitivity (0.92) & specificity (0.85), differentiating children with ASD (100%) from children with other developmental disorders (97%) Concurrent validity (w/Autistic Diagnostic Observation Schedule) K = 0.95
TITLE: Systematic Observation of Red Flags for Autism Spectrum Disorders in Young Children (SORF) RELATED REFERENCE: Wetherby, A.M., & Woods, J. (2002). *Systematic Observation of Red Flags for Autism Spectrum Disorders (SORF).* Tallahassee, FL: Florida State University.	12–36 months	Screening	Review of videotaped communication or behavior samples between child and caregiver	Probe areas: • Reciprocal social interaction • Unconventional gestures • Unconventional sounds & words • Repetitive behaviors & restricted interests • Emotional regulation	Inter-rater reliability • Mean 97.1% • Range 89.7–100% across children • Range 83–100% across items

From Autism and related disorders: Trends in diagnosis and neurobiologic considerations, by P.A. Prelock and S.H. Contompasis, 2006, *Autism spectrum disorders: Issues in assessment and intervention* (pp. 43–48). P.A. Prelock (Ed.), Austin, TX: PRO-ED. Copyright 2006 by PRO-ED; reprinted with permission.

The Individuals with Disabilities Education Improvement Act (IDEA) of 2004 (PL 108-446) stipulates that all children have a right to an education and that accommodations must be made so that children with disabilities can access their education. Because a great deal of the intervention for ASDs is educational, IDEA is a critical piece of legislation. It has been revised several times since 1990 (PL 101-476), but the primary intent and focus remains the same. IDEA has several parts: Part C addresses the needs of children age birth to 3, whereas Part B addresses children age 3–21.

This section describes early intervention services for children birth to 3, followed by a description of services and intervention for children throughout the school years. Next is information on adulthood, followed by health care considerations and information on complementary and alternative medicine (CAM).

Early Intervention

Part C of IDEA stipulates that children with ASDs qualify for an individualized family service plan (IFSP). Services are usually home based and the goals are family focused. A wide variety of services are offered in most disciplines. Because it is often during these years that developmental delays are noticed, it is important that an appropriate diagnosis be made so that the child can begin receiving early intervention services (Volkmar & Wiesner, 2004). ASDs are not the sort of disability with which a provider should take a "wait and see" approach. Early intervention is shown to be important in the outcomes for most children on the spectrum. Nurses have a critical role in shepherding the diagnostic process and supporting families through it. At age 3, children transition from Part C of IDEA to Part B, the school-age years. Refer to chapters 3, 4, and 6 for more information.

School-Age Years

Children who were served through an IFSP will now transition to an individualized education program (IEP). There is a distinct shift from a family focus to an individual focus, with the family participating as a fully functioning team member and focusing on school-based services. The responsibility for evaluating children with ASDs now falls to the education team. There are some differences between medical diagnostic labels and special educational eligibility labels (Volkmar & Wiesner, 2004). Some states use the *autism* label as a separate special education category. Others do not and may use a different category for special education eligibility, such as *other health impaired*. Medical labels as noted earlier can be autism, Asperger syndrome, PDD-NOS, Rett syndrome, or CDD. It is important that the autism diagnosis be made clear to educational teams, even if their special education category is different.

Education-related interventions focus on identified impairment areas critical to the student's ability to learn. Areas of intervention may include play, social-emotional development, and communication (Prelock, 2006). A variety of disciplines are involved in the education and care of children with ASDs, offering their expertise to support the goals as delineated in the child's IEP. Often, the primary health care provider is invited to a school team meeting to discuss health care issues and their impact on learning, such as the use of medications and their side effects. Nurses have a critical role in working closely with the family, school team, and primary care provider in managing data, including medication trials and effects, creating safety plans (e.g., for the management of seizures), and acting as a liaison between all parties (Volkmar & Wiesner, 2004).

Adolescence

Adolescents with ASDs experience the same physical and emotional changes as typically developing adolescents, and also have some unique characteristics (Volkmar & Wiesner, 2004). Because of social communication difficulties, managing effects of adolescence, such as mood swings and transitions, may be more challenging. For those who are functionally nonverbal, there may be an increase in self-injurious or aggressive behaviors. Some adolescents with ASDs may have intense feelings of sexuality, whether they are high or low functioning, whereas others may not (Volkmar & Wiesner, 2004). It is important to begin teaching adolescents about sexuality, starting at their developmental level. For example, instructional content on gender awareness may be indicated if students do not understand those differences yet. Other issues needing attention are privacy, self-care skills, masturbation, physical changes, menses and premenstrual syndrome (for girls), nocturnal emissions (for boys), and most important, teaching about boundaries.

Individuals with ASDs are at greater risk for developing seizure disorders than the general population (25% versus 5%) (Volkmar & Wiesner, 2004). Often, seizures present during adolescence. Individuals with autism do not usually outgrow their seizure disorder and will likely require treatment from a neurologist.

Transition planning to adult services usually begins at age 16 and is lead by the child's IEP team (Betz & Nehring, 2007; IDEA, 2004; Myers & Johnson, 2007). Usually representatives of agencies that provide adult services, such as vocational rehabilitation, participate in the transition planning meetings. The transition teams focus on movement from a secondary educational setting to a work setting or college, and from living at home to independent or community-based living arrangements (Betz & Nehring, 2007; Myers & Johnson, 2007). A young adult's transition to adult medical care, however, is something that the youth may need the assistance from the family to handle (Volkmar & Wiesner, 2004). Finding an internist or family practice physician who is knowledgeable about ASDs may be a challenge. Speaking to other families affected by ASDs may help. Nurses can act as a resource to families during this transition by researching experienced physicians and sharing information with them on caring for individuals with ASDs.

Adulthood

For adults, most supports are received through the vocational rehabilitation system administered through the U.S. Department of Education (Lawer, Brusilovskiy, Salzer, & Mandell, 2009). Assessment and diagnosis, counseling, on-the-job training, job search, and assistive technology are offered through the Office of Vocational Rehabilitation and are available to those with a disability who require supports.

However, adults with ASDs still face many challenges in finding suitable employment and living situations (AUCD, 2008). Social interaction challenges continue to persist throughout adulthood, necessitating the need for ongoing intervention and care (Wilkins & Matson, 2009). Adults with ASDs would benefit from targeted interventions particularly in social interaction and nonverbal behaviors, as these behaviors tend to be more prevalent than other behaviors associated with ASDs in adults. Research by Shattuck et al. (2007) suggests that there is overall improvement in certain behaviors in adults with ASDs, particularly repetitive behaviors and interests, while social reciprocity remains most challenging. They found that many of the behaviors of adults with ASDs remained stable or improved over time, with behavior deterioration occurring in only a minority of individuals.

It is evident that individuals with ASDs continue to make gains in symptoms and behaviors throughout their life span, yet there is less treatment available for adolescents and adults (Shattuck et al., 2007). There is also a lack of research on effective program models for adolescents and adults with ASDs (Betz & Nehring, 2007; Myers & Johnson, 2007). Required supports and interventions are needed to help adults with ASDs succeed in independent living situations, their social lives, and employment. Nurses are poised to act as resources for families seeking information and assistance in accessing available services. Nurses can also seek out respite resources in the state, ensuring families receive the necessary relief from the exhaustion associated with chronic care giving.

HEALTH CARE CONSIDERATIONS

It is critical to provide appropriate health care to individuals with ASDs across their life span and to understand the unique features of each life phase. Pediatricians and other primary health care providers have a key role in caring for children on the autism spectrum (Myers & Johnson, 2007). In addition to screening, diagnosis, and referral, the primary care role also includes ongoing care and management. Health challenges unique to individuals on the spectrum are gastrointestinal problems, sleep disturbance, and nutritional challenges (Contompasis & Prelock, 2006; Myers & Johnson, 2007). Particularly important is management of potential coexisting conditions, such as the onset of psychiatric or seizure disorders.

Gastrointestinal Problems

Gastrointestinal issues are far more frequent for individuals with ASDs and may include chronic constipation, frequent vomiting, and abdominal pain (Myers & Johnson, 2007). Endoscopy has shown the presence of significant inflammation and may be indicated if an individual presents with persistent symptoms. Medical and dietary management of gastrointestinal problems is indicated (Contompasis & Prelock, 2006).

Sleep Disturbance

Sleep disturbance is common among individuals with ASDs. It not only interferes with their ability to function effectively, but it contributes greatly to overall family stress (Myers & Johnson, 2007). It may persist until adulthood (Volkmar & Wiesner, 2004). Unfortunately, there is little evidence for the most effective pharmacological approaches; therefore, providers usually make clinical decisions based upon their experiences. It is important to try and ascertain the cause of the sleep disturbance, such as pain (e.g., esophageal reflux). Providing a consistent bedtime routine can be very effective in establishing a good sleep pattern (Volkmar & Wiesner, 2004).

Because children with ASDs crave routine and have difficulty with spontaneity, it is important for care providers to ensure the child adheres to the routine. That said, it is also important to build in some variances, such as different book choices, to help with the times that things cannot be exactly the same. Environmental noise and light levels can also impact sleep.

Nutritional Issues

Children with ASDs may have rigidity associated with food preferences, such as taste, color, and texture (Contompasis & Prelock, 2006; Volkmar & Wiesner, 2004). These food issues may contribute to growth and energy level problems. Growth parameters need to be followed closely as part of well-child visits. An interdisciplinary approach, including a nutritionist specializing in children with special needs, is effective in resolving nutritional problems (Contompasis & Prelock, 2006). The OT can offer expertise on increasing tolerance to different textures and the SLP may help with attaching language and stories to meals. The nutritionist can provide the overall guidance to ensuring adequate nutrition. Of course, the family is at the core and contributes its rituals and values around mealtimes.

Psychiatric Comorbidities

Individuals with ASDs are likely to develop mental health, behavioral, or psychiatric conditions. However, because of their ASD symptoms, they are at risk for not receiving an accurate diagnosis (Contompasis & Prelock, 2006). Depression is the most common psychiatric condition associated with ASDs, usually occurring in adolescence and adulthood with the incidence rising with age (Sterling, Dawson, Estes, & Greenson, 2008). Sterling et al. (2008) found that those with higher cognitive levels and social functioning seem more vulnerable to depression. Depression was also correlated with anxiety and OCD, both of which are expressed more in individuals with ASDs than the general population. Although the efficacy of pharmacological therapy medications is still unknown in managing the core impairments of ASDs, they may be useful in the presence of psychiatric comorbidities or maladaptive behaviors (Myers & Johnson, 2007). Traditional medical treatments for anxiety, OCD, and depression are effective for individuals with ASDs, along with other types of counseling and therapy (Volkmar & Wiesner, 2004). With any new drug regimen, careful data needs to be kept regarding behavioral changes and side effects across environments.

Care providers should watch for the emergence of depression in adolescents and adults with higher cognitive functioning who increase their social skills through intervention (Sterling et al., 2008). An increase in symptoms may include aggression, self-injurious behavior, and OCD behavior, and may indicate a depressive episode. Nurses can function as important members of the team in bringing a mental health and well-being perspective to teams and families grappling with a rise in challenging behaviors.

Seizure Disorders

As mentioned earlier, individuals with ASDs are more susceptible to developing seizure disorders than the general population (Contompasis & Prelock, 2006; Volkmar & Wiesner, 2004). There seem to be two critical times in a child's life when seizures may present: before 5 years of age and during adolescence (Myers & Johnson, 2007). Aside from the dramatic clonic-tonic symptoms, more subtle ones include confusion and staring spells (Contompasis & Prelock, 2006).

If seizure activity is suspected, a referral may be made to a neurologist and an evaluation plan made. The primary care provider can act as a central point for gathering information, calling upon those who have extended contacts with the child to do some specific observations and data keeping. The school nurse can set up the observational protocol and data system, acting as a liaison between all parties. The protocol should include date, time, activity, antecedent event, suspected seizure behavior, and consequent event (Contompasis & Prelock, 2006). Once seizures are verified, medical treatment needs to be carefully considered, including drug side effects and risk of more seizures (Volkmar & Wiesner, 2004). The school nurse will create a safety plan should seizures occur at school, monitor medicines and their efficacy, and continue to act as a liaison between family, school, and primary care.

TREATMENT OPTIONS

Many treatment options are available for individuals with ASDs, including use of medications, health care surveillance, and CAM.

Use of Medications

The use of medications may be warranted at times in treating behavior problems associated with ASDs when other approaches seem not to be working adequately (Volkmar & Wiesner, 2004). It is important to continue with a full array of approaches using medicine to supplement the treatment, not replace it. The primary medications considered for use are neuroleptics (major tranquilizers) and stimulants (Volkmar & Wiesner, 2004). First-generation neuroleptics such as Thorazine and Haldol are still used, but are not as commonly prescribed for individuals with ASDs because of their problematic side effects, especially tardive dyskinesia or involuntary body movements. Antianxiety medications such as Librium, Valium, and Xanax seem to be effective for children with ASDs and have fewer side effects, especially tardive dyskinesia (Contompasis & Prelock, 2006). Second-generation neuroleptics are more commonly used because they have fewer side effects, especially tardive dyskinesia. Stimulant medicine may be used to help increase attention in children with ASDs; however, the research is inconclusive about the efficacy of this treatment (Volkmar & Wiesner, 2004). Whenever a new medical regimen is instituted, a data and evaluation plan needs to be implemented; this is a task well suited to the school nurse, who can coordinate across the child's settings.

Health Care Surveillance

Regular medical care is essential for individuals of all ages with ASDs, ideally within a medical/health care home (Contompasis & Prelock, 2006; Volkmar & Wiesner, 2004). It is important for health care providers to be experienced in the care of individuals with ASDs and their families—or at least be willing to learn. Because of the complexity of health and medical concerns requiring multiple consultants and resources, the provider or nurse must act as a care coordinator for the family in order to achieve optimal health outcomes (Contompasis & Prelock, 2006).

The best approach to providing comprehensive health care to individuals with ASDs is to use preventive health checklists and problem-oriented records (Contompasis & Prelock, 2006). When caring for individuals with ASDs, it is crucial to not only provide good preventive medical/health care but to ascertain their level of participation and activity in their lives. Periodic care conferences can be very effective in providing streamlined care and an opportunity for an interdisciplinary conversation about challenges and successes. Assuming the role of care coordinator, the nurse can be a liaison to all providers and the family, facilitate care conferences, link families to resources and programs, and follow up on action plans.

In addition to routine screening, early detection of dental problems, scoliosis, vision problems, hearing problems, poor growth, and hypertension is critical (Volkmar & Wiesner, 2004). The interdisciplinary team can ascertain the need for further testing, such as genetic testing for fragile X syndrome, and examine the child for signs of tuberous sclerosis and seizure disorder, both known to be associated with ASDs. As the service coordinator, the nurse can maintain a master list of medical problems and the consultants involved, as well as oversee a problem list that includes the current challenges and the care plan (Contompasis & Prelock, 2006). A health care checklist can guide the office visit ensuring that critical issues are not overlooked (Contompasis & Prelock, 2006; see Figure 15.2). Pain or illness assessment can be difficult with individuals with ASDs, especially if they are nonverbal. Differences in gestures, behavior, facial expressions, vocalizations, and physiological behaviors can indicate the presence of pain or illness (Contompasis & Prelock, 2006).

Providing medical/health care to an individual with ASD requires patience and flexibility (Volkmar & Wiesner, 2004). Optimal interactions between providers and the child should be characterized by a calm and careful approach, initially without instruments. Procedural preparation will be needed, whether it is for an intrusive or nonintrusive procedure. Intrusive and painful procedures, such as a blood draw, should be accompanied by the use of a topical anesthetic cream. It is best to minimize time spent in the waiting room given the child's issues with sensory processing.

A few things can be done before the visit to ensure its success (Volkmar & Wiesner, 2004):

1. Work with the family to establish a routine in the visit and have family members review it with the individual before each visit

2. Try to accommodate the individual's particular sensory issues

3. Use the individual's specific interests to engage them (e.g., if a child is passionate about dinosaurs, have some toys available)

4. Contact the school nurse prior to seeing a child with ASD to get up-to-date information and after the visit to provide an update

Note that the disclosure of information between the health care system and school settings will require the signed permission of the family or youth.

Complementary and Alternative Medicine

CAM is broadly defined as healing practices outside of the domain of Western conventional medicine. It is reported that parents with children with ASDs may use CAM more than those with typical children (Wong, 2008). Reported reasons were to improve quality of life, reduce toxicities of medicines, or to improve overall health

Child's Name: _____   Health Care Provider: _____

List identified Clinical Concerns:

General _____   Internal _____

Facial _____   _____

Skeletal _____   Neural _____

Surface _____   _____

Health Care Activity	Target Date (s)	Accommodations Needed	Outcomes	Follow-up Needed
Monitor growth				
Review nutritional status & eating patterns				
Assess seizure activity				
Review medications				
Review sleep patterns				
Review toileting needs				
Assess vision				
Assess hearing				
Assess communication development				
Review opportunities for social experiences				
Assess behavior				

Figure 15.2.   Health care checklist for children with ASD. *(From Health-care considerations for children with ASD, by S.H. Contompasis and P.A. Prelock, 2006, Autism spectrum disorders: Issues in assessment and intervention [p. 549], P.A. Prelock [Ed.], Austin, TX: PRO-ED. Copyright 2006 by PRO-ED; reprinted with permission.)*

outcomes. Some families may use CAM in search of a cure for ASDs (Contompasis & Prelock, 2006). Care providers need to listen carefully to family concerns and discuss current research and thinking regarding the etiology of ASDs. Because families may not disclose their use of CAM, it is prudent to ask families what other healing modalities they are using and their reasoning, and have an open discussion with them about how they may integrate with other treatments (Wong, 2008). This discussion may be most successful if it is approached in a culturally competent manner and as an opportunity for mutual learning.

CONCLUSION

ASDs are a group of disorders, including classic autism, Asperger syndrome, PDD-NOS, Rett syndrome, and CDD (APA, 2000). ASDs are neurologically and genetically based with no known etiology as yet (Szpir, 2006; Zilbovicius et al., 2006). It is anticipated that within the next few years, genetic and brain research will unveil an etiology for ASDs. With the latest incidence reports of 1 in 150 children having ASDs, there is much debate about whether ASDs are actually on the rise (Fombonne, 2008; Rutter, 2005). The question is still not answered to the satisfaction of the science community, nor is the genetic-environmental interplay understood. Perhaps when these questions are answered, more will be known about the prevalence, etiology, prevention, and treatment of ASDs.

ASDs are a lifelong condition requiring lifelong care. An interdisciplinary, family-centered approach to intervention and care assures the best outcomes for individuals with ASDs and their families and the greatest satisfaction for providers (Beatson, 2008; Beatson & Prelock, 2002; Prelock, 2006). Interventions extend across several care systems, including health, education, and vocational rehabilitation. Nurses have a vital role in the primary care system as well as the school system (Volkmar & Wiesner, 2004). In the primary care office, they can make real the vision of a medical/health care home, especially with facilitating care conferences and care coordination—two critical aspects of the medical/health care home practice (Contompasis & Prelock, 2006). In the education system, school nurses can provide the link between families, IEP teams, and primary care offices by offering a cohesive approach to implementation and evaluation of care plans.

Fewer developmental disabilities cause as much debate and public discourse as ASDs. The many unanswered questions regarding etiology, environmental toxins, and prevalence cause stress for families, providers, and policy makers, so much so that new legislation such as the Combating Autism Act of 2006 (PL 109-416) is now being implemented. The act calls for more research, surveillance, and education in the area of ASDs. Hopefully, with additional resources being poured into ASDs, the compelling unanswered questions of ASDs will be answered. Until that time, nurses and other care providers must resolve to stay abreast of the research, engaging with families and individuals with ASDs so that they can realize the best outcomes possible.

REFERENCES

American Academy of Family Physicians. (2008). *Definition of patient-centered medical home*. Retrieved on July 3, 2009, from http://www.aafp.org/online/en/home/policy/policies/p/patientcenteredmedhome.html.

American Academy of Pediatrics. (2004). *Autism A.L.A.R.M.* Retrieved on October 25, 2008, from http://www.medicalhomeinfo.org/health/Autism%20downloads/AutismAlarm.pdf.

American Psychiatric Association. (2000). *Diagnostic and statistical manual of mental disorders* (4th ed., text rev.). Washington, DC: Author.

Association of University Centers on Disability. (2008). *AUCD statement on autism awareness month*. Silver Spring, MD: Author.

Autism Society of America. (2008). *Autism prevalence in the U.S. rises to 1 in 150*. Retrieved on July 3, 2009, from http://www.autism-society.org/site/News2?page=NewsArticle&id=9289.

Beatson, J.E. (2006). Preparing speech-language pathologists as family-centered practitioners in assessment and program planning for children with autism spectrum disorder. *Seminars in Speech and Language, 27*, 1–9.

Beatson, J.E. (2008). Walk a mile in their shoes: Implementing family-centered care in serving children and families affected by autism spectrum disorder. *Topics in Language Disorders, 28*, 307–320.

Beatson, J., & Prelock, P.A. (2002). The Vermont Rural Autism Project: Sharing experiences, shifting attitudes. *Focus on Autism and Other Developmental Disabilities, 17*, 48–54.

Betz, C.L., & Nehring, W.M. (2007). *Promoting health care transition planning for adolescents with special health care needs and disabilities*. Baltimore: Paul H. Brookes Publishing Co.

Centers for Disease Control and Prevention. (2009). *Prevalence of autism spectrum disorders in multiple areas of the United States, surveillance years 2000 and 2002*. Retrieved on June 16, 2009, from http://www.cdc.gov/ncbddd/dd/addmprevalence.htm.

Contompasis, S.H., & Prelock, P.A. (2006). Health-care considerations for children with ASD. In P.A. Prelock (Ed.), *Autism spectrum disorders: Issues in assessment and intervention* (pp. 541–568). Austin, TX: PRO-ED.

Combating Autism Act. (2006). *Fact sheet: Combating autism act of 2006*. Retrieved on November 7, 2008, from www.whitehouse.gov/news/2006/12/20061219-3.

Dennis, R., Edelman, S., & Prelock, P.A. (2006). Sensory and motor considerations in the assessment of children with ASD. In P.A. Prelock (Ed.), *Autism spectrum disorders: Issues in assessment and intervention* (pp. 303–345). Austin, TX: PRO-ED.

Doja, A., & Roberts, W. (2006). Immunizations and autism: A review of the literature. *The Canadian Journal of Neurological Sciences, 33*, 341–346.

Dunst, C.J., Trivette, C.M., & Hamby, D.W. (2007). A meta-analysis of family-centered helpgiving practices research. *Mental Retardation and Developmental Disabilities Research Reviews, 13*, 370–378.

Fadiman, A. (1997). *The spirit catches you and you fall down: A Hmong child, her American doctors, and the collision of two cultures*. New York: Farrar, Straus, & Giroux.

Filipek, P.A., Accardo, P.J., Ashwal, S., Baranek, G.T., Cook, E.H., Dawson, G., et al. (2000). Practice parameter: Screening and diagnosis of autism: Report of the Quality Standards Committee of the American Academy of Neurology and the Child Neurology Society. *Neurology, 55*, 468–479.

Fitzpatrick, M. (2007). The end of the road for the campaign against MMR. *The British Journal of General Practice, 57*, 679.

Fombonne E. (2003). Epidemiologic surveys of autism and other pervasive developmental disorders: An update. *Journal of Autism and Other Developmental Disorders, 33*, 365–382.

Fombonne, E. (2008). Is autism getting commoner? *The British Journal of Psychiatry, 193*, 1.

Individuals with Disabilities Education Improvement Act (IDEA) of 2004, PL 108-446, 20 U.S.C. §§ 1400 *et seq.*

Individuals with Disabilities Education Improvement Act (IDEA) of 1990, PL 101-476, 20 U.S.C §§ 1400 *et seq.*

Jarbrink, K., McCrone, P., Fombonne, E., Zanden, H., & Knapp, M. (2007). Cost-impact of young adults with high functioning autistic spectrum disorder. *Research in Developmental Disabilities, 28,* 94–104.

Kalyanpur, M., & Harry, B. (1999). *Culture in special education: Building reciprocal family-professional relationships.* Baltimore: Paul H. Brookes Publishing Co.

Kanner, L. (1943). Autistic disturbances of affective contact. *Nervous Child, 2,* 217–250.

Lawer, L., Brusilovskiy, E., Salzer, M.S., & Mandell, D.S. (2009). Use of vocational rehabilitative services among adults with autism. *Journal of Autism and Developmental Disorders, 39,* 487–494.

Myers, S.M., & Johnson, C.P. (2007). *Management of children with autism spectrum disorders.* Retrieved on November 4, 2008, from http://aappolicy.aappublications.org/cgi/reprint/pediatrics;120/5/1162.pdf

O'Rourke, D., & Dennis, R. (2004). Community-based interdisciplinary assessment: Considering the context for a child with spina bifida. In C.M. Vargas & P.A. Prelock (Eds.), *Caring for children with neurodevelopmental disabilities and their families: An innovative approach to interdisciplinary practice* (pp. 147–182). London: Lawrence Erlbaum.

Prelock, P.A. (2006). *Autism spectrum disorders: Issues in assessment and intervention.* Austin, TX: PRO-ED.

Prelock, P.A., & Contompasis, S.H. (2006). Autism and related disorders: Trends in diagnosis and neurobiologic considerations. In P.A. Prelock (Ed.), *Autism spectrum disorders: Issues in assessment and intervention* (pp. 3–63). Austin, TX: PRO-ED.

Prelock, P.A., & Vargas, C.M. (2004). A different kind of challenge. In C.M. Vargas & P.A. Prelock (Eds.) *Caring for children with neurodevelopmental disabilities and their families: An innovative approach to interdisciplinary practice* (pp. 1–34). London: Lawrence Erlbaum.

Rutter, M. (2005). Incidence of autism spectrum disorders: Changes over time and their meaning. *Acta Paediatric 2, 94,* 2–15.

Shattuck, P.T., Seltzer, M.M., Greenberg, J.S., Orsmond, G.I., Bolt, D., Kring, S., et al. (2007). Change in autism symptoms and maladaptive behaviors in adolescents and adults with autism spectrum disorder. *Journal of Autism and Developmental Disorders, 37,* 1735–1747.

Shelton, T.L., & Stepanek, J.S. (1995). Excerpts from family-centered care for children needing specialized health and developmental services. *Pediatric Nursing, 21,* 362–364.

Silverman, R.D. (2009). Litigation, regulation, and education—protecting the public's health through childhood immunization. *New England Journal of Medicine, 360,* 2500–2501.

Smith, V.K., & Dillenbeck, A. (2006). Developing and implementing early intervention plans for children with autism spectrum disorders. *Seminars in Speech and Language, 27,* 10–20.

Sterling, L., Dawson, G., Estes, A., & Greenson, J. (2008). Characteristics associated with presence of depressive symptoms in adults with autism spectrum disorder. *Journal of Autism and Developmental Disorders, 38,* 1011–1018.

Szpir, M. (2006). Tracing the origins of autism: A spectrum of new studies. *Environmental Health Perspectives, 114,* A412–A418.

Vargas, C.M., & Beatson, J.E. (2004). Cultural competence in differential diagnosis: Posttraumatic stress disorder and reactive attachment disorder. In C.M. Vargas & P.A. Prelock (Eds.), *Caring for children with neurodevelopmental disabilities and their families: An innovative approach to interdisciplinary practice* (pp. 69–112). London: Lawrence Erlbaum.

Volkmar, F.R., & Wiesner, L.A. (2004). *Healthcare for children on the autism spectrum: A guide to medical, nutritional, and behavioral issues.* Bethesda, MD: Woodbine House.

Whalen, C., & Schreibman, L. (2003). Joint attention training for children with autism using behavior modification procedures. *Journal of Child Psychology and Psychiatry, 44,* 456–468.

Wilkins, J., & Matson, J.L. (2009). A comparison of social skills in intellectually disabled adults with and without ASD. *Behavior Modification, 33* 143–155.

Wright, L.M., & Leahey, M. (2005). *Nurses and families: A guide to family assessment and intervention* (4th ed.). Philadelphia: F.A. Davis.

Wong, V.C.N. (2008). Use of complementary and alternative medicine (CAM) in autism spectrum disorders (ASD): Comparison of Chinese and Western culture. *Journal of Autism and Developmental Disorders, 39,* 454–463.

Yeargin-Allsopp, M., Rice, C., Karapurkar, T., Doernberg, N., Boyle, C., & Murphy, C. (2003). Prevalence of autism in a US metropolitan area. *JAMA, 289,* 49–55.

Zilbovicius, M., Meresse, I., & Boddaert, N. (2006). Autism: Neuroimaging. *Revista Brasileira de Psiquiatria, 28,* S21–S28.

CHAPTER 16

Fragile X Syndrome

Rebecca Kronk and Janice S. Dorman

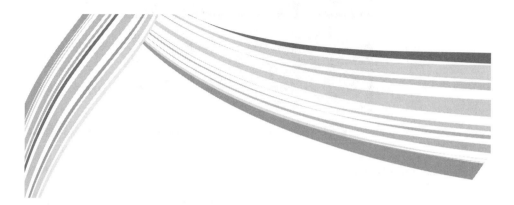

The number of identified X-linked causes of intellectual and developmental disability (IDD) has grown significantly over the years. In 1990, the total count was 39 conditions, with no genes mapped or cloned. By 2007, a total of 215 conditions had been identified and linked to a specific syndrome (98), neuromuscular condition (51), or a nonspecific condition (66; Chiurazzi, Schwartz, Gecz, & Neri, 2008). The gene responsible for fragile X (FX) was discovered in 1991; it is known as the *fragile X mental retardation 1 gene* or *FMR1*. FX continues to be the most recognized X-linked cause of IDD and is almost always introduced as the leading inherited genetic cause of IDD. FX represents three known genetic conditions that affect families across the life span, including fragile X syndrome (FXS), fragile X-associated tremor/ataxia syndrome (FXTAS), and fragile X-associated primary ovarian insufficiency (FXPOI).

This chapter provides a genetic and molecular explanation of each condition of FX, followed by a section that describes the phenotypical and functional presentation of individuals affected by FX. The chapter concludes with a discussion of interventions based on a multidisciplinary approach that emphasizes the role of nursing within a biopsychosocial model of disability.

GENETIC PICTURE OF FRAGILE X

In 1943, Martin and Bell published an article titled "A Pedigree of Mental Defect Showing Sex-Linkage," wherein they described a family of 11 males with IDD and a few less affected females (Sherman, 2002). The related syndrome was called *fragile X* in the 1970s after cell culture media deficient in folic acid portrayed the chromosome material in the distal arm of the X chromosome as barely held by the remainder of the chromosome (see Figure 16.1). This visualization method was the diagnostic test for FX until 1991, when the actual gene was identified on site Xq27.3 (Visootsak, Warren, Anido, & Graham, 2005).

The unstable area contains an increased number of cytosine-guanine-guanine (CGG) trinucleotide repeats in the 5' untranslated region of the FMR1 gene. This

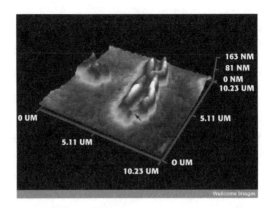

Figure 16.1.   Fragile distal arm of X chromosome. (From Dr. Ben Oostra/Wellcome Images [1998]. London: The Wellcome Trust Medical Photographic Library; reprinted by permission.)

alteration is responsible for over 95% of FXS cases (Hagerman & Hagerman, 2002; see Figure 16.2). Because FXS is an X-linked disorder, the prevalence is higher in males (1 in 4,000) than females (1 in 6,000; Walker & Johnson, 2006). Mutation status for FXS is based on the number of CGG repeats. According to the American College of Medical Genetics, normal FMR1 alleles have < 45 CGG repeat (Maddalena et al., 2001). The premutation or carrier status is associated with 56–200 repeats, and the full mutation occurs with more than 200 repeats (Visootsak et al., 2005).

When a full mutation of greater than 200 CGG repeats occurs, the FMR1 gene is highly methylated. As a result, messenger ribonucleic acid (mRNA) levels are reduced and the gene product, which is known as the fragile X mental retardation protein (FMRP), is absent or deficient. This causes many of the physical, behavioral, and cognitive characteristics of FXS (Hagerman, 2002; Hart, 1998; Loehr, Synhorst, Wolfe, & Hagerman, 1986; Musumeci et al., 1995).

Hagerman and Hagerman (2002, p. 278) reported that "there is not yet universal agreement as to the number of repeats that should define the lower limit for the premutation range," so the above-mentioned parameters can vary by a few repeats. When a maternal premutation is transmitted, it will expand in the next generation; therefore, if an unaffected mother has a premutation with more than 100 repeats, there is a high probability that her children will inherit the full FMR1 mutation with more than 200 repeats. The FMRP level in the premutation allele can be normal or not; therefore, it is possible to exhibit many features of FXS even as a carrier. Recently, a gray or intermediate zone has been described as occurring with 45–55 repeats, but significance of this expansion is yet undetermined (Lashley, 2005).

In 2008, at the request of the National Institutes of Health, the term *premature ovarian failure (POF)* was changed to *FXPOI*. POF itself can have both genetic and environmental etiologies; the occurrence rate is 1% in the general population. FXPOI refers to ovarian insufficiency in women younger than 40 and who are carriers of the FMR1 premutation; the occurrence rate in this group is approximately 20%. The size of the premutation appears to have an association with ovarian dysfunction; the risk for FXPOI begins to decrease at repeats of 100 and is not observed in women with a full mutation (Allingham-Hawkins et al., 1999; Giovannucci Uzielli et al., 1999; Sherman, 2000; Sullivan et al., 2005; Welt, Smith, & Taylor, 2004).

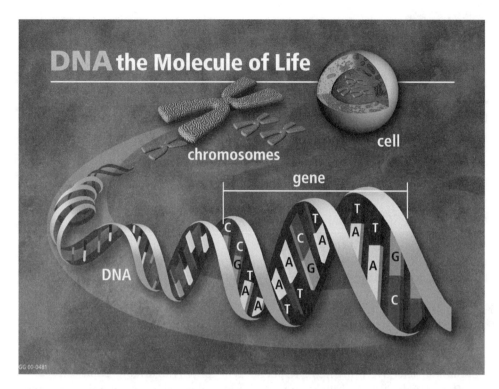

Figure 16.2. DNA with typical CGG arrangements. (From the U.S. Department of Energy Genome Programs, Genome Management Information System. *DNA: The molecule of life.* Oak Ridge, TN: Oak Ridge National Laboratory. Retrieved December 29, 2008, from http://genomics.energy.gov/gallery/basic_genomics/detail.np/detail-17.html).

A subgroup of male carriers and a few less female carriers between age 50 and 70 years have developed the neurologic syndrome of FXTAS. A study by Jacquemont et al. (2004) identified FXTAS in 17% of males with premutation alleles in their 50s, 38% of males with premutation alleles in their 60s, 47% of males with premutation alleles in their 70s, and 75% of males with premutation alleles in their 80s. Interestingly, these individuals did not have a history of IDD, were typically higher educated, and had professional careers. None of the females who presented with FXTAS had dementia, whereas 20% of their male counterparts demonstrated cognitive changes (Hagerman, 2006). It has been hypothesized that the clinical features of FXTAS are caused by abnormally high levels of mRNA (2 to 10 times higher than normal; Hessl, Rivera, & Reiss, 2004).

DIAGNOSTIC TESTING

Diagnostic testing involves a combination of Southern blot and polymerase chain reaction (PCR) analyses (Strom et al., 2007). PCR includes primer sets that flank the CGG repeat and are capable of amplifying genes with up to 100 repeats. Larger repeats are unstable and cannot be amplified by PCR. Southern blot analysis is used to analyze pre- and full mutations, and to determine the methylation status of the FMR1 gene using a restriction enzyme that will not cleave to DNA if the recognition site contains methlyated cytidine residues. Premutations with 56–200 mutations are not methylated, whereas alleles with more than 200 repeats are methylated. Molecular genetic testing for fragile X is 99% sensitive and 100% specific (McConkie-Rosell et al., 2005).

In addition to diagnostic testing for FXS, the American College of Medical Genetics recommends preconceptional testing for individuals with a family history of FXS and prenatal testing for known FMR1 carriers (McConkie-Rosell et al., 2005). However, genetic testing and subsequent counseling for FX remains challenging because of the extremely variable expression of the disorders, particularly in females, the need for an interpretation of the number and methylation status of the CGG repeats, and complexity of the pattern of inheritance. Daughters of a male with a premutation should be individually tested rather than inferring their status based on their fathers' mutations.

CLINICAL PRESENTATION OF FRAGILE X

The extent to which FMRP is deficient influences the severity of clinical presentation, particularly in males with the full mutation (Hagerman et al., 2009). Another biological factor that influences cognitive and behavioral outcomes is mosaicism, either of methylation or allele size.

The behavioral presentation of children with a full mutation of FXS can be highly variable. They may have inattention, hyperactivity, impulsivity, gaze avoidance, or social anxiety accompanied by environmental sensitivities. Coexisting psychiatric diagnoses may also occur, including generalized anxiety disorder, social phobia, selective mutism, or Asperger syndrome (Hagerman, 2006).

Both children and adults with premutation allele sizes are emerging as a new clinical group previously thought to be unaffected. Lowered levels of FMRP and/or heightened levels of mRNA can lead to behavioral features of FXS, even as a carrier. These conditions include brain dysfunction, anxiety, social phobia, and depression, as well as disorders such as autism, attention-deficit/hyperactivity disorder (ADHD), and learning disabilities (Farzin et al., 2006; Goodlin-Jones, Tassone, Gane, & Hagerman, 2004; Hagerman, 2006; Jacquemont et al., 2004; Visootsak et al., 2005). Johnston and colleagues (2001) reported a positive association between allele size and depression in adult female carriers. Additionally, Coffey and colleagues (2008) observed an increase of thyroid disease (50%), hypertension, seizures, peripheral neuropathy, and fibromyalgia, in addition to FXTAS symptoms of tremor and ataxia in female carriers of premutation alleles. FXTAS symptoms include a progressive intention tremor and/or balance problems and Parkinsonian symptoms, such as a masked facies, intermittent resting tremor, and mild rigidity (Hagerman & Hagerman, 2004; Visootsak et al., 2005).

The clinical or phenotypic presentation of FX has broadened over the last decade. Hagerman called FX a "portal disorder" that will open pathways to understanding other complex genetic conditions, including autism, ADHD, anxiety, mood instability, epilepsy, and neurodegenerative disorders (2006, p. 63). Physical features of FXS are related to connective tissue changes and 80% of individuals with FXS will have one or more features; however, presentation can vary with age (Hagerman & Hagerman, 2002). Table 16.1 provides a summary of clinical and medical conditions and prevalence rates associated with FXS.

The following sections present research findings within the biological and cognitive areas primarily affected by FXS. When treatment interventions are listed, they reflect current practice and are not based on intervention studies within the FX population.

Table 16.1. Prevalence of characteristic physical, cognitive, and behavioral symptoms in children with fragile X syndrome and prevalence of fragile X syndrome among individuals with clinical presentation of these symptoms

Characteristic/symptom	Percent of condition in all individuals with fragile X syndrome	Percent of fragile X cases among individuals with condition	Percent of individuals without fragile X syndrome but with condition
Epilepsy	13–20[a] 23[b] 0[c]	No studies found	
Cardiac abnormalities	1[a]	No studies found	
Macroorchidism	68[d]	39[e]	
Mental retardation	70[a] 50–70 (full mutation females)[f] 100[g]	0.9-8.9[h] 0.3-1[h] 2-3[n]	
Elongated face	50[g]	No studies found	
Large ears	100[g]	No studies found	
Language delay	75[a]	0.56[i]	
Speech problems	70[a]	No studies found	
Attention and concentration difficulties	100[a]	No studies found	
Autism	24–33[j] 15–33[k]	2–16[j]	
Autism-like features	90[a] 58[g]	75[l]	
Attention-deficit/ hyperactivity disorder	80[m] 67[g]	1[m]	
Social anxiety and hyperarousal	100[a]	No studies found	
Mental retardation	51[d]		7[d]
Elongated face	27[d]		11[d]
Large ears	41[d]		23[d]
Hyperextensible finger joints	22[d]		4[d]
Soft/smooth skin	68[d]		16[d]
Macroorchidism			27[n]
Characteristic personality	63[d]		4[d]

From Mazzocco, Michèle M, and Judith Ross, eds., *Neurogenetic developmental disorders: Variation of manifestation in childhood,* Table 3.1, © 2007 Massachusetts Institute of Technology, by permission of The MIT Press.

[a]Hagerman, R.J., & Cronister, A. (Eds.). (1996). *Fragile X syndrome: Diagnosis, treatment and research* (2nd ed.). Baltimore: Johns Hopkins University Press.

[b]Wisniewski, K.E., Segan, S.M., Miezejeski, C.M., Sersen, E.A., & Rudelli, R.D. (1991). The fragile X syndrome: Neurological, electro-physiological, and neuropathological abnormalities. *American Journal of Medical Genetics, 38,* 476–480.

[c]Vieregge, P., & Froster-Iskenius, U. (1989). Clinico-neurological investigations in the fragile X form of mental retardation. *Journal of Neurology, 236,* 85–92.

[d]de Vries, B.B.A., Mohkamsing, S., van den Ouweland, A.M.W., Mol, E., Gelsema, K., van Rijn, M., et al. (1999). Screening for the fragile X syndrome among the mentally retarded: A clinical study. *Journal of Medical Genetics, 36,* 467–470.

[e]Vatta, S., Cigui, I., Demon, E., Morgutti, M., Pecile, V., Benussi, D.G., et at. (1998). Fragile X syndrome, mental retardation and macroorchidism [Letter to the Editor]. *Clinical Genetics, 54,* 366–367.

[f]de Vries, B.B.A., Wiegers, A.M., Smits, A.P.T., Mohkamsing, A., Duivenvoorden, H.J., Fryns, J.-P., et al. (1996). Mental status of females with an FMR1 gene full mutation. *American Journal of Human Genetics, 58,* 1025–1032.

[g]Giangreco, C.A., Steele, M.W., Aston, C.E., Cummins, J.H., & Wenger, S.L. (1996). A simplified six-item checklist for screening for fragile X syndrome in the pediatric population. *Journal of Pediatrics, 129,* 611–614.

[h]Pooled data, numerous worldwide studies, 1983–2005.

[i]Mazzocco, M.M., Myers, G.F., Hamner, J.L., Panoscha, R., Shapiro, B.K., & Reiss, A.L. (1998). The prevalence of the FMR1 and FMR2 mutations among preschool children with language delay. *Journal of Pediatrics, 132,* 795–801.

[j]Pooled data, reviewed in the following: Demark, J.L., Feldman, M.A., & Holden, J.J.A. (2003). Behavioral relationship between autism and fragile X syndrome. *American Journal on Menial Retardation, 108,* 314–326.

[k]Pooled data, reviewed in this chapter.

[l]Sherman, S. (1996). Epidemiology. In R.J. Hagerman & A. Cronister (Eds.), *Fragile X syndrome: Diagnosis, treatment and research* (2nd ed., pp. 165–192). Baltimore: Johns Hopkins University Press.

[m]Bastain, T.M., Lewczyk, C.M., Sharp, W.S., James, R.S., Long, R.T., Eagen, P.B., et al. (2002). Cytogenetic abnormalities in attention-deficit/hyperactivity disorder. *Journal of the American Academy of Child and Adolescent Psychiatry, 41,* 806–810.

[n]Slaney, S.F., Wilkie, A.O.M., Hirst, M.C., Chariton, R., McKinley, M., Pointon, J., et al. (1995). DNA testing for fragile X syndrome in schools for learning difficulties. *Archives of Disease in Childhood, 72,* 33–37.

Connective Tissue Changes

In 1987, Waldstein and colleagues observed abnormal elastin fibers in the skin, aorta, and cardiac valves of males with FXS. However, the exact causes of the specific connective tissue problems remains unknown (Hagerman & Hagerman, 2002). Musculoskeletal abnormalities may include umbilical or inguinal hernias (15%), joint dislocations (3%), and flat feet in the majority of cases. Occurrence rates of strabismus in children with FXS (8%) are higher than the general population (0.5% to 1%; Hatton, Buckley, Lachiewicz, & Roberts, 1998). Hagerman, Altshul-Stark, and McBogg (1987) reported the frequency of middle ear infections to be excessive in 30 boys with FXS (63%) compared to 15% of their siblings and 38% of other children with developmental disabilities, suggesting hypotonia and connective tissue dysplasia as the possible culprits. Although more common in adults with FXS, Loehr et al. (1986) evaluated 40 patients with FXS and diagnosed 55% with mitral valve prolapse and 18% with dilation of the aortic root. Gastro-esophageal reflux is not uncommon and should be suspected in infants with frequent vomiting, irritability, those unable to tolerate feedings, and infants with poor weight gain (Rudolph et al., 2001). Overall hypotonia and a relaxed gastroesophageal sphincter may exacerbate the symptoms of gastroesophageal reflux (Hagerman & Hagerman, 2002).

Endocrine Issues

A Prader-Willi phenotype (PWP) has emerged in a subgroup of males with FXS (Fryns, Haspeslagh, Dereymaeker, Volcke, & Van den Berghe, 1987). Typical presentation includes extreme obesity, short stature, broad hands and feet, and obsessive eating patterns. Symptoms of autism are also more common in this subgroup compared to children with FXS without PWP (Nowicki et al., 2007). As with other children with autism, early and intensive behavioral interventions must be incorporated. In addition, behavior programs—proven successful for individuals with Prader-Willi syndrome—that address diet management, exercise, environmental modifications, and family lifestyle need to be added (Chen, Visootsak, Dills, & Graham, 2007; Hagerman et al., 2009; Nowicki et al., 2007). Psychopharmalogical medications that cause significant weight gain (e.g., risperidone) should be avoided in these individuals. If left untreated, PWP can result in complications of early obesity, such as hypertension, type 2 diabetes, dyslipidemias, and obstructive sleep apnea (Hagerman et al., 2009; Nowicki et al., 2007).

Seizures

Although a wide range of seizures have been documented in children with FXS, complex partial seizures are the most common type (Musumeci et al., 1999). Overall reported occurrence rate in FXS is 20%. The prevalence rate is 13%–18% in males and approximately 5% in females (Berry-Kravis, 2002; Incorpora, Sorge, Sorge, & Pavone, 2002). Age of onset of seizures has been reported between ages 6 months to 4 years, with mean age of onset around 2 years of age (Berry-Kravis, 2002; Incorpora et al., 2002; Musumuci et al., 1999).

A wide variety of safe and effective anticonvulsants exists. Pharmacological treatment in individuals with FXS must avoid further impairment of cognitive and behavioral functioning, as well as consider associated symptoms (e.g., hypotonia) and drug interactions. Phenytoin (Dilantin), phenobarbital, and gabapentin are contraindicated in FXS because of specific side effects. Gum hypertrophy and tissue overgrowth are side effects of phenytoin; therefore, it exacerbates dental issues in children who may already be oversensitive to oral stimulation. Phenobarbital and gabapentin increase hyperactivity and may worsen behavioral problems (Hagerman et al., 2009).

Attention–Deficit/Hyperactivity Disorder

All types of ADHD including inattentive, hyperactive, or combined type are reported at higher rates in the majority of males with FXS (Sullivan et al., 2006). Overall, the prevalence of ADHD symptoms (see Table 16.1) is higher in FXS compared to other genetic conditions or to individuals with nonspecific IDD (Cornish et al., 2004; Farzin et al., 2006; Munir, Cornish, & Wilding, 2000).

Compared with a group of controls, Farzin et al. (2006) found higher rates of autism (79%) and ADHD (93%) in boys with a premutation, whereas 13% of sibling controls had ADHD symptoms and none had autism. IQ scores were not significantly different between groups. However, psychotropic medication use was more prevalent in the premutation group.

Stimulant medications are first-line treatment to help control target symptoms of inattention, hyperactivity, and impulsivity. Their exact mechanism of action is unknown; however, these medications may increase the concentration of dopamine and norepinephrine in areas of the brain that mediate arousal in the cortex (Barkley, 2004). Current stimulant medications include short-acting (3–4 hours), intermediate-acting (3–8 hours), and long-acting (8–12 hours) methylphenidate or amphetamine formulations. Atomoxetine is the only nonstimulant medication approved for the treatment of ADHD in children. Preparations include lisdexamfetamine (Vyvanse), a new amphetamine prodrug, and Daytrana, a methylphenidate transdermal patch. Dosing should begin at the lowest level for each preparation then titrated upward, not surpassing maximum recommended dose, until target symptoms are controlled without significant side effects. Treatment is monitored via parent and teacher reports and routine clinical follow-up, with particular attention to side effects such as weight loss, sleep problems, transient stomachaches, and headaches. Prescribing these medications should always be based on American Academy of Pediatrics (AAP) practice guidelines, which provide the most current evidence-based recommendations (AAP, 2001). These same guidelines are typically followed for adults with FXS.

Sleep

Advances in developmental neuroscience reveal that sleep plays an essential role in learning and memory consolidation, especially during early periods of development. Thus, optimal sleep is essential to support learning and development, especially in individuals with developmental impairments such as FXS. In the clinical setting, sleep issues are commonly reported (e.g., resistance to bedtime, early rising, multiple night awakenings) and often cause stress and hardship within the family. Sleep disturbances may have a detrimental impact on the caregiver–child relationship as well as functional, behavioral, and cognitive outcomes of the child;

therefore, sleep is an essential area to assess regularly (Bates, Viken, Alexander, Beyers, & Stockton, 2002; Fredrikson, Rhodes, Reddy, & Way, 2004; Fuligni & Hardway, 2006; Sadeh, Gruber, & Raviv, 2002, 2003).

A few studies have described sleep patterns in children with FXS; they discovered, by parent report, that 48%–77% of children with FXS have problematic sleep behaviors (Kronk, 2008; Richdale, 2003). By using polysomnography, Musumeci and colleagues (1995) investigated the neurophysiology of sleep in FXS. They observed that the individuals with FXS had significantly less total and REM sleep times, an increase in the first REM latency and slow-wave sleep, and a significant increase in twitch movements during REM.

Gould et al. (2000) investigated a possible association between melatonin levels, sleep patterns, and hyperactivity. The study revealed disturbed sleep patterns in boys with FXS. Interestingly, the mean melatonin level was higher for the boys with FXS. The fact that the individuals with FXS had both increased melatonin levels and significant sleep problems was quite unexpected. The authors suggested that the higher daytime levels may eliminate a threshold level that triggers sleep onset or possibly diminished melatonin receptor activation. Sleep and endocrine abnormalities may be associated with dysregulation of the hypopituitary axis (HPA). Because the HPA is the primary stress response system, it may significantly contribute to the many facets of the FXS phenotype (Hessl, Rivera, & Reiss, 2004).

There are few investigations of pharmacotherapy in treating sleep disturbances of children in general, and even fewer involving children and adults with developmental disabilities. Melatonin appears to be the most widely investigated medication in children with IDD to enhance sleep (Giannotti, Cortesi, Cerquiglini, & Bernabei, 2006; Jan, 2000; Pillar et al., 2000; Sajith & Clarke, 2007; Turk, 2003; Wirojanan et al., 2007). Hagerman, Riddle, Roberts, Breese, and Fulton (1995) surveyed parents of 35 patients with FXS who were prescribed clonidine. They found that 37% of the children received clonidine to treat sleep issues and 54% of the parents were satisfied with its use for this purpose. To further investigate the efficacy of sleep medications, there is a need for double-blind, crossover design studies that enroll significant numbers of children so that families and clinicians have scientific data on which to make informed treatment decisions.

Autism

With the consistent implementation of diagnostic tools, such as the Autism Diagnostic Observation Schedule (Lord et al., 1989) and the Autism Diagnostic Interview, Revised (Lord, Rutter, & LeCouter, 1994), the percentage of children with FXS and autism has increased from 15% in the 1980s to 35% in the 2000s (Hagerman, 2006). Overall, children with both FXS and autism demonstrate behavioral patterns very similar to children with only autism who display social aversion, repetitive behaviors and interests, and altered communication. These children generally demonstrate more severe adaptive, cognitive, language, and social impairments (Hatton et al., 2002). Hyperarousal may occur in response to auditory, visual, or tactile stimuli within the environment, resulting in such behaviors as hand flapping, hand biting, and head banging. Lack of eye contact, especially accompanied by tangential or perseverative speech, seems to be related to social anxiety (Belser & Sudhalter, 1995).

Several researchers suggest an association between lower levels of FMRP and prevalence of autistic behaviors (Goodlin-Jones et al., 2004; Hessl, Glaser, Dyer-Friedman, & Reis, 2006; Mazzocco, Kates, Baumgardner, Freund, & Reis, 1997). Goodlin-Jones et al. (2004) reported on six children, within the premutation range, who also had autism spectrum disorder and cognitive abilities that ranged from normal to moderate IDD. The underlying neurobiological mechanisms are yet to be determined. However, molecular pathways resulting from the lack of FMRP or mRNA toxicity may be causative, or the autism features may be the result of gene–environment interactions as posited in most other autism spectrum disorders.

Hessl et al. (2006) measured cortisol changes and anxiety-related behaviors of 90 children with FXS and 90 of their unaffected siblings. Although the study could not determine whether gaze aversion was due to anxiety or autism, the authors posited that treatment choices to improve social reciprocity relied on this answer. Mazzocco et al. (1997) examined autistic behaviors in 30 school-age girls with FXS. The authors reported that girls with FXS possessed a pattern of autistic behaviors similar in quality, but not quantity, to boys with FXS. Lower FMR1 gene expression was associated with more severe and varied types of autistic behaviors. Bailey, Hatton, Skinner, and Mesibov (2001) found autistic behaviors strongly associated with lower developmental levels and slower developmental trajectories of growth as measured on the Batelle Developmental Inventory (Newborg, 2005), whereas FMRP levels and autistic behaviors were not associated in their sample.

COGNITIVE/FUNCTIONAL PROFILE

As mentioned previously, the degree of cognitive impairment seen with FXS correlates with the amount of FMRP produced by each individual, ranging from normal to mild learning disabilities to severe intellectual impairments. Hagerman (2006) noted that studies with large samples find a significant association between IQ and FMRP level. Typically only 15% of males, but 70% of females, with FXS have an IQ greater than or equal to 70 (Hagerman, 2006). Older children with FXS show a steeper decline in IQ scores compared to age-matched peers with autism only; both genders show a decline in IQ scores and adaptive functioning as they age. Decline occurs in all areas: verbal reasoning, abstract/visual ability, quantitative skills, and short-term memory. Adaptive behavior also declines in all areas: communication, daily living skills, and socialization. This decline is not due to regression in abilities, but more likely reflects a slower rate of acquisition and inability to keep pace with peers (Fisch, Simensen, & Schroer, 2002; Fisch et al., 1996).

Hatton and colleagues (2003) found that age has a significant positive association with adaptive behavior scores in boys with fragile X without autistic behavior. A steady and gradual increase in adaptive behavior skills was observed in all individuals; however, those with less autistic behaviors and children with a higher level of FMRP demonstrated better performance in all adaptive areas than those with more severe autism. In addition, nonverbal IQs of children with FXS were higher than their adaptive behavior scores until age 10, when the scores merged.

Hatton, Bailey, Hargett-Beck, Skinner, and Clark (1999) studied the behavioral styles of 45 boys with the full mutation of FXS, ages 47–88 months, in a prospective longitudinal study in which nine dimensions of temperament were examined: activity level, rhythmicity, approach, adaptability, intensity, mood, persistence/attention span, distractibility, and sensory threshold. In five of the nine dimensions, there were significant findings in which boys with FXS were more active and less approachable, adaptable, intense, and persistent. Only 16 boys with FXS were categorized as easy, difficult, or slow to warm up, indicating that these traditional categories "do not adequately describe the temperament of boys with FXS" (Hatton et al., 1999, p. 630). Severity of IDD was not significantly linked to temperament score. Temperament scores also remained stable over time.

Dyer-Friedman et al. (2002) identified both biology (e.g., X activation, FMRP levels, mean parent IQ) and the quality of the home environment as significant predictors of IQ for both boys and girls with FXS. Interestingly, parent ratings of the effectiveness of special education services and therapies were not significantly associated with cognitive outcomes.

Speech and Language

Children with FXS have delayed language acquisition. Belser and Sudhalter investigated the linguistic competency of males with FXS who were chronologically and verbally matched to individuals with IDD and individuals with autistic disorder. One study looked at patterns of repetitive speech (Belser & Sudhalter, 2001), which revealed the fragile X group producing significantly more repetitions. Their other study revealed tangential language occurring significantly more in males with FXS (Sudhalter & Belser, 2001). These authors recognized that the cause of social anxiety and atypical behaviors in children with FXS may be directly related to dysregulation of the sympathetic nervous system (Miller et al., 1999). Their knowledge stemmed from previous work examining greater skin conductance levels in males with FXS when looking directly at their partner during conversation. These individuals demonstrated a greater reactivity to environmental stimuli (e.g., loud voices, crowds, direct eye contact) and had more difficulty returning to a prestimulus level of functioning (Belser & Sudhalter, 1995).

Philofsky, Hepburn, Hayes, Hagerman, and Rogers (2004) proposed that higher receptive language skills may be an early marker to differentiate children with nonautistic FXS from children with FXS and autism. Children with FXS and autism and children with autism alone scored similarly in receptive language; children with autism alone showed no discrepancy between expressive and receptive language.

Roberts, Mirrett, and Burchinal (2001) examined whether cognitive skills or characteristics of autism would explain discrepancies in the acquisition of receptive and expressive language skills in males with FXS. Males with FXS demonstrated individual differences in the acquisition of both expressive language and receptive language. Over time, expressive language was acquired more slowly than receptive language. At the mean chronological age of 66 months, the average expressive language was at 29 months and receptive language was at 30 months. Cognitive skills were a significant predictor of language skills and rate of acquisition. Children with autism and FXS had lower language scores overall. The authors referred to the characteristic anxiety and hyperarousal of this syndrome, the level of FMRP correlating to cognitive development, and responsiveness of the home environment as key factors influencing language development.

Price, Roberts, Vandergrift, and Martin (2007) examined language comprehension skills including vocabulary, grammatical morphology (i.e., prepositions and plurals), and syntax (i.e., arrangement of words). The receptive language of boys with FXS did not differ with or without autism after controlling for nonverbal cognition and maternal education. Nonverbal cognitive skills correlated with receptive language skills, but less in boys with FXS.

NURSING AND THE BIOPSYCHOSOCIAL MODEL OF DISABILITY

The clinical presentation of FXS can be complex and variable, resulting in multisystem effects on the development of the individual. Despite the small number of participants, limited use of standardized assessments, and varied presentation of children and adults with FX, behavioral research has provided some insight into the phenotypical presentation and functional outcomes of individuals with FX.

The genomic mutation of FX may vary among family members and phenotypic expression can emerge during various developmental periods along the life span (e.g., FXS, FXTAS, FXPOI). The psychological and social effects of FX influence all family members regardless of their genotype and can be experienced even prior to a confirmed diagnosis. Therefore, the biopsychosocial model of disability as proposed by the World Health Organization (2002) can synthesize a coherent approach to this disability. Known as the International Classification of Functioning (ICF), this model posits that a disability is "always an interaction between features of the person and features of the overall context in which a person lives" (WHO, 2002, p. 9). This view integrates biology with individual and environmental factors (see Figure 16.3). Figure 16.4 briefly highlights applicability of ICF to FXTAS. This model can also serve as a universal framework to integrate the involvement of various disciplines (e.g., speech and language, occupational therapy) that work with the families to plan and assess functional progress.

Kearney and Pryor (2004) presented a review of the ICF and concluded that the classification system is a useful conceptual framework for nursing education, practice, and research. The authors also posited that the ICF has the potential to expand nursing practice by broadening an awareness of the many dimensions of disability. Figures 16.4, 16.5, and 16.6 present ways the nurse can approach each

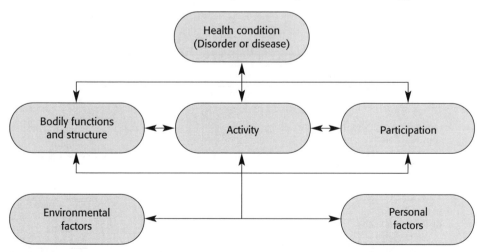

Figure 16.3.   Psychosocial model of disability based on the International Classification of Functioning. (From World Health Organization [2002]. Towards a common language for functioning, disability and health ICF [p. 9]. Geneva: Author; reprinted by permission.)

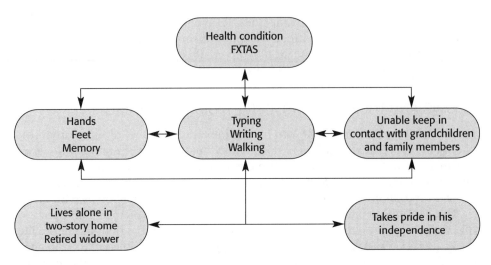

Figure 16.4.   Applying the International Classification of Functioning model to fragile X-associated tremor/ataxia syndrome.

varied condition of FX based on the ICF model. For example, a male with FXTAS may have limited functioning and participation in activities due to bilateral hand weakness and tremors, ataxia when walking, and memory loss. This individual will need supportive care in the form of home health nursing, physical therapy, and occupation therapy interventions. Keeping in contact with his children is of utmost importance to him, so assistive technology support options will need to be explored (e.g., audiotapes, larger keyboard).

Although children with FXS may be delayed or have divergent developmental trajectories, it is important to remember that children's lives are not static and their developmental and psychosocial progress within a family and within their typical and unique environments need to be assessed. The implementation and on-

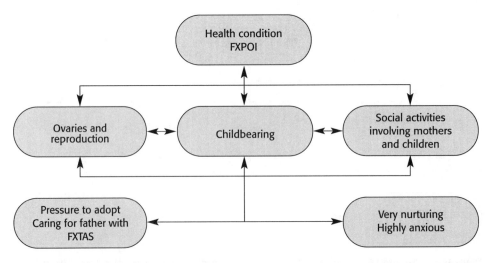

Figure 16.5.   Applying the International Classification of Functioning model to fragile X-associated primary ovarian insufficiency.

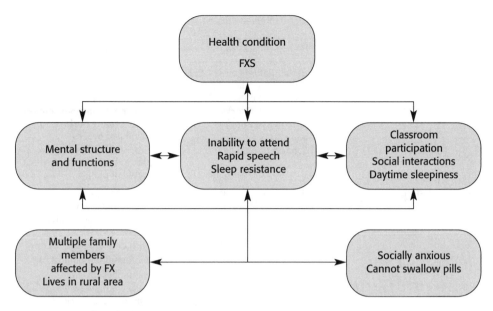

Figure 16.6. Applying the International Classification of Functioning model to fragile X syndrome.

going support of an interdisciplinary team is crucial. Treatment plans must be highly individualized and monitored for success, in whatever way that may be defined by the family or dictating situation. Comprehensive treatment plans and goals involve family members, educational professionals, and community supports.

There is no cure for FXS. A multidisciplinary team is essential to support families and individuals, to enhance functioning, and minimize secondary conditions. It is most helpful that a medical/health home be established to coordinate services, including (but not limited to) professionals in the fields of nursing, developmental-behavioral pediatrics, genetics, education, occupational therapy, physical therapy, speech therapy, psychology, and neurology. The professional nurse has the ideal training to understand the complex biological, social, and psychiatric affects of this condition. The nursing professional also has the capability to comprehend, coordinate, and direct the efforts of team members.

There are specific treatment concerns for women at risk of carrying a full or premutation. These include implications for future children, as well as their own possible expression of clinical features of FXS, FXTAS, or FXPOI. One study reported negative feelings about self and coping in all women who were identified as FXS mutation carriers (McConkie-Rosell, Spiridigliozzi, Dawson, Sullivan, & Lachiewicz, 2001). Therefore, genetic counseling interventions—including provision of coping, social/family support, and psychological resources—should be considered for carrier women with FXS. This emphasizes the importance of a genetic counselor as part of a multidisciplinary team. Prenatal diagnosis and genetic counseling for FX requires full explanations of the benefits and limitations of the test results so that women can make the choice that is right for them. Moreover, it is necessary for the couple to fully understand the range of possible outcomes for male and female fetuses with pre- and full mutations.

Although not exhaustive, Table 16.2 highlights assessments, evaluations, and interventions that can be considered when screening or evaluating for coexisting

Table 16.2.   Assessments, evaluations, and interventions for coexisting conditions

Common secondary behavioral/cognitive conditions	Evaluation/assessments tools	Nonpharmacological interventions
Attention-deficit/hyperactivity disorder	Vanderbilt Rating Forms (Wolraich, Feurer, Hannah, Baumgaertel, & Pinnock, 1998) Child Behavior Checklist (Achenbach, 2001) Connors' Rating Scales-Revised (Connors, 2000)	Behavior modification plan Environmental modification plan (e.g., minimize stimulation and distractions, preferential seating in classroom, scheduled breaks) Educational plans (e.g., 504 plan or individualized education plan [IEP])
Adaptive functioning	Vineland Adaptive Behavior Scales II (Sparrow, Balla, & Cicchetti, 2005) Adaptive Behavior Assessment System (Harrison & Oakland, 2003)	Physical therapy Occupational therapy (e.g., activities of daily living, sensory issues) Speech and language therapy Environmental modifications Community supports Adaptive equipment (e.g., orthotics, visual schedule)
Anxiety	Multidimensional Anxiety Scale for Children (March, 1997) Screen for Childhood Anxiety Related Emotional Disorders (Birmaher, Khetarpal, Cully, Brent, & Mckenzie, 1995)	Cognitive behavior therapy Social skills group therapy Planning ahead for overwhelming events Not forcing eye contact; sit side by side rather than face to face
Speech and language	Connors' Rating Scales-Revised (Connors, 2000) Speech and language evaluation, including oral motor assessment Audiology evaluation	Augmentative/alternative communication Speech and language therapy for • Articulation: aired auditory and visual stimuli, imitation, practice • Pragmatics: verbal rehearsals, role playing • Syntax: modeling, slowing speech, picture sentences • Semantics: visual cues, meaningful connections, acting
Autism	Autism Diagnostic Observation Schedule (Lord et al., 1989) Autism Diagnostic Interview-Revised (Lord, Rutter, & LeCouteur, 1994)	TEACCH Model (Service program) Denver Model Pivotal response training Applied behavior analysis Visual schedules and cues
Intellectual Impairment	Mullen Scales of Early Learning (Mullen, 1995) Stanford-Binet Intelligence Scales, 5th ed. (Roid, 2003) Behavior Rating Inventory of Executive Function (Gioia, Isquith, Guy, & Kenworthy, 2000)	Building on cognitive strengths Visual prompts, supplementing auditory directions IEP Learning support/special education Peer buddies Tutoring

Common secondary behavioral/ cognitive conditions	Evaluation/ assessments tools	Nonpharmacological interventions
Sleep	*Subjective measures* Two-week sleep diary Child Sleep Habits Questionnaire (Owens, Spirito, & McGuinn, 2000) Pediatric Sleep Questionnaire (Chervin, Hedger, Dillon, & Pituch, 2001) *Objective measures* Polysomnography Actigraphy	Implement calming, regular bedtime routine Eliminate stimulating or anxiety provoking activities Electronic curfew Fading

conditions with FXS. The cognitive, speech and language, and autism evaluations require clinicians with specific training and clinical expertise. The remaining assessments listed are accessible, cost effective, and based primarily on parent and/or teacher reports; they can be implemented within the primary care setting. Accurate coexisting behavioral, educational, and medical diagnoses and implementation of evidenced-based treatments may necessitate consultation and/or referral to a specialist; however, scant research is available regarding the effectiveness of specific behavioral interventions in the FXS population.

The National Fragile X Foundation has developed a consortium of FXS clinics throughout the United States, Canada, and internationally that work to advance the treatment of FXS based on research and clinical expertise. Also, the AAP (1996) has issued standards of care for FXS. These standards are meant to serve as practice guidelines for the primary care provider regarding specific considerations at each well-child visit, including anticipatory guidance pertaining to the prevention of secondary conditions. The FXS Clinic Consortium has compiled an excellent review of current treatment options based on neurobiological and behavioral investigations (Hagerman et al., 2009).

FUTURE PHARMACOLOGICAL TREATMENTS

The single-gene alteration that occurs with FXS serves as an important genetic model. The deficiency of FMRP causes a chain reaction in the production of other proteins that are essential for synapse development and pruning. Understanding the molecular basis and neurobiology of FXS has resulted in extensive testing of medications that effect metabotropic glutamate receptor 5 (mGluR5) and gamma-aminobutyric acid (GABA) pathways in the brain of animal models. Clinical trials involving human subjects are beginning to take place. Berry-Kravis et al. (2008) conducted an add-on trial of lithium because it plays a role in certain molecular pathways used by mGluRs. A randomized double-blind placebo controlled clinical trial of the AMPA receptor CX516 was completed by Berry-Kravis et al. in 2006. Most recently, a pilot trial of Minocycline has been funded by the FRAXA Research Foundation. Minocylcine in the mouse model inhibited a protein called matrix metalloproteinase-9 (MMP) and corrected brain abnormalities in the dendritic spines (Bilousova et al., 2009).

GABA$_A$ receptors are the major inhibitory receptors in the brain involved in anxiety, depression, insomnia, learning, memory, and epilepsy. D'Hulst et al. (2006) significantly lowered expression of these receptor subunits in the *Dorsophils melanogastor* model. Ganaxolone, a neurosteroid GABAergic agonist anticonvulsant, may play a future role in treating epilepsy, anxiety, and certain cognitive factors in FXS (Hagerman et al., 2009). In FX, mGluR pathways are overactive or upregulated and cause weakened synaptic connections (Dölen et al., 2007). Treatment trials will include the mGluR5 antagonist fenobam, which in mouse models reduced the production of mGluR5 and the formation of excessive neuronal connections.

CONCLUSION

FX continues to lead the way in the understanding of the complexity of X-linked causes of IDD. FX demonstrates how minute molecular changes can impact generations in a family with an X-linked syndrome that causes IDD. The professional nurse is uniquely qualified to understand the biological, psychological, and social impacts of FX across the life span. Nurses have the skills to manage the multidisciplinary nature of interventions and treatments. Most important, nurses can educate family members and advocate for their clients within each system of service.

REFERENCES

Achenbach, T.A. (2001). *Child behavior checklist.* Burlington, VT: Achenbach System of Empirically Based Assessment.

Allingham-Hawkins, D., Babul-Hirji, R., Chitayat, D., Holden, J., Yang, K., Lee, C., et al. (1999). Fragile X premutation is a significant risk factor for premature ovarian failure: The international collaborative POF in fragile X study—preliminary data. *American Journal of Medical Genetics, 83,* 322–325.

American Academy of Pediatrics. (1996). Health supervision for children with fragile X syndrome. *Pediatrics, 98,* 297–300.

American Academy of Pediatrics. (2001). Clinical practice guidelines: Treatment of the school-aged child with attention-deficit/hyperactivity disorder. *Pediatrics, 108,* 1033–1044.

Bailey, D., Hatton, D., Skinner, M., & Mesibov, G. (2001). Autistic behavior, FMR1 protein, and developmental trajectories in young males with fragile X syndrome. *Journal of Autism and Developmental Disorders, 31,* 165–174.

Barkley, R.A. (2004). Adolescents with attention-deficit/hyperactivity disorder: An overview of empirically based treatments. *Journal of Psychiatric Practice, 10,* 39–56.

Bates, J., Viken, R., Alexander, D., Beyers, J., & Stockton, L. (2002). Sleep and adjustment in preschool children: Sleep diary reports by mothers relate to behavior reports by teachers. *Child Development, 73,* 62–75.

Belser, R., & Sudhalter, V. (1995). Arousal difficulties in males with fragile X syndrome: A preliminary report. *Developmental Brain Dysfunction, 8,* 252–269.

Belser, R., & Sudhalter, V. (2001). Conversational characteristics of children with fragile X syndrome: Repetitive speech. *American Journal of Mental Retardation, 106,* 28–38.

Berry-Kravis, E. (2002). Epilepsy in fragile X syndrome. *Developmental Medicine and Child Neurology, 44,* 724–728.

Berry-Kravis E., Krause, S.E., Block, S.S., Guter, S., Wuu, J., Leurgans, S., et al. (2006). Effect of CX516, an AMPA-modulating compound, on cognition and behavior in fragile X syndrome: A controlled trial. *Journal of Adolescent Phycopharmacology, 16,* 525–540.

Berry-Kravis E., Sumis, E., Hervey, C., Nelson, M., Porges, S.W., Weng, N., et al. (2008). Open-label treatment trial of lithium to target the underlying defect in fragile X syndrome. *Journal of Developmental and Behavioral Pediatrics, 29,* 293–302.

Bilousova, T., Danise, L., Ngo, M., Aye, J., Charles, J., Ethell, D., et al. (2009). Minocycline promotes dendritic spine maturation and improves behavioral performance in the fragile X mouse model. *Journal of Medical Genetics, 46,* 94–102.

Birmaher, B., Khetarpal, S., Cully, M., Brent, D., & Mckenzie, S. (1995). *Screen for Child Anxiety Related Disorders (SCARED).* Pittsburgh: Western Psychiatric Institute and Clinic, University of Pittsburgh.

Chen, C., Visootsak, J., Dills, S., & Graham, J. (2007). Prader-Willi syndrome: An update and review for the primary pediatrician. *Clinical Pediatrics, 46,* 580–591.

Chervin, R.D., Hedger, K.M., Dillon, J.E., & Pituch, K.J. (2001). Pediatric Sleep Questionnaire (PSQ): Validity and reliability of scales for sleep disordered breathing, snoring, sleepiness, and behavioral problems. *Sleep Medicine, 1,* 21–32.

Chiurazzi, P., Schwartz, C., Gecz, J., & Neri, G. (2008). XLMR genes: Update 2007. *European Journal of Human Genetics, 16,* 422–434.

Coffey, S., Cook, K., Tartaglia, N., Tassone, F., Nguyen, D., Bronsky, H., et al. (2008). Expanded clinical phenotype of women with FMR1 premutation. *American Journal of Medical Genetics, 146,* 1009–1016.

Connors, K.C. (2000). *Connors' rating scales–revised.* North Tonawanda, NY: Multi Health Systems.

Cornish, K., Turk, J., Wilding, J., Sudhalter, V., Munir, F., Kooy, F., et al. (2004). Annotation: Deconstructing the attention deficit in fragile X syndrome: A developmental neuropsychological approach. *Journal of Child Psychology and Psychiatry, 45,* 1042–1053.

D'Hulst, C., De Geest, N., Reeve, S., Van Dam, D., Deyn, P., Hassan, B., et al. (2006). Decreased expression of GABA receptor in fragile X syndrome. *Brain Research, 1121,* 238–245.

Dölan, G., Osteraeil, B., Rao, S., Smith, G., Auerbach, B., Chattarji, S., et al. (2007). Correction of fragile X syndrome in mice. *Neuron, 56,* 955–962.

Dyer-Friedman, J., Glaser, B., Hessl, D., Johnston, C., Taylor, A., Wisbeck, J., et al. (2002). Genetic and environmental influences on cognitive outcomes of children with fragile X syndrome. *Journal of the American Academy of Child and Adolescent Psychiatry, 41,* 237–244.

Farzin, F., Perry, H., Hessl, D., Loesch, D., Cohen, J., Bacalman, S., et al. (2006). Autism spectrum disorders and attention-deficit/hyperactivity disorder in boys with the fragile X premutation. *Developmental and Behavioral Pediatrics, 27,* S137–S144.

Fisch, G.S., Simensen, R., & Schroer, R. (2002). Longitudinal changes in cognitive and adaptive behavior scores in children and adolescents with fragile X mutation or autism. *Journal of Autism and Developmental Disorders, 32,* 107–114.

Fisch, G.S., Simensen, R., Tarleton, J., Chalifoux, M., Holden, J.J.A., Carpenter, N., et al. (1996). Longitudinal study of cognitive abilities and adaptive behavior in fragile X males: A prospective multicenter analysis. *American Journal of Medical Genetics, 64,* 356–361.

Fredrikson, K., Rhodes, J., Reddy, R., & Way, N. (2004). Sleepless in Chicago: Tracking the effects of adolescent sleep loss during the middle years. *Child Development, 75,* 84–95.

Fryns, J., Haspeslagh, M., Dereymaeker, A., Volcke, P., & Van den Berghe, H. (1987). A peculiar subphenotype in the FRA(X) syndrome: Extreme obesity, short, stature, stubby hands and feet, diffuse hyperpigmentation. Further evidence of disturbed hypothalamic function in the FRA(X) syndrome? *Clinical Genetics, 32,* 388–392.

Fuligni, A., & Hardway, C. (2006). Daily variations in adolescents' sleep, activities, and psychological well-being. *Journal of Research on Adolescence, 16,* 353–378.

Giannotti, F., Cortesi, F., Cerquiglini, A., & Bernabei, P. (2006). An open label study of controlled-release melatonin in treatment of sleep disorders in children with autism. *Journal of Autism and Developmental Disorders, 36,* 741–752.

Gioia, G.A., Isquith P.K., Guy, S.C., & Kenworthy, L. (2000). *Behavior Rating Inventory of Executive Function (BRIEF).* Minneapolis, MN: Pearson.

Giovannucci Uzielli, M., Guarducci, S., Lapi, E., Cecconi, A., Ricci, U., Ricotti, G., et al. (1999). Premature ovarian failure (POF) and fragile X premutation females: From POF to fragile X carrier identification, from fragile X carrier diagnosis to POF association data. *American Journal of Medical Genetics, 84,* 300–303.

Goodlin-Jones, B.L., Tassone, F., Gane, L.W., & Hagerman, R.J. (2004). Autism spectrum disorder and the fragile X premutation. *Developmental and Behavioral Pediatrics, 25,* 392–398.

Gould, E.L., Loesch, D.Z., Martin, M.J., Hagerman, R.J., Armstrong, S.M., & Huggins, R.M. (2000). Melatonin profiles and sleep characteristics in boys with fragile X syndrome: A preliminary study. *American Journal of Medical Genetics, 95,* 307–315.

Hagerman, P., & Hagerman, R.J. (2004). Fragile X-associated tremor/ataxia syndrome (FXTAS). *Mental Retardation and Developmental Disabilities, 10,* 25–35.

Hagerman, R.J. (2002). The physical and behavioral phenotype. In R.J. Hagerman & Hagerman P.J. (Eds.), *Fragile X syndrome diagnosis, treatment, and research* (3rd ed., pp. 3–109). Baltimore: The Johns Hopkins University Press.

Hagerman, R.J. (2006). Lessons from fragile X regarding neurobiology, autism, and neurodegeneration. *Developmental and Behavioral Pediatrics, 27,* 63–74.

Hagerman, R.J., Altshul-Stark, D., & McBogg, P. (1987). Recurrent otitis media in boys with fragile X syndrome. *American Journal of Disease in Children, 141,* 184–187.

Hagerman, R.J., Berry-Kravis, E., Kaufmann, W., Ono, M., Tartaglia, N., Lachiewicz, A., et al. (2009). Advances in the treatment of fragile X syndrome. *Pediatrics, 123,* 378–390.

Hagerman, R.J., & Hagerman, P.J. (2002). The fragile X premutation: Into the phenotypic fold. *Current Opinions in Genetics & Development, 12*, 278–283.

Hagerman, R.J., Riddle, J.E., Roberts, L.S., Breese, K., & Fulton, M. (1995). Survey of efficacy of clonodine in fragile X syndrome. *Development and Brain Dysfunction, 8*, 336–344.

Harrison, P., & Oakland, T. (2003). *Adaptive Behavior Assessment System-Second Edition (ABAS).* Minneapolis, MN: Pearson.

Hart, C. (1998). Not an easy diagnosis to make: 50% of fragile X patients lack telltale signs, *AAP News, 14(6)*, 1–17.

Hatton, D.D., Bailey, D.B., Hargett-Beck, M.Q., Skinner, M.L., & Clark, R.D. (1999). Behavioral style of young boys with fragile X syndrome. *Developmental Medicine and Child Neurology, 41*, 625–632.

Hatton, D.D., Buckley, E., Lachiewicz, A., & Roberts, J. (1998). Ocular status of boys with fragile X syndrome: A prospective study. *Journal of AAPOS: American Association for Pediatric Ophthalmology & Strabismus, 2*, 298–302.

Hatton, D.D., Hooper, S., Bailey, D., Skinner, M., Sullivan, K., & Wheeler, A. (2002). Problem behavior in boys with fragile X syndrome. *American Journal of Medical Genetics, 108*, 105–116.

Hatton, D.D., Wheeler, A.C., Skinner, M.L., Bailey, D.B., Sullivan, K.M., Roberts, J.E., et al. (2003). Adaptive behavior in children with fragile X syndrome. *American Journal of Mental Retardation, 108*, 373–390.

Hessl, D., Glaser, B., Dyer-Friedman, J., & Reis, A. (2006). Social behavior and cortisol reactivity in children with fragile X syndrome. *Journal of Child Psychology and Psychiatry, 47*, 602–610.

Hessl, D., Rivera, S., & Reiss, A. (2004). The neuroanatomy and neuroendocrinology of fragile X syndrome. *Mental Retardation and Developmental Disabilities, 10*, 17–24.

Incorpora, G., Sorge, G., Sorge, A., & Pavone, L. (2002). Epilepsy in fragile X syndrome. *Brain & Development, 24*, 766–769.

Jacquemont, S., Hagerman, R.J., Leehey, M.A., Hall, D., Levine, R., Brunberg, J.A., et al. (2004). Penetrance of the fragile X-associated tremor/ataxia syndrome in a premutation carrier population. *JAMA, 291*, 460–469.

Jan, M. (2000). Melatonin for the treatment of handicapped children with severe sleep disorders. *Pediatric Neurology, 23*, 229–232.

Johnston, C., Eliez, S., Dyer-Friedman, J., Hessl, D., Glaser, B., Blasey, C., et al. (2001). Neurobehavioral phenotype in carriers of fragile X premutation. *American Journal of Medical Genetics, 103*, 314–319.

Kearney, P., & Pryor, J. (2004). The international classification of functioning, disability, and health (ICF) and nursing. *Journal of Advanced Nursing, 46*, 162–170.

Kronk, R. (2008). *Are children with fragile X syndrome losing their Zzzz's and Y . . . ?* Unpublished doctoral dissertation, University of Pittsburgh. Retrieved June 15, 2009, from http://etd.library.pitt.edu/ETD/available/etd-04082008-111106/.

Lashley, F.R. (2005). *Clinical genetics in nursing practice* (3rd ed.). New York, Springer.

Loehr, J.P., Synhorst, D.P., Wolfe, R.R., & Hagerman, R.J. (1986). Aortic root dilatation and mitral valve prolapse in the fragile X syndrome. *American Journal of Medical Genetics, 23*, 189–194.

Lord, C., Rutter, M., Goode, S., Heemsbergen, J., Jordan, H., Mawhood, L., et al. (1989). Autism diagnostic observation schedule: A standardized observation of communicative and social behavior. *Journal of Autism and Developmental Disorders, 19*, 185–212.

Lord, C., Rutter, M., & LeCouteur, A. (1994). Autism diagnostic interview-revised: A revised version of a diagnostic interview for caregivers of individuals with possible pervasive developmental disorders. *Journal of Autism and Developmental Disorders, 5*, 659–685.

Maddalena, A., Richard, C.S., McGinniss, M.J., Brothman, A., Desnick, R.J., Grier, R.E., et al. (2001). Technical standards and guidelines for fragile X. The first of a series of disease-specific supplements to the Standards and Guidelines for Clinical Genetics Laboratories of the American

College of Medical Genetics. Quality Assurance Subcommittee of the Laboratory Practice Committee. *Genetic Medicine, 3,* 200–205.

March, J. (1997). *Multidimensional Anxiety Scale for Children (MASC).* Minneapolis, MN: Pearson.

Martin, J.P., & Bell, J. (1943). A pedigree of mental defect showing sex-linkage. *Journal of Neurology and Psychiatry, 6,* 154–157.

Mazzocco, M., Kates, W., Baumgardner, T., Freund, L., & Reis, A. (1997). Autistic behaviors among girls with fragile X syndrome. *Journal of Autism and Developmental Disorders, 27,* 415–436.

McConkie-Rosell, A., Finucane, B., Cronister, A., Abrams, L., Bennett, R.L., & Petterson, B.J. (2005). Genetic counseling for fragile X syndrome: Updated recommendations of the National Society of Genetic Counselors. *Journal of Genetic Counseling, 14,* 249–270.

McConkie-Rosell, A., Spiridigliozzi, G.A., Dawson, D.V., Sullivan, J.A., & Lachiewicz, A.M. (2001). Longitudinal study of the carrier testing process for fragile X syndrome: Perceptions and coping. *American Journal of Medical Genetics, 98,* 37–45.

Miller, L., McIntosh, D., McGrath, J., Shyu, V., Lame, M., Taylor, A., et al. (1999). Electrodermal responses to sensory stimuli in individuals with fragile X syndrome: A preliminary report. *American Journal of Medical Genetics, 83,* 268–279.

Mullen, E. (1995). *Mullen Scales of Early Learning: AGS Edition.* Bloomington, MN: AGS Publishing.

Munir, F., Cornish, K., & Wilding, J. (2000). A neuropsychological profile of attention deficits in young males with fragile X syndrome. *Neuropsychologia, 38,* 1261–1270.

Musumeci, S.A., Hagerman, R., Ferri, R., Bosco, P., Dalla Bernardina, B., Tassinari, C., et al. (1999). Epilepsy and EEG findings in males with fragile X syndrome. *Epileplsia, 40,* 1092–1099.

Musumeci, S.A., Ferri, R., Elia, M., Grecco, S.D., Scuderi, C., Stefanini, M.C., et al. (1995). Sleep neurophysiology in fragile X patients. *Development and Brain Dysfunction, 8,* 218–222.

Newborg, J. (2005). *Batelle Developmental Inventory* (2nd ed). Rolling Meadows, IL: Riverside Publishing.

Nowicki, S., Tassone, F., Ono, M., Ferranti, J., Croquette, M., Goodlin-Jones, B., & Hagerman, R. (2007). The Prader-Willi phenotype of fragile X syndrome. *Journal of Developmental & Behavioral Pediatrics, 28,* 133–138.

Oostra, B. (1998). *Fragile X.* London: The Wellcome Trust Medical Photographic Library.

Owens, J.A., Spirito, A., & McGuinn, M. (2000). The Children's Sleep Habits Questionnaire (CSHQ): Psychometric properties of a survey instrument for school-aged children. *Sleep, 23,* 1043–1051.

Philofsky, A., Hepburn, S., Hayes, A., Hagerman, R., & Rogers, S. (2004). Linguistic and cognitive functioning and autism symptoms in young children with fragile X syndrome. *American Journal of Mental Retardation, 109,* 208–218.

Pillar, G., Shahar, E., Peled, N., Ravid, S., Lavie, P., & Etzioni, A. (2000). Melatonin improves sleep-wake patterns in psychomotor retarded children. *Pediatric Neurology, 23,* 225–228.

Price, J., Roberts, N., Vandergrift, N., & Martin, G. (2007). Language comprehension in boys with fragile X syndrome and boys with Down syndrome. *Journal of Intellectual Disability Research, 51,* 318–326.

Richdale, A. (2003). A descriptive analysis of sleep behaviour in children with fragile X. *Journal of Intellectual and Developmental Disability, 28,* 135–144.

Roberts, J., Mirrett, P., & Burchinal, M. (2001). Receptive and expressive communication development of young males with fragile X syndrome. *American Journal of Mental Retardation, 106,* 216–230.

Roid, G.H. (2003). *Stanford-Binet Intelligence Scales* (5th ed.). Rolling Meadows, IL: Riverside Publishing.

Rudolph C.D., Mazur, L.J., Liptak, G.S., Baker, R.D., Boyle, J.T., Colletti, R.B., et al. (2001). Guidelines for evaluation and treatment of gastroesophageal reflux in infants and children: Recommendations of the North American Society for Pediatric Gastroenterology and Nutrition. *Journal of Pediatric Gastroenterology and Nutrition, 32,* S1–S31.

Sajith, S.G., & Clarke, D. (2007). Melatonin and sleep disorders associated with intellectual disability: A clinical review. *Journal of Intellectual Disability Research, 51,* 2–13.

Sadeh, A., Gruber, R., & Raviv, A. (2002). Sleep, neurobehavioral functioning, and behavior problems in school-age children. *Child Development, 73,* 405–417.

Sadeh, A., Gruber, R., & Raviv, A. (2003). The effects of sleep restriction and extension on school-age children: What a difference an hour makes. *Child Development, 74,* 444–455.

Sherman, S. (2000). Premature ovarian failure in the fragile X syndrome. *American Journal of Medical Genetics, 97,* 189–194.

Sherman, S. (2002). Epidemiology. In R.J. Hagerman & P.J. Hagerman (Eds.), *Fragile X syndrome: Diagnosis, treatment, and research* (3rd ed., pp. 136–186). Baltimore: The Johns Hopkins University Press.

Sparrow, S.S., Balla, D.A., & Cicchetti, D.V. (2005). *Vineland Adaptive Behavior Scales, Second Edition (Vineland-II).* Minneapolis, MN: Pearson.

Strom, C.M., Crossley, B., Redman, J.B., Buller, A., Quan, F., Peng, M., et al. (2007). Molecular testing for fragile X syndrome: Lessons learned from 119,232 tests performed in a clinical laboratory. *Genetics in Medicine, 9,* 46–51.

Sudhalter, V., & Belser, R. (2001). Conversational characteristics of children with fragile X syndrome: Tangential language. *American Journal of Mental Retardation, 106,* 389–400.

Sullivan, A., Hatton, D., Hammer, J., Sideris, J., Hooper, S., Ornstein, P., et al. (2006). ADHD symptoms in children with FXS. *American Journal of Medical Genetics, 140A,* 2275–2288.

Sullivan, A., Marcus, M., Epstein, M., Allen, E., Anido, A., Paquin, J., et al. (2005). Association of FMR1 repeat size with ovarian dysfunction. *Human Reproduction, 20,* 402–412.

Turk, J. (2003). Melatonin supplementation for severe and intractable sleep disturbance in young people with genetically determined developmental disabilities: Short review and commentary. *Journal of Medical Genetics, 40,* 793–796.

U.S. Department of Energy Genome Programs, Genome Management Information System. *DNA: The Molecule of Life.* Oak Ridge, TN: Oak Ridge National Laboratory.

Visootsak, J., Warren, S.T., Anido, A., & Graham, J.M. (2005). Fragile X syndrome: An update and review for the primary pediatrician. *Clinical Pediatrics, 44* 371–381.

Waldstein, G., Mierau, G., Ahmad, R,. Thibodeau, S.N., Hagerman, R.J., & Caldwell, S. (1987). Fragile X syndrome: Skin elastin abnormalities. *Birth Defects, 23,* 103–114.

Walker, W.O., & Johnson, C.P. (2006). Mental retardation: Overview and diagnosis. *Pediatric Reviews, 117,* 204–212.

Welt, C., Smith, P., & Taylor, A. (2004). Evidence of early ovarian aging in fragile X premutation carriers. *Journal of Endocrinology and Metabolism, 89,* 4569–4574.

Wirojanan, J., Jacquemont, S., Goodlin-Jones, B., Diaz, R., Anders, T.F., & Hagerman, R. (2007). *The efficacy of melatonin treatment for sleep problems in children with autism and fragile X syndrome.* Paper presented at the Annual Meeting of the Society for Developmental and Behavioral Pediatrics, Providence, RI.

Wolraich, M.L., Feurer, I.D., Hannah. J.N., Baumgaertel, A., & Pinnock, T.Y. (1998). Obtaining systematic teacher reports of disruptive behavior disorders utilizing DSM-IV. *Journal of Abnormal Child Psychology, 26,* 141–152.

World Health Organization. (2002). *Towards a common language for functioning, disability, and health: ICF.* Geneva: Author.

CHAPTER 17

Sensory Impairment

Joni Bosch and Sandie M. Bass-Ringdahl

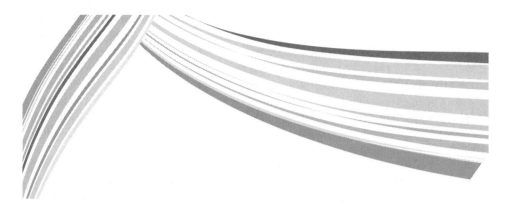

Though sensory impairment presents many challenges across the life span—uncertainty for parents of a newborn, limited expectations of the adolescent, employment barriers for the adult, fear for the senior newly diagnosed with macular degeneration—it is not a death sentence. Those of us who have learned to live with sensory impairment enjoy productive, busy lives and seldom think about its presence. Every single deaf, blind, or visually impaired person, and every person who cares about someone with a sensory impairment, *must* know that there is hope and look forward to the future. Just as for the sighted or hearing person, life won't be perfect—but it will be good.

Mike Hoenig (personal communication, March 16, 2008)

Vision and hearing are major senses by which people interact with the world. Not only do the sense organs provide people with the opportunity for interactions with others and enjoyment of the environment, but these organs also warn of danger. However, many conditions that are associated with developmental disabilities include comorbid sensory impairments. Half of all children with significant vision impairment have associated impairments in other areas (Boulton, Haines, & Smyth, 2006). In this chapter, the incidence of sensory impairment, development of sensory systems, development of a sensory impairment, and types of sensory impairments, including vision, hearing, and deafblindness are discussed. The chapter concludes with a discussion of the nursing role in caring for individuals with sensory impairments.

INCIDENCE OF SENSORY IMPAIRMENT

Globally, more than 161 million individuals are estimated to experience significant visual impairments, and 36.8 million are blind. Most visual impairment occurs in adults over 50 years of age; however, children constitute about 4% of the visually impaired. Worldwide, 278 million people are estimated to have moderate to profound hearing impairment (World Bank Group, 2006).

DEVELOPMENT OF SENSORY SYSTEMS

Sensory input can be divided into two major categories: the general senses of pain, temperature, touch, pressure, vibration, and proprioception; and the special senses of smell, vision, taste, equilibrium, and hearing (Martini, Ober, Garrison, Welch, & Hutchings, 1989). A given stimulus must be transmitted to the central nervous system (CNS), which requires intact and functioning nerve fibers and neurotransmitters. The stimuli must be passed through the brain to the appropriate processing sites, which require both pathways and processing sites to be intact and functional.

Many activities occur during each developmental stage of early life, and insults during specific stages of development can affect multiple tissues and sites. If a disruption occurs, organs—including the brain, eye, and ear—may be affected. Some sensory problems may have their origin in the prenatal period and will be present at birth (Galaburda, 2003). Other prenatal problems may manifest after birth. Depending on the condition, the impairment may remain stable, improve, or worsen over time. For instance, the vision impairment associated with cytomegalovirus (CMV) infection is usually stable over time, whereas CMV-related hearing impairment can worsen over time. Even if the eye and ear develop normally themselves, their signals must be interpreted by the brain in a meaningful manner. Cortical blindness and cortical deafness are obvious examples of sensory problems that result from CNS abnormalities, but dyslexia and visual spatial impairments are also related to abnormal brain development of vision and hearing centers (Galaburda, 2003).

DEVELOPMENT OF SENSORY IMPAIRMENT

In addition to general developmental problems, specific genetic syndromes, illness, trauma, aging, or the treatment of medical conditions may affect multiple

Table 17.1.   Common causes of visual impairment

Type	Cause
Congenital	Congenital malformations (aniridia)
	Congenital toxoplasmosis
	Cataract
	Retinal or macular genetic disorders
	Optic atrophy
	Micro-ophthalmia
	Retinitis pigmentosa
Acquired	Retinopathy of prematurity
	Degenerative myopia
	Amblyopia/Strabismus
	Aphakia
	Self-injury
Adult	Cataract
	Keratoconus
	Age-related macular degeneration
	Glaucoma
	Diabetic retinopathy

Sources: Ingelse and Steele (2001); Warburg (2001).

Table 17.2.   Risk factors for visual impairment

Risk factor	Example
Prematurity	
Intracranial bleed	
Infection	Rubella
	Varicella
	Meningitis
	Human immunodeficiency virus
	Toxoplasmosis
Genetic syndromes	Down syndrome
	Trisomy 13
	Stickler syndrome
	Marfan syndrome
	Neurofibromatosis
	Noonan syndrome
	De Lange syndrome
	Lysosomal storage disorders
	Fabry's disease
	Hurler syndrome
	Maroteaux-Lamy syndrome
	Morquio syndrome
	Aniridia-Wilms' tumor association
	Bardet-Biedl syndrome
	CHARGE syndrome
	Usher syndrome
Head injury	

organ systems, including the sensory systems (see Tables 17.1 and 17.2). Waardenberg syndrome, for instance, is a genetic syndrome that can be associated with a profound sensorineural hearing impairment at birth (Venes, Biderman, Adler, Fenton, & Enright, 2005). Other genetic abnormalities may leave an individual more susceptible to later problems, such as hearing loss and cataracts associated with Down syndrome.

Prenatal and postnatal infections (e.g., rubella or CMV) can impair vision or hearing. Again, these impairments may be present at birth (e.g., congenital rubella syndrome) or progressive (e.g., hearing impairment secondary to CMV). Other postnatal generalized CNS infections, such as meningitis, can lead to central or cortical sensory impairment. Trauma may be central (e.g., traumatic brain injury) or peripheral (e.g., injury to an eye or ear). Injuries to specific parts of the brain associated with sensory processing can cause specific sensory impairment. Injuries to the eyeball can cause loss of vision peripherally (Martini et al., 1989).

Medical interventions can adversely affect vision and hearing as well. Oxygen has been implicated in retinopathy of prematurity (Smith, 2004). Certain antibiotics, such as gentamycin, can cause permanent hearing impairment. Sometimes the medical intervention itself will reliably result in sensory impairment, such as when an eye is removed because of retinoblastoma.

In summary, sensory impairment can be a result of genetic factors, prenatal or postnatal infections, trauma, the consequence of a medical intervention, or any combination thereof. The impairment may be present at birth or may develop later. It is important for the nurse to know and understand the diagnoses of the patient or consumer in order to anticipate and prepare for potential problems.

HYPERSENSITIVITY TO SENSORY INPUT

Although impaired ability to see or hear well can interfere with activities of daily living, individuals with some disabilities may experience impairment due to hypersensitivity to the environment. Children with autism may be thought to have hearing impairments because they may not respond even to their own names. However, there is evidence that individuals with autism may be extremely sensitive to noise (Khalfa et al., 2004). Because loudness can be irritating, individuals with autism may experience behavioral problems in the presence of sound levels that are not bothersome to their caregivers. Controlling noise levels may have a significant impact on behavior, education, social interactions, and work performance.

OTHER CONSIDERATIONS IN ALTERATION OF SENSES

Vision and hearing are not the only sources of sensory input. Smell and taste are intimately related. When sense of smell is impaired or is hyperacute, individuals may not be interested in eating. Likewise, touch is essential for triggering safe swallowing. Individuals with Asperger syndrome may have increased sensitivity to touch, which may affect their tolerance of some clothing (Blakemore et al., 2006). Inability to feel hot, cold, or pressure as associated with spinal cord problems (e.g., spina bifida, spinal cord injury, other peripheral neuropathy) can contribute to skin breakdown. Individuals with impairments of their kinesthetic sense are at risk for injury from falls because they have difficulty locating themselves in space. Injuries to the CNS as a result of trauma, infection, or developmental problems have consequences in terms of health, development, and socialization.

VISUAL IMPAIRMENT

Visual interactions between parents and their infants and children are an important part of communication (Papousek & Papousek, 1983). However, although there are stylistic differences in parenting, parents of congenitally blind children do bond with their children, and their children typically do not experience long-term difficulties as a result. The new parents may benefit from learning more physical and vocal ways of interacting with their infant (Mills & Ciolofi Murphy, 2007).

Congenitally blind infants may face other challenges. They may be delayed in self-initiated mobility. Setting up a safe environment in which to move around and orient is critical. Parents should also be aware of behavior such as rocking or eye poking. These types of self-stimulation may be seen if the child is bored or frustrated and can lead to further eye damage if the behavior is severe.

The facial expressions of individuals with blindness may accurately reflect their emotional state, although the expressions may not be as pronounced as those of sighted individuals (Galati, Scherer, & Ricci-Bitti, 1997). It may be that the habitual facial expressions that sometimes may be adopted by those who are blind, particularly those with congenital blindness, distract others from accurately assessing their emotional responses and may impair their ability to be fully integrated into social groups. It is important, therefore, to remember that individuals with significant vision impairment may be dealing with more than just an inability to see well.

Causes and Types of Visual Impairments

Visual impairment can be secondary to genetic problems, developmental problems, infections, or trauma (See Table 17.1 and 17.2). Some problems, such as anophthalmia (lack of development of an eye) are clearly identifiable at birth. Other problems, such as vision loss related to Usher syndrome or age-related macular degeneration, develop over time. Vision loss can range from complete absence of response to light to myopia or hyperopia, which is easily corrected by lenses or eye surgery (e.g., laser-assisted in situ keratomileusis or Lasik).

Assessment and Diagnosis of Visual Impairment

Diagnosis of a visual impairment can be difficult, but not impossible, in a child or adult with preexisting disabilities. Diagnosis is important not only to provide adequate corrections and accommodations, but also to access appropriate educational, vocational, and social services. Routine screening can also prevent the development of or the worsening of vision impairments, such as the impaired vision that arises from untreated glaucoma or diabetes. All children should have a vision screen before the age of 5 years (National Institutes of Health, 2001).

A vision examination usually includes attention, fixation, and position and movement of the eyes, as well as a general assessment of how the eyes look (Van Splunder, Stilma, & Evenhuis, 2003). Although all individuals with disabilities should have routine screening by a professional, nurses can play a key role in identifying the need for a more complete examination or earlier follow-up appointment.

Treatment and Habilitation or Rehabilitation of Visual Impairment

Low-vision habilitation or rehabilitation may be helpful for individuals who require more than corrective lenses. This requires an interdisciplinary approach and early intervention to be most effective (Wilkinson, 2003). A low-vision team includes a low-vision specialist who provides diagnosis, development of a plan, and prescriptions for assistive devices. Occupational therapists assess capabilities and barriers; make recommendations for further assistive devices, such as kitchen equipment that can be used by those who are blind; and provide training in their use. A rehabilitation teacher or vocational rehabilitation specialist adds specialization in compensating for the visual impairment in the classroom or workplace. Orientation and mobility specialists teach special ambulation techniques, such as the use of a cane or guide dog. A social worker can help with accessing resources and support systems such as waiver programs. Psychologists, adaptive technology consultants, speech and hearing specialists, and itinerant teachers for the vision and hearing impaired may also be helpful in dealing with individual problems that have been identified by nurses or other members of the health care team, such as behavioral problems or individualized needs for adaptive equipment not acquired by the occupational therapist. Assessments should occur in the individual's home, school, and work settings in order to best assess strengths and barriers. Specialists in vision impairment can also provide training and information for family and care providers, allowing them to better understand the needs of individuals with vision impairment and assist in meeting their needs.

Visual and adaptive magnification strategies can help those with low residual vision (National Institutes of Health, 2001). Visual devices include lenses, such as spectacles, magnifying glasses, closed-circuit television, or computer screens to facilitate visual input. Holding materials closer to the eyes is another magnification strategy. Adaptive devices include large print and high-contrast materials (Wilkinson, 2003). It is possible that some individuals who do not tolerate corrective lenses are not finding them helpful, particularly since it may be very difficult to obtain adequate feedback about the correction provided. While glass lenses are less likely to scratch, polycarbonate or plastic lenses may be safer, particularly for those individuals with behavior problems.

Braille is another modality that can allow people with vision impairment to read by means of touch. Individuals with intellectual disabilities also can learn braille. Books are available to help families or care providers learn braille, and there are web sites with helpful information as well. Many assistive devices are available, but it is critical that patients and their care providers all know how to use the devices for successful use. A significant contribution to the failure rate for assistive devices is related to lack of understanding of their proper use (Markowitz, 2006).

Nursing Assessment of Individuals with Vision Impairment

Nurses should assess individuals for visual problems. Complaints of difficulty seeing, double vision, eye pain, blurriness, or headache may be associated with vision problems. The nurse should observe if the eyes track together, if there is any deviation of one or both eyes, or if cloudiness is evident on the lens. The observation of "red eye" in photographs can be helpful. If one eye is red and the other is not, or if there are white or black spots on the pupil in photographs, the individual should be seen promptly. Some nystagmus is normal at the very extreme lateral gaze but should not normally be present otherwise. Wandering eyes are a cause for concern. Sclerae that are reddened or bluish may indicate problems, as can tearing or exudate. It is also easy to assess whether the pupils are equal, round, and react equally to light. Hemangiomas or ptosis may block part of the visual field and lead to amblyopia, so partial occlusion of the eye is of concern as well (Miller & Apt, 2003).

Individuals with visual problems may also hold their heads in different positions, such as tipped to one side, in order to see more clearly. Some may hold objects very close to their face, squint, or miss objects placed in a specific part of their visual field. Some children with vision impairment may poke their eyes with their thumb, fingers, or hand. This type of self-stimulation is not unusual in children with visual impairment but can cause further eye damage. Rubbing of the eyes can be another indication of a vision problem (Miller & Apt, 2003).

The following are questions to consider when assessing visual impairment (Salati, Schiavulli, Giammari, & Borgatti, 2001):

1.   How functional is the individual's vision?

2.   Does the individual actually look at others in the environment?

3. Can the individual follow an object with his or her eyes? (Be sure that the person is not actually orienting to noise or voices.)

4. Can the ambulatory individual avoid obstacles in his or her path?

5. Can the individual look at, reach for, or indicate something of interest?

6. Are there any changes in participation in activities, ability to recognize people from a distance, or perform close work?

Problems noted in the eyes may also be a sign of a problem elsewhere. Sunset eyes (sclera visible above the irises), for instance, can be a sign of hydrocephalus. Proptosis (bulging eyes) may indicate a thyroid problem (Miller & Apt, 2003).

Nursing Interventions for Visual Impairment

Illumination can be very important in enhancing visual function. Multiple incandescent lights may provide the best lighting with the least amount of photo stress (Markowitz, 2006). Enhancing contrast is helpful. Light-colored objects are seen more clearly against dark backgrounds.

When working with an individual with low vision, the plan of care should take into consideration both visual strengths and weaknesses. When distance vision is decreased, the environment should be kept clear of hazards, and caution should be used in repositioning furniture. High-contrast colors on the walls and floors can make it easier to see corners and doors. Painting door jambs with colors that contrast with the walls and doors is helpful. Changes in floor coverings can help an individual identify the room in which they are located. Textured stickers can be used to identify knobs and buttons. Bars and guide rails can help protect against falls. Posts or bushes by the sidewalk in front of a home can help with identifying it when the individual is out in the community (Spruyt-Rocks, 2007).

An additional concern, particularly for those who are totally blind, is the impairment of the ability to synchronize to a 24-hour day. Light is a major zeitgeber (time cue), although social cues such as breakfast and work or school also play a role (Skene & Arendt, 2007). Individuals with absent light perception often develop a more free-running circadian rhythm, typically based on a day closer to 24.5–25 hours in length. Those with a free-running cycle may have periods of good sleep and no naps, followed by periods of poor sleep with a need for frequent daytime naps. To the degree possible, individuals should be allowed their own biorhythms.

Traditional sleep medications have been of little help. Melatonin has been shown to be helpful, although the timing is important. It works best if started when the individual is staying up later. Dosing may start with 5 mg at 2:00 a.m., providing it 1 hour earlier for each of the next 5 days, and finally holding it at 10:00 p.m. If it is unclear where the individual is in their circadian cycle, an alternative is to start the melatonin right at the end of a good sleep phase, taking the melatonin at bedtime.

Peer support and community inclusion can make a big difference in the sense of well-being of individuals with sensory impairment (Kef & Dekovic, 2004). Blindness does not preclude an individual from participating in sports. There are national and international programs in a variety of areas (Open Directory Project, n.d.). Those with residual vision in only one eye need to be careful to use protection during sporting events. Individuals who are blind should not be inactive simply because they have vision impairments.

There are a number of interpersonal strategies that facilitate positive and appropriate interactions with individuals who have visual impairments. These strategies may include the following:

1. Begin with introductions

2. Explain what is going to happen

3. Let the individual feel any instruments that may be used in their care

4. Have health care information available in braille or auditory formats, or have the information translated into an accessible format

5. It is acceptable to use words that refer to vision (http://www.afb.org)

6. Be precise and thorough when describing the environment/situation

7. Remember that service animals are working; they should not be petted

8. Speak out calmly and clearly describe any potentially dangerous situations (e.g., "There is a curb right in front of you.")

9. Don't leap in to perform tasks individuals can do for themselves (e.g., ask if assistance is actually needed; offer your arm, but do not grab, push, or pull)

10. Walk at a comfortable pace about one step ahead when serving as a walking guide; on steps, curbs, or changes in direction, stop and wait for the individual to catch up

Prevention of Visual Impairment

Sunglasses that block UVA and UVB should be provided to prevent visual problems such as cataracts. If one eye has significantly impaired vision, protective glasses may be needed to preserve vision in the other eye. Management of medical problems, such as diabetes and glaucoma, can prevent or delay progression of visual impairment. Routine follow-up vision care is important.

HEARING IMPAIRMENT

Hearing impairment can develop at any point during the life span. While the presence of hearing impairment at any point in time has implications for an individual's ability to communicate, special attention must be paid to hearing impairment presenting in infancy and early childhood as they are critical periods in the development of speech and language (Meadow-Orlans, 1997). For a family in which caregivers have normal hearing, the presence of a hearing impairment in a newborn or young child can create challenges in communication, especially if the child's hearing impairment is severe enough to require the use of a sign system. In this case, successful communication and caregiver–child interaction is dependent upon the learning of a new system (or language) of communication (e.g., signs). The ability to communicate fluently with a newborn or young child greatly enhances caregiver–child interaction and thus, language acquisition (Meadow-Orlans, 1997). Families should be supported and encouraged to develop a system of communication that is congruent with the child's needs and family goals.

Studies indicate that at least 30% of children who are deaf or hard of hearing have some additional health problems or disability (Moores, 2001). For young infants and children who are deaf or hard of hearing and also have additional disabilities, the use of an augmentative system of communication (e.g., sign language) is often necessary regardless of the degree of hearing impairment. For example, it is common for a child with Down syndrome to use a sign system to support the growth of speech and language, regardless of the etiology or degree of hearing loss.

Language, Academic, and Social Implications of Hearing Impairment

As with vision impairment, hearing loss may influence the individual's function and integration into society. Development of a shared system of language is important. For the majority of children and adults with hearing impairment, the language of the family and community is likely to be spoken. In fact, 90% of children born with congenital hearing impairment are born to parents without hearing impairment (National Dissemination Center for Children with Disabilities, 2004).

The development of spoken language is often a priority for these families (Erting, 2003). A smaller number of children born with congenital hearing impairment will be born to families who use a form of sign language to communicate and who may be part of the Deaf community. The Deaf community is a unique culture with a shared sign language. In the United States, this shared language is American Sign Language (ASL). Communicating in shared language (spoken or signed) is the primary means by which a child becomes part of the family (Bodner-Johnson, 2003). In addition, early language experiences of children at home and at school relate to literacy development in the school years (Hart & Risley, 1995; 1999).

Until the early 1990s, the average age of identification of congenital hearing impairment was 2–2.5 years of age. With the widespread adoption of universal newborn hearing screening, the average age of identification of congenital hearing loss is rapidly declining (Vohr, Carty, Moore, & Letourneau, 1998). Early identification and early intervention of hearing impairment have been shown to increase the likelihood that a child can develop normal or near normal language ability (Moeller, 2000; Yoshinaga-Itano, Sedey, Coulter & Mehl, 1998). Even in the presence of cognitive impairment, early identification and intervention of hearing impairment is related to better language outcomes (Yoshinaga-Itano et al., 1998). Moeller (2000) found that a highly involved family could overcome some of the negative consequences of late identification and intervention of the child with a hearing impairment in the areas of language, vocabulary, and verbal reasoning.

Although research clearly supports the importance of early intervention in determining outcomes for children with hearing impairment, intervention is still often delayed for children with multiple disabilities. The presence of a hearing impairment may sometimes delay or even mask the identification of additional impairments (Moeller, 1985). Likewise, the presence of certain impairments may mask the identification of a hearing impairment. The difficulty with identifying hearing impairment in the presence of additional disabilities stems from the fact that many disabilities (e.g., autism) include significant delays in speech and language development (Jones & Jones, 2003). Finally, for some caregivers, the diagnosis of a second disability may be more difficult to accept than the first resulting in delayed intervention for the second disability (Meadow-Orlans, Smith-Gray, & Dyssegaard, 1995).

Academically, children who are deaf or hard of hearing are at risk for delays in vocabulary, word learning, syntax, morphology, and social communication development (Moeller, Tomblin, Yoshinaga-Itano, Connor, & Jerger, 2007). Overall academic performance of children with hearing impairment has been shown to be well below that of children without hearing impairment (Davis, Elfenbein, Schum, & Bentler, 1986; Wake, Hughes, Poulakis, Collins, & Rikards, 2004). Behavioral problems are also evident in children who are deaf or hard of hearing, including aggression, impulsivity, immaturity, and resistance to discipline and structure. Language ability—specifically, receptive communication skill—may play a role in the increased problem behaviors sometimes reported in children who are deaf or hard of hearing (Marshall, 1997).

Causes and Types of Hearing Impairments

There are three basic types of hearing impairment: conductive, sensorineural, and mixed. *Conductive hearing impairment* occurs when one or more structures of the outer or middle ear are affected. For example, conductive hearing impairment may be the result of excessive wax buildup in the ear canal, a hole in the eardrum, fluid in the middle ear, or disruption of the bones or ossicles of the middle ear. This type of hearing loss is typically medically treatable.

Sensorineural hearing loss may result from damage to the cochlea, auditory nerve, or higher auditory centers in the brain. This type of hearing impairment is permanent and typically not treatable by medication. Auditory neuropathy or auditory dyssynchrony refers to a constellation of auditory symptoms similar to optic neuropathy or cortical blindness (Sininger & Trautwein, 2002).

Mixed hearing impairment refers to a combination of conductive and sensorineural hearing impairment. For example, an individual with a sensorineural hearing impairment may have an additional impairment due to a middle ear infection.

Hearing impairment is described not only by the type of impairment, but also by degree of impairment. More information can be found in Table 17.3. It should be noted that a hearing impairment can occur in one or both ears. *Bilateral hearing impairment* refers to hearing impairment in both ears, whereas *unilateral hearing impairment* refers to hearing impairment in one ear.

Risk Factors and Signs of Hearing Impairment

As discussed previously, hearing impairment can occur at any point during the life span, yet special attention must be paid to hearing impairment present in infancy and early childhood. This attention is necessary because infancy and early childhood are critical periods for the development of speech and language. Parental concerns regarding hearing, speech, language, or developmental delay should be taken seriously.

In general, the prevalence of hearing impairment increases with advancing age. The majority of those with hearing impairment are elderly adults. Hearing impairment due to aging is usually a gradual process; therefore, a gradual withdrawal from participation in the many activities of everyday life may be observed. The hearing impairment associated with aging is bilateral sensorineural, typically affecting hearing first in higher pitches and then progressing over time to affect the lower pitches. As the degree of hearing impairment increases, the ability to under-

Table 17.3.   Degrees of hearing impairment

Classification of hearing	Threshold (softest sound) that a person can hear
Normal hearing	−10 to 20 decibels (dB)
Mild hearing loss	21–40 dB Difficulty with whispers, increasing school problems
Moderate hearing loss	41–55 dB Difficulty with normal speech, school problems early
Moderate to severe hearing loss	56–70 dB May hear loud speech, difficulty acquiring language
Severe hearing loss	71–90 dB May hear loud noise 12 inches from ear, difficulty acquiring language
Profound hearing loss	91–120 decibels Usually unable to understand amplified speech, primarily visual communicator

From Iowa's Early Hearing Detection and Intervention System. (2008). *Iowa family resource guide: For parents of children who are deaf or hard of hearing* (3rd ed., p.18). Des Moines, IA: Iowa Department of Public Health; adapted by permission.
Source: Schlesinger (1995).

stand speech becomes more difficult. Many illnesses can be associated with adult-onset hearing impairment. Ménière disease is one such illness that can be debilitating. It involves a fluctuating, often progressive, sensorineural hearing impairment in combination with tinnitus and vertigo.

Common signs and symptoms of hearing impairment include (Trychin, 2003):

• Frequently asking people to repeat

• Inappropriate response to what is said

• Difficulty understanding in groups

• Puzzled expression when listening

• Intently watching the speaker's mouth

• Strained expression around the eyes

Assessment and Diagnosis of Hearing Impairment

Newborn hearing screening (screening after birth and prior to discharge from the hospital) is considered the standard of care in the majority of the states in the United States. Screening for hearing impairment in infancy is conducted either with otoacoustic emissions (OAE) or auditory brainstem response (ABR) testing. (The latter may also be referred to as the *brainstem auditory evoked response, brainstem auditory evoked potential,* or *brainstem evoked response.*)

The OAE screening measures the function of the cochlea or inner ear. OAE screening is conducted by placing a small, soft earphone into the child's ear canal and playing sounds into the ear. Positive OAEs usually indicates normal inner ear function. If OAEs are not present, several causes, such as middle ear effusion and excessive wax, must be ruled out. OAEs do not determine degree of hearing impairment.

ABR screening is conducted by playing sounds through earphones to the infant's ears. The brain's response to these sounds is measured by surface electrodes placed on the infant's head. It is important for the infant to be still and/or asleep during these screening procedures. For infants who receive care in the neonatal intensive care unit, ABR is the recommended screening method due to an increased incidence of auditory neuropathy or dyssynchrony in this population (Joint Committee on Infant Hearing, 2007).

The screening result can be either a *pass* or a *refer*. A pass indicates that the screen is consistent with normal auditory function. A refer indicates the need for further testing; it does not necessarily indicate the presence of a hearing impairment. Only diagnostic testing can determine the presence of a hearing impairment. Regardless of the results of the screening test, caregivers should be encouraged to monitor their child for the development of speech and language milestones (discussed in the sections on risk factors and signs of hearing impairment) and to consult the child's physician if any concerns arise. Hearing impairment can develop following a passed hearing screen.

Treatment, Habilitation, and Rehabilitation of Hearing Impairment

Following the diagnosis of hearing impairment and prior to beginning a course of treatment, medical follow-up is essential. Following medical clearance, a course of habilitation or rehabilitation is often necessary. This habilitation or rehabilitation may take the form of the fitting of hearing aids, a frequency modulated system (allows speaker's voice to be heard over background noises), an assistive listening device or alerting device, and/or the provision of individual or group therapy. For those with severe or profound sensorineural hearing impairment, an implantable device known as the *cochlear implant* may be an option. The cochlear implant provides for electrical stimulation of the auditory nerve.

The course of treatment will be determined by many variables, including (but not limited to) the individual's age, degree of hearing loss, communication ability, cognitive and developmental status, employment or vocational setting, and academic environment. Many different professionals may be involved in the individual's treatment plan (e.g., audiologist, speech-language pathologist, teacher of the deaf and hard of hearing). For those who develop hearing impairment in later childhood or in adulthood, the goal is one of rehabilitation. Rehabilitation will be provided to maintain the individual's current quality of life and communication ability, or to improve/restore functional communication as related to hearing impairment. For a hearing impairment present at birth (congenital) or a hearing impairment that develops during early childhood, the goal is one of habilitation or the fostering of new skill development (e.g., speech and language).

Hearing aids are typically the first technology tried for a young child if the goal is to develop spoken language. Depending on the degree of hearing impairment, hearing aids alone may or may not make sounds loud enough for the child to hear. Sometimes parents without hearing impairment or caregivers who are members of the Deaf community choose not to have their children use hearing aids. The decision not to use hearing aids is usually associated with the use of a signed language, such as ASL, as the primary mode of communication. Some members of the Deaf community do choose for their children to use hearing aids. If a child does not benefit enough from the use of hearing aids to develop spoken language and if spoken language development is the goal of the caregiver(s), then a cochlear implant may be an option. Candidacy requirements for the cochlear implant are continually evolving. Currently, children must be at least 12 months of age, with severe/profound sensorineural hearing impairment and demonstrated lack of benefit from hearing aid use. The most current candidacy requirements for the provision of cochlear implants in children and adults can be located at the U.S. Food and Drug Administration web site (www.fda.gov/cdrh/cochlear).

Nursing Assessment of Individuals with Hearing Impairments

A hearing impairment may develop at any time during a child's or an adult's life (see Table 17.4.). Diagnosis and intervention will serve to minimize the impact of hearing impairment at any point in an individual's life. If hearing impairment is suspected, the individual should be referred to an audiologist for an audiological evaluation. The presence of multiple sensory impairments and/or developmental delay does not preclude audiological assessment. Audiologists use a battery of tests to determine the degree and etiology of hearing loss and can assess difficult patients.

The typical test battery may consist of objective as well as behavioral tests of hearing. ABR and OAE testing are considered objective testing because the individual is not required to provide a response. Tympanometry, which is a measure of how the middle ear functions, is also considered an objective test. Behavioral

Table 17.4. Risk factors for hearing impairment

Risk factor	Example
Neonatal intensive care unit stay of 5 days or more	Extracorporeal membrane oxygenation
	Assisted ventilation
	Exposure to ototoxic medications (gentamicin and tobramycin) or loop diuretics (furosemide/Lasix)
	Hyperbilirubinemia that requires exchange transfusion
Physical findings	Craniofacial anomalies, including those that involve the pinna, ear canal, ear tags, ear pits, and temporal bone anomalies
	Physical signs, such as white forelock, that are associated with a syndrome known to include a sensorineural or permanent conductive hearing loss
Infection	In utero infections, such as cytomegalovirus, herpes, rubella, syphilis, and toxoplasmosis
	Postnatal infections, such as meningitis
Genetic syndromes	Neurofibromatosis
	Osteopetrosis
	Usher syndrome
	Waardenburg syndrome
	Alport syndrome
	Pendred syndrome
	Jervell and Lange-Nielson syndrome
	Hunter syndrome
	Friedreich's ataxia
	Charcot-Marie-Tooth syndrome
Head injury	Basal skull/temporal bone fracture
Other	Chemotherapy
	Aging
	Exposure to noise

Source: Joint Committee on Infant Hearing (2007).

tests are used to determine threshold or the softest sounds that an individual can hear. Behavioral tests of hearing require that the individual provide a response to sound (e.g., hand raise, head turn, vocalization). Visual reinforcement audiometry, conditioned play audiometry, and conventional audiometry are all examples of behavioral tests that may be included in an audiological test battery.

Signs of early childhood hearing impairment include delayed speech and language. The lack of well-formed syllables, known as canonical babble (e.g., /baba/), and delayed speech are milestones that serves as red flags for hearing impairment. The National Institute on Deafness and Other Communication Disorders provides an excellent interactive website for caregivers to monitor speech and language developmental milestones (www.nidcd.nih.gov/health/voice/speechandlanguage). In addition, caregiver concerns regarding hearing status should be taken seriously and the child should be referred for immediate evaluation.

Nursing Interventions for Hearing Impairment

There are helpful ways to assist the child or adult to maximize the communication exchange. Some of these suggestions serve to improve visual communication, whereas others aim to minimize background noise and thus enhance the auditory signal. For young children, the following recommendations serve to promote language growth by enhancing the listening and visual environment (Estabrooks & Marlowe, 2000; Swisher, 2000):

- Sit beside the child, on the side of the better hearing ear
- Speak close to the child's hearing aids and/or cochlear implant microphone
- Use speech that is repetitive and rich in melody, expression, and rhythm
- Use acoustic highlighting to enhance the audibility of spoken language
- Use touch to gain the child's attention
- Use exaggerated facial expressions
- Sign in the child's line of vision or peripheral field of vision

For school-age children, the following are recommendations for use in the classroom or other educational settings (Johnson, Benson, & Seaton, 1997):

- Promote acceptance of the student
- Be sure hearing aids and other amplification devices are used when recommended
- Provide preferential seating
- Increase visual information
- Minimize classroom or other background noise
- Use clear speech (see next paragraph) and encourage others to do so
- Modify teaching techniques
- Have realistic expectations

For adults or any person with hearing impairment, the use of clear speech can be helpful (Oticon, n.d.). Clear speech is speech that is

- Accurate and fully formed
- Naturally slower

- Naturally louder
- Lively with inflection and stress
- Characterized by pauses between all phrases and sentences

Cultural Implications of Hearing Impairment

Some individuals with hearing impairment may be members of the Deaf community. American Deaf culture is considered a unique linguistic minority that communicates primarily through the use of ASL (National Technical Institute for the Deaf, 2004). The terms *deaf* and *hard of hearing* are preferred over the term *hearing impaired*. It is important to realize that members of the Deaf community may include individuals with mild to profound hearing impairment because Deaf culture is defined by a shared language and experiences and not solely by degree of hearing impairment.

The majority of children with deafness are born to parents without hearing impairment. Therefore, Deaf culture is primarily passed on through contact with Deaf people in the community and not through families (Iowa Department of Public Health, 2008).

Prevention of Hearing Impairment

The Joint Committee on Infant Hearing (2007) has identified several risk factors associated with permanent congenital, delayed-onset, or progressive hearing loss in childhood. Some hearing loss may be preventable if diagnosed early through the following steps:

- Monitoring ototoxic medications
- Minimizing exposure during pregnancy to certain infections associated with congenital hearing impairment using simple steps, such as frequent hand-washing
- Preventing head trauma through the use of appropriate car restraints as well as helmets during activities, such as bicycling
- Receiving vaccinations for preventable infections, such as meningitis

Great strides, however, can be made in the prevention of hearing impairment due to noise exposure with increased awareness and the use of hearing protection.

DEAFBLINDNESS

The diagnosis of deafblindness does not require complete loss of vision or hearing. However, the impairment in both vision and hearing, even when corrected, is such that these individuals have severe difficulties with communication, mobility, and access to information (Scott, 1998). Ninety percent of children with deafblindness have at least one other disability or chronic health problem (National Consortium on Deafblindness, n.d.). As with vision and hearing impairments alone, deafblindness can be a result of genetic problems, prematurity, brain injury, or illness. Early diagnosis is critical but may be missed because of comorbidities experienced by many children. Touch is the primary means of interacting with the world for an individual who is deafblind. An infant with deafblindness alone in a crib is essentially alone in the world.

A support service provider (SSP) is a person who works with an individual who is deafblind and acts as a link between that person and the community. The SSP provides access to the community, either by acting as a human guide or by arranging transportation. The SSP also provides information about visual, auditory, and other environmental conditions. The adult with deafblindness should ultimately be the person making decisions, not the SSP, who is merely acting as a guide. SSPs are not necessarily expected to provide direct care, teach, or run errands. However, they can help the individual with deafblindness interact socially with others, without which help the individual may be very isolated.

It is important for others in the environment to reach out to the person with deafblindness rather than waiting for them to make the first move. People interacting with individuals with deafblindness should pay attention to subtle cues, such as changes in movements, to indicate emotional status, wants, and needs. People who know the individual well may be particularly adept at identifying problems or needs based on behavior; these people should be taken seriously when they identify concerns or changes in the behavior of the deafblind individual that may be indicative of medical problems requiring further investigation. Consistency also helps impose order on an environment that otherwise can be lacking in useful information.

In addition to communication, safety is a concern for those who are deafblind. They are unable to access alarms and warnings in the usual manner. They may be unable to communicate with health care providers in an emergency (Scott, 1998). Individuals with deafblindness may have some residual hearing or vision and may be able to respond to voices, particularly with a hearing aid, or to visual cues. When interacting with a deafblind person in an emergency, try each ear. Likewise, vision may be best at a set distance, such as 1 foot, 2 feet, or 3 feet (Scott, 1998). Touch cues, such as an arm or hand to let the individual know someone is there, are helpful. This includes a touch to signify one's presence, allowing the individual to feel instruments that may be used, or communication through use of the deaf-blind alphabet or signs. It may also be possible to slowly write block alphabet characters into the hand of the person who is deafblind.

NURSING ROLE IN THE CARE OF INDIVIDUALS WITH SENSORY IMPAIRMENT

Nurses remain an integral part of the team when caring for individuals with sensory impairments. They may be responsible for helping individuals with sensory impairments learn to manage their own health care, training direct care providers, coordinating team care, and case management. Although the nurse may be responsible for training direct care providers, the individual nurse caring for a person with a sensory impairment may not be an expert in sensory impairment. It is therefore critical to be in close contact with the specialists on the team. It may be possible to organize in-service education provided by the experts. Safety considerations are a significant concern. In addition to providing information and helpful hints to direct care providers, the experts can also help nurses learn ways to adapt health care procedures for the individual with impaired vision. Nurses, in turn, can then provide further opportunities for practice and learning in independent health care management, such as accessing medications, wound care, and activities such as insulin management. Empowering patients or consumers in learning self-advocacy is an important aspect of nursing care.

Case management is another critical component of nursing care. Patients or consumers need to get to scheduled appointments or have recommended consultations scheduled. Different clinicians have been known to give contradictory advice; nurses can help to clarify these discrepancies and facilitate communication between providers. An individual with limited communication ability in addition to a sensory impairment may need an advocate when dealing with others in the health care system or the community in general, although it is important to support the individual in their attempts to advocate for themselves.

EMERGENCY PREPAREDNESS FOR INDIVIDUALS WITH SENSORY IMPAIRMENT

Nurses may be providing care for individuals with sensory impairments in their own homes, community-based supported living, or intermediate care facilities. In these settings, nurses may be directly responsible for managing the safety of individuals facing an emergency evacuation.

Nurses need to consider how individuals with sensory impairment will be notified of emergencies, how and where they will be evacuated, and who will act as an interpreter for the emergency. Having a buddy system may be helpful. Practice sessions, such as fire drills or responding to tornado warnings, prior to an emergency may be useful.

A copy of medical records should be available, including guardianship papers if appropriate, as well as a supply of medication. There should be extra batteries for hearing aids, cochlear implants, or other battery-operated sensory or communication devices. An extra pair of glasses or other visual aids should be available. A dark pen and high-contrast paper may be useful. Mobility canes need to be accessible. Braille or other communication cards should be in the emergency kit, along with contacts for those who can interpret (American Association of the Deaf-Blind, 2007; Bourquin et al., 2006). Communication cards contain commonly used sentences, questions, or information that can be handed to others in situations in which an interpreter is not available. There should be specific information on the individual's needs (e.g., the type of sign language they use, what devices they use to communicate). If individuals have service animals, water and food will be needed and should be readily accessible. Other items appropriate to the care of the individual, which may include formula, feeding bags, and catheters, should be available.

CONCLUSION

Vision and hearing are integral parts of communication and socialization, as well as a source of information about dangers in the environment. Significant vision or hearing impairment can be a primary source of disability or can be associated with other types of disability. Nurses should consider the following points when caring for individuals with sensory impairment:

- Be aware of the individual's diagnoses for anticipatory guidance and care planning

- Early identification and intervention is critical to promote optimal outcomes
- Consider sensory impairments if there are changes in behavior or problem behaviors
- Functional data, such as the ability to see something small and pick it up, are helpful
- Obtain help from those with expertise in vision impairment, hearing impairment, or deafblindness
- Structure and routine can be very important for those with sensory impairments
- Do not make assumptions about cognitive status based on sensory impairment
- Be in touch with your own responses so as not to isolate or exclude the individual
- Include emergency planning in care plans
- Make use of the Internet to find information about leisure activities, assistive devices, and support groups
- Ensure consumers, families, and direct care staff know how assistive devices are to be used
- Reinforce skills taught by occupational therapists, physical therapists, mobility and orientation specialists, and other specialists in sensory impairment so these skills can be practiced in all settings
- Base nursing practice on a "people first" philosophy, recognizing that people with sensory impairments are people first and are not defined by having a sensory impairment

In this chapter, sensory impairments have been discussed. Practical advice for the nursing care of individuals with vision or hearing impairments or deafblindness has been highlighted.

REFERENCES

American Association of the Deaf-Blind. (2007). *Building an emergency kit: Checklist*. Retrieved July 17, 2008, from http://www.aadb.org/information/emergency_preparation/emerg_kit.html.

Blakemore, S., Tavassoli, T., Calo, S., Thomas, R., Catmur, C., Frith, U., et al. (2006). Tactile sensitivity in Asperger syndrome. *Brain and Cognition, 61,* 5–13.

Bodner-Johnson, B. (2003). The deaf child in the family. In B. Bodner-Johnson & M. Sass-Lehrer (Eds.), *The young deaf or hard of hearing child: A family-centered approach to early education* (pp. 3–37). Baltimore: Paul H. Brookes Publishing Co.

Boulton, M., Haines, L., & Smyth, D. (2006). Health-related quality of life of children with vision impairment or blindness. *Developmental Medicine & Child Neurology, 48,* 656–661.

Bourquin, E., Gasaway, M., Jordan, B., Pope, R., Rosensweig, N., & Spiers, E. (2006). *Support service providers for people who are deaf-blind.* American Association of the Deaf-Blind. Retrieved July 16, 2008, from http://aadb.org/pdf/SSP%20White%20Paper%20FINAL%20NOV%2006.pdf.

Davis, J.M., Elfenbein, J., Schum, R., & Bentler, R. (1986). Effects of mild and moderate hearing impairments on language, educational, and psychosocial behavior of children. *Journal of Speech and Hearing Disorders, 51,* 53–62.

Erting, C. (2003). Language and literacy development in deaf children. In B. Bodner-Johnson & M. Sass-Lehrer (Eds.), *The young deaf or hard of hearing child: A family-centered approach to early education* (pp. 373–398). Baltimore: Paul H. Brookes Publishing Co.

Estabrooks, W., & Marlowe, J. (2000). *The baby is listening: An educational tool for professionals who work with children who are deaf or hard of hearing* (pp. 1–78). Washington, DC: Alexander Graham Bell Association for the Deaf and Hard of Hearing.

Galaburda, A. (2003). Developmental disorders of vision. *Neurologic Clinics of North America, 21,* 687–707.

Galati, D., Scherer, K., & Ricci-Bitti, P. (1997). Voluntary facial expression of emotion: Comparing congenitally blind with normally sighted encoders. *Journal of Personality and Social Psychology, 73,* 1363–1379.

Hart, B., & Risley, T.R. (1995). *Meaningful differences in the everyday experiences of young American children.* Baltimore: Paul H. Brookes Publishing Co.

Hart, B., & Risley, T.R. (1999). *The social world of children learning to talk.* Baltimore: Paul H. Brookes Publishing Co.

Ingelse, J., & Steele, G. (2001). Characteristics of the pediatric/adolescent low-vision population at the Illinois school for the visually impaired. *Optometry, 72,* 761–766.

Iowa Department of Public Health. (2008). *Iowa's early hearing detection and intervention family resource guide: For parents of children who are deaf or hard of hearing* (3rd ed.). Retrieved August 4, 2009, from http://www.idph.state.ia.us/iaehdi/common/pdf/iaehdi_family_resource_guide_english.pdf.

Johnson, C.D., Benson, P.V., & Seaton, J. (Eds.). (1997). Assessment practice. In C.D. Johnson, P.V. Benson, & J.B. Seaton (Eds.). *Educational audiology handbook* (pp. 49–66). San Diego: Singular Thomson Learning.

Joint Committee on Infant Hearing. (2007). *Year 2007 position statement: Principles and guidelines for early hearing detection and intervention programs.* Retrieved August 4, 2008, from http://www.asha.org/docs/html/PS2007-00281.html.

Jones, T.W., & Jones, J.K. (2003). Educating young deaf children with multiple disabilities. In B. Bodner-Johnson & M. Sass-Lehrer (Eds.), *The young deaf or hard of hearing child: A family-centered approach to early education* (pp. 297–29). Baltimore: Paul H. Brookes Publishing Co.

Kef, S., & Dekovic, M. (2004). The role of parental and peer support in adolescents well-being: A comparison of adolescents with and without a visual impairment. *Journal of Adolescence, 27,* 453–466.

Khalfa, S., Bruneau, N., Roge, B., Georgieff, N., Veuillet, E., Adrien, J., et al. (2004).

Increased perception of loudness in autism. *Hearing Research, 198,* 87–92.

Markowitz, S. (2006). Principles of modern low vision rehabilitation. *Canadian Journal of Ophthalmology, 41,* 289–312.

Marshall, L.A. (1997). *Communication accessibility, behavioral ratings, and childhood deafness: Investigation of three modes of communication.* Unpublished doctoral dissertation, Gallaudet University.

Martini, F., Ober, W., Garrison, C., Welch, K., & Hutchings, R. (1989). *Fundamentals of anatomy and physiology* (4th ed.). Upper Saddle River, NJ: Prentice Hall.

Meadow-Orlans, K. (1997). Effects of mother and infant hearing status on interactions at twelve and eighteen months. *Journal of Deaf Studies and Deaf Education, 2,* 26–36.

Meadow-Orlans, K.P., Smith-Gray, S., & Dyssegaard, B. (1995). Sources of stress for mothers and fathers of deaf and hard of hearing infants. *American Annals of the Deaf, 140,* 352–357.

Miller, K., & Apt, L. (2003). The eyes. In C. Rudolph & A. Rudolph (Eds.), *Rudolph's pediatrics* (21st ed., pp. 2351–2419). New York: McGraw-Hill.

Mills, D., & Ciolofi Murphy, A. (2007). Sensory alterations. In N. Potts & B. Mandelco (Eds.), *Pediatric nursing: Caring for children and their families* (pp. 1007–1043). Clifton Park, NY: Thompson.

Moeller, M.P. (1985). Developmental approaches to communication assessment and enhancement. In E. Cherow (Ed.), *Hearing impaired children and youth with developmental disabilities: An interdisciplinary foundation for service* (pp. 171–198). Washington, DC: Gallaudet University Press.

Moeller, M.P. (2000). Early intervention and language development in children who are deaf and hard of hearing. *Pediatrics, 106,* 1–9.

Moeller, M.P., Tomblin, J.B., Yoshinaga-Itano, C., Connor, C.M., & Jerger, S. (2007). Current state of knowledge: Language and literacy of children with hearing impairment. *Ear and Hearing, 28,* 740–753.

Moores, D. (2001). *Educating the deaf: Psychology , principles, and practices* (5th ed.). Boston: Houghton Mifflin.

National Consortium on Deaf-Blindness. (n.d.). *Overview of deaf-blindness.* Retrieved July 17, 2008, from http://www.nationaldb.org/NCDBProducts.php?prod ID=38.

National Dissemination Center for Children with Disabilities. (2004). *Deafness and hearing loss.* Retrieved October 1, 2008, from http://old.nichcy.org/pubs/factshe/fs3txt.htm.

National Institutes of Health. (2001). *Healthy people 2010: Vision and hearing.* Retrieved July 17, 2008, from http://www.healthy-people.gov/document/HTML/Volume2/28Vision.htm.

National Technical Institute for the Deaf. (2004). *Deaf culture.* Retrieved October 1, 2008, from http://www.netac.rit.edu/publication/tipsheet/deafculture.html.

Open Directory Project. (n.d.). *Top: Sports: Disabled: Blind.* Retrieved August 4, 2008, from http://www.dmoz.org/Sports/Disabled/Blind/.

Oticon. (n.d.). *Clear speech.* Retrieved October 1, 2008, from http://otikids.oticonus.com/eprise/main/Oticon/US_en/SEC_AboutHearing/LearnAboutHearing/Products/SEC_OtiKids/Parents/Networking/90642810pf1_cbr_clspeech.pdf.

Papousek, H., & Papousek, M. (1983). Biological basis of social interactions: Implications of research for an understanding of behavioral deviance. *Journal of Child Psychology and Psychiatry, 24,* 117–129.

Salati, R., Schiavulli, O., Giammari, G., & Borgatti, R. (2001). Checklist for the evaluation of low vision in uncooperative patients. *Journal of Pediatric Ophthalmology and Strabismus, 38,* 90–94.

Schlesinger, H. (1995). Hearing loss. In S. Parker & B. Zuckerman (Eds.), *Developmental and behavioral pediatrics* (pp. 174–179). Boston: Little, Brown.

Scott, J. (1998). Communicating with a deaf-blind patient in an emergency. *Accident and Emergency Nursing, 6,* 164–166.

Sininger, Y.S., & Trautwein, P. (2002). Electrical stimulation of the auditory nerve via cochlear implants in patients with auditory neuropathy. *The Annals of Otology, Rhinology, and Laryngology, 111,* 29–31.

Skene, D., & Arendt, J. (2007). Circadian

rhythm sleep disorders in the blind and their treatment with melatonin. *Sleep, 8,* 651–655.

Smith, L.E.H. (2004). Pathogenesis of retinopathy of prematurity. *Growth Hormone & IGF Research, 14,* 140–144.

Spruyt-Rocks, R. (2007). Right at home: Homes for deaf-blind adults designed to be "senseable." *Abilities, 21, 1–2.*

Swisher, M.V. (2000). Learning to converse: How deaf mothers support the development of attention and conversational skills in their young deaf children. In P.E. Spencer, C. Erting, & J. Marschark (Eds.), *The deaf child in the family and at school: Essays in honor of Kathryn P. Meadow-Orlans* (pp. 21–40). Mahwah, NJ: Lawrence Erlbaum.

Trychin, S. (2003). *Living with hearing loss workbook.* Erie, PA: Author.

Van Splunder, J., Stilma, J., & Evenhuis, H. (2003). Visual performance in specific syndromes associated with intellectual disability. *European Journal of Ophthalmology, 13,* 566–574.

Venes, D., Biderman, A., Adler, E., Fenton, B., & Enright, A. (2005). *Taber's cyclopedic medical dictionary.* Atlanta, GA: F.A. Davis.

Vohr, B.R., Carty, L.M., Moore, P.E., & Letourneau, K. (1998). The Rhode Island Hearing Assessment Program: Experience with statewide hearing screening (1993–1996). *The Journal of Pediatrics, 133,* 353–357.

Wake, M., Hughes, E.K., Poulakis, Z., Collins, C., & Rikards, F.W. (2004). Outcomes of children with mild-profound hearing loss at 7 to 8 years: A population study. *Ear & Hearing, 25,* 1–8.

Warburg, M. (2001). Visual impairment in adult people with moderate, severe, and profound intellectual disability. *ACTA Ophthalmological Scandinavica, 79,* 450–454.

Wilkinson, M. (2003). Low vision rehabilitation: A concise overview. *Journal of the American Society of Ophthalmic Registered Nurses, 28,* 111–119.

World Bank Group, Disease Control Priorities Project. (2006). *Loss of vision and hearing.* Retrieved July 17, 2008, from http://www.dcp2.org/pubs/DCP/50/Section/7535.

Yoshinaga-Itano, C., Sedey, A., Coulter, D.K., & Mehl, A.L. (1998). Language of early and later identified children with hearing loss. *Pediatrics, 102,* 1161–1171.

CHAPTER 18

Policies, Legislation, and Ethical/Legal Issues

Kathryn Smith and Teresa A. Savage

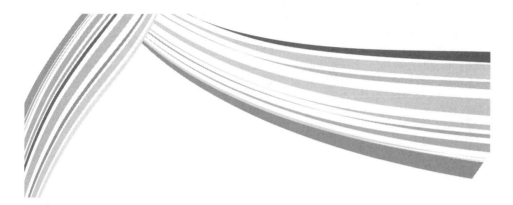

T his chapter provides an overview of the major legislation affecting the lives of individuals with intellectual and developmental disabilities (IDD) and their families; ethical and legal issues related to care of the population; and nursing implications for practice, research, and policy. Nurses have an obligation to keep current with legislation in order to provide optimal care and assistance to individuals with IDD and their families, as well as to impact the communities in which they reside.

LEGISLATION

Various pieces of legislation over the years have helped to ensure the rights and full inclusion into society of individuals with IDD. These laws form the basis of our special education and developmental disabilities service systems, and are therefore important to understand in the context of advocating for services on behalf of individuals with IDD and their families. While the focus of this chapter will be major federal legislation, there are numerous other federal and state laws and statutes that provide protection and direct the services of individuals with specials needs; these should be known to anyone serving the population in a specific locale.

The Americans with Disabilities Act

The Americans with Disabilities Act (ADA) of 1990 (PL 101-336) is civil rights legislation governed by the U.S. Department of Justice. It ensures that people with disabilities have equal opportunities to participate in programs, services, and activities related to employment, public services, public accommodations, and services operated by private entities, communications, and public health and welfare (U.S. Department of Justice, 2008). The purpose of the legislation is to provide a clear national mandate for the elimination of discrimination against those with disabilities, provide enforceable standards addressing discrimination, ensure that the federal government plays a central role in enforcing the standards, and address major areas of discrimination faced by people with disabilities. The ADA mandates changes to an environment, including reasonable accommodation for those with disabilities in schools, hospitals, physicians' offices, and community businesses. Similar to the Rehabilitation Act of 1973 (PL 93-112), an individual with a disability is defined as someone who has a physical or mental impairment that substantially limits one or more major life activities; has a record of such an impairment; or is regarded as having such an impairment.

The ADA contains five titles. Title I of the Act prohibits

> No covered entity (i.e., private employers, state and local governments, employment agencies and labor unions [sic]) shall discriminate against a qualified individual with a disability because of the disability of such individual in regard to job application procedures, the hiring, advancement, or discharge of employees, employee compensation, job training, and other terms, conditions and privileges of employment (ADA, 1990).

Reasonable accommodations in the workplace are required, such as making existing facilities usable by someone with a disability, job restructuring, modifying work schedules, acquiring or modifying equipment or devices, adjusting or modifying examinations, training materials or policies, or providing qualified readers or interpreters, although the reasonable accommodation need not impose an undue hardship on the employer (U.S. Equal Opportunity Commission, 2009). Furthermore, an employer is not required to lower quality or production standards to make an accommodation. That being said, there are numerous accommodations that can be made to assist qualified individuals with disabilities to be successful in the workplace. Job coaches, vocational specialists, physical and occupational therapists, and ergonomics experts can assist in identifying necessary modifications to assure accommodation.

Title II addresses public entities, including any state or local government and telecommunications and public transportation. It also prohibits exclusion or denial of public service benefits based on disability, and assures access to such private public facilities as hotels, restaurants, theaters, and transportation modalities (U.S. Department of Justice, 2008).

Title III of the Act describes various public facilities and accommodations that are included in the Act, including hotels, restaurants, recreational facilities, and stores. Title IV requires states to have telephone relay systems to promote communication between hearing and nonhearing users. Individuals with disabilities are entitled to programs and services generally available to other members of the public, such as restaurants, banks, stores, and medical offices (American Academy of Pediatrics, 1996). Title V refers to other provisions of the law related to federal jurisdiction, legal fees, and categories of individuals not covered. Full inclusion and accessibility to the world at large is the goal of these provisions.

In 2008, the ADA Amendments Act of 2008 (PL 110-325) was passed. This act provides clear and comprehensive national mandate for the elimination of discrimination and clear, strong, enforceable standards. Specifically, this Act seeks to restore the 1990 act to its original intent and address court proceedings that have occurred, limiting the scope of the act, and giving businesses a clearer understanding of what they need to do to comply with the bill (Mitka, 2008).

The Developmental Disabilities Assistance
and Bill of Rights Act Amendments of 2000

The Developmental Disabilities Assistance and Bill of Rights Act Amendments of 2000 (PL 106-402) was originally authorized in 1963 as the Mental Retardation Facilities and Community Mental Health Centers Construction Act of 1963 (PL 88-164) and later reauthorized as the Developmental Disabilities Assistance and Bill of Rights Act of 1975 (PL 94-103). It begins with some important words that frame the discussion for many of the pieces of legislation discussed in this chapter:

> Congress finds that... disability is a natural part of the human experience that does not diminish the right of individuals with developmental disabilities to live independently, to exert control and choice over their lives, and to fully participate in and contribute to their communities through full integration and inclusion in the economic, political, social, cultural, and educational mainstream of United States society. (S. 1809, H.R. 4920).

As such, the purpose of the Developmental Disabilities Assistance and Bill of Rights Act Amendments of 2000 is, in part, to

> Assure that individuals with developmental disabilities and their families participate in the design of, and have access to needed services, supports, and assistance to promote self-determination, independence, productivity, integration, and inclusion in all facets of community life through culturally competent programs authorized under this title (S. 1809, H.R. 4920).

The Act further specifies that this will be achieved in a number of ways, including the following:

1. State councils on Developmental Disabilities, which are charged with advocacy, capacity building, and systems change related to a coordinated, consumer, and family-directed comprehensive system that includes services, supports, and other assistance. State councils are to be consumer and family directed, with not less than 60% who are individuals with developmental disabilities, parents, or guardians of children with developmental disabilities, or immediate relatives or guardians of adults with mentally impairing developmental disabilities (Association of University Centers on Disabilities [AUCD], 2007). Individual state councils can be found by using a web search engine and typing in the state's name and the term *state council on developmental disabilities*. These sites will often provide a link to other resources for individuals and families related to developmental disabilities and the state's service system.

2. A Protection and Advocacy system in each state, charged with protecting the legal and human rights for individuals with disabilities. The National Disability Rights Network (http://www.napas.org) is a nonprofit membership organization for the federally mandated protection and advocacy systems and provides links to specific state offices.

3. University Centers for Excellence in Developmental Disabilities Education, Research, and Service (commonly known as UCEDDs) provide training, community services, conduct research, and disseminate information related to developmental disabilities. Information about UCEDDs, which are located in each state, can be found at www.aucd.org.

4. The Family Support Program provides grants to states to help them provide supports and services to help families caring for members with severe disabilities (AUCD, 2007).

5. Projects of National Significance are funded to collect data to provide technical assistance and support promising projects that will contribute to the Act's goals of independence, productivity, integration, and inclusion of those with developmental disabilities (AUCD, 2007).

While the Developmental Disabilities Assistance and Bill of Rights Act Amendments of 2000 provides overall direction in terms of services for individuals with developmental disabilities, each state develops its own system for serving the population. These agencies can be located within health, developmental services, mental health, or other systems within the state, and therefore can be difficult to find. Using the above links and search strategies will enable the nurse to learn more about a specific state's system, and promote successful advocacy on behalf of individuals with IDD and their families. For those working directly with individuals as care managers, nurse practitioners, and in other similar roles, it is essential to become knowledgeable about the local service system in order to work effectively on behalf of individuals with IDD, in either an advocacy and/or care coordination role.

The Individuals with Disabilities Education Act

Children and youth with disabilities have not always been entitled to a free appropriate public education. Although compulsory education laws were in place in all states by 1918, the exclusion of students with disabilities was upheld in courts as recently as 1969. By the late 1960s and early 1970s, most states had passed laws requiring states to educate students with disabilities. In 1975, President Gerald Ford signed the Education of All Handicapped Children Act (EAHCA) of 1975 (PL 94-142), providing federal funding to states to assist them in educating students with disabilities, wherein states would provide a free appropriate public education to students with disabilities in return for federal funding. The 1990 amendments of the EAHCA renamed the legislation the Individuals with Disabilities Education Act (IDEA) of 1990 (PL 101-476) and was altered again in 2004 as the Individuals with Disabilities Education Improvement Act of 2004 (IDEA 2004; PL 108-446). IDEA 2004 is administered by the Office of Special Education Programs in the U.S. Department of Education. For additional information on early intervention programs, refer to Chapters 3 and 4.

For children birth to age 3, IDEA 2004 provides the requirement for early intervention services for children with or at risk for a developmental delay in one or more of the following developmental areas: cognitive, physical, communication, social/emotional, or adaptive. The process begins with a multidisciplinary evaluation and assessment of the child's strengths, delays or difficulties, and a determination of whether or not the child is eligible for early intervention services. After the evaluation is complete, the team and parents meet together to review the findings and develop the individual family service plan (IFSP), used to map out needed services for the child and family. The IFSP provides specific information about the child's developmental level and needs, family information, goals, services to be provided, where, by whom, and payment source, and the steps to take to transition the child out of early intervention. The IFSP must be reviewed every 6 months and updated annually (National Dissemination Center for Children with Disabilities [NICHCY], 2009a).

Early intervention services can include special instruction, therapies, parent support and training, transportation, equipment, and service coordination. Services are to be provided in natural settings whenever possible, such as the home, a child care setting, or a preschool. Some services are free, while others may require that families use their health insurance, Medicaid, or cash on a sliding scale basis (NICHCY, 2009a).

For children 3 to 21 years, the cornerstone of the day-to-day operation of IDEA is the individualized education program (IEP). The IEP is a written document of the educational plan designed to meet the needs of the individual child. The plan has two purposes: to set learning goals for the child and to document the services that the school district will provide to assist the child in meeting the goals. The IEP is developed by a team, including the parents, the child's regular education teacher, the special education teacher, any providers of related services, and a school administrator who can commit to resources on behalf of the district, and may include the student as well. Parents may bring additional supports as they wish, including advocates, family members, friends, or professionals who provide care to the child. The IEP must include the child's present level of academic performance and functioning, measurable annual goals, the special education, and related services that are to be provided. The IEP specifies how much of the day the child will spend separately from children without disabilities, how the child will participate in district and state-wide testing, how often services will be provided, and how progress will be measured (NICHCY, 2009b; U.S. Department of Education, 2008a). In addition, beginning with the first IEP after the child turns 16, the IEP must include appropriate postsecondary goals related to training, education, employment, and independent living skills, and the services needed to assist the youth in reaching these goals (U.S. Department of Education, 2008a, b).

The process for development of the IEP begins with a comprehensive assessment to determine the child's need for services and determine that the child has an eligible condition. Eligible conditions include intellectual disabilities, hearing, speech, language or visual impairments, serious emotional disturbance, orthopedic impairments, autism, traumatic brain injury, other health impairments, or specific learning disabilities. An evaluation, or assessment, can be requested by school personnel or by a parent, although parents must provide their consent before the evaluation can take place. The school has 60 days from the time of parental consent to complete the evaluation. An IEP meeting must be held within 30 days of the completion of the assessment to determine if the child is eligible for special education. The IEP must then be reviewed annually to ensure that it meets the child's needs in achieving goals, and is revised as needed, although parents may request more frequent reviews of the IEP if desired. At least every 3 years, the child must be reevaluated, but again, this can occur more frequently if the parents have cause for concern (NICHCY, 2009b).

If the child has health concerns that impact the child's learning, often a nurse will be included on the IEP team. The nurse brings valuable information to the rest of the team about the health issues and needed services. In addition, the nurse can serve as an advocate and a support person for the child and parents during the IEP process. For more information on special education and IEPs, see Chapters 3 and 5.

Rehabilitation Act of 1973

The Rehabilitation Act of 1973 (PL 93-112), amended as the Rehabilitation Act Amendments of 1993 (PL 103-73) and 1998 (PL 105-220) provides a range of services for individuals with physical and cognitive disabilities (WebAIM, 2008), including state plans for rehabilitation, evaluations, studies of methods of providing rehabilitation services, construction of rehabilitation facilities, development of new and innovative methods for services, and expansion of services to those previously underserved. Other provisions of the bill include the promotion and expansion of employment opportunities, increasing rehabilitation personnel, evaluating existing approaches to architectural and transportation barriers, and enforcing existing statutory and regulatory standards and requirements. It was signed into law by President Richard Nixon and is a civil rights law, aimed at protecting individuals with disabilities from discrimination based on their disabilities (Yell, Rogers, & Rogers, 1998). It applies to employers as well as any entity that receives federal financial assistance, including all government agencies, federally funded projects, K-12 schools, and postsecondary educational institutions (Web AIM, 2008).

Section 504 of the Rehabilitation Act is one of the features of great importance to those serving and advocating on behalf of individuals with disabilities. Section 504 of the specifies that

> No otherwise qualified individual with a disability in the United States... shall solely by reason of her or his disability, be excluded from the participation in, be denied the benefits of, or be subjected to discrimination under any program or activity receiving Federal financial assistance (H.R. 8070).

Section 504 requires recipients of federal funds to provide to students with disabilities appropriate educational services, supplementary services, and/or special education and related services designed to meet their individual needs within a regular classroom setting.

To be protected under Section 504, a student must be determined to 1) have a physical or mental impairment that substantially limits one or more major life activities, 2) have a record of such an impairment, or 3) be regarded as having such an impairment (U.S. Department of Education, 2008b; U.S. Department of Health and Human Services, 2008). The law is designed to ensure that those with disabilities are not discriminated against because of their disability. Title II of the ADA extends the prohibition against discrimination to a full range of state or local services, including public schools, whether or not they receive federal funding (U.S. Department of Education, 2008b).

Most important, Section 504 allows for reasonable accommodations for students with disabilities, even if they are not receiving special education services. This allowance is important for those students who have a special need, but who do not qualify for special education. This may include a youth with spina bifida who needs extra time to get from one classroom to the next due to limitations in mobility, or a child with diabetes who needs to be able to eat a snack in the classroom or leave class to check blood sugar.

The school's Section 504 coordinator—often an assistant principal, counselor, or a clerk—is responsible for facilitating the Section 504 process including plan development and implementation. The plan, consisting of the identified disability and the accommodations, is ideally developed by a committee composed of individuals

Table 18.1.   Comparison of a Section 504 plan and an individualized education program (IEP)

Section 504 plan	IEP
Has a disability and does not require special education services	Has a disability and requires special education services
General education	Special education
Does not include clearly established procedural safeguards	Includes system of procedural safeguards
Developed collaboratively between parent and school administrator	Rules regarding inclusion of specific team members
Requires school districts to conduct impartial hearings for parents who disagree with the school's decision	Requires school districts to conduct impartial hearings for parents who disagree with the school's decisions
Addresses the need for specific accommodations	Provides a comprehensive plan for services
No specific timelines	Specific timelines

Source: Nonverbal Learning Disorders Association (2008).

involved in the student's education, and includes the parents. Accommodations can include such things as extra time to take a test, taking tests orally or in a separate location, or preferential seating. If families believe that their child has needs that can be met through special education versus accommodations, parents may then initiate the IEP process. See Table 18.1 for a comparison of Section 504 and IEP plans.

This section provided basic information about key laws protecting those with IDD in their pursuit of full inclusion in our society. Ethical and legal issues are described below and provide a context for the application of these laws.

ETHICAL/LEGAL ISSUES

Nurses working with individuals with IDD encounter a myriad of ethical issues. Many of the ethical issues center around the person's capacity to make decisions or when and/or how much paternalism is appropriate. Four ethical issues, embedded in the language of rights, will be discussed in this section: the right to community inclusion, the right to bodily integrity (growth attenuation), the right to sexual expression and reproduction, and the freedom to participate in research.

The Right to Community Inclusion

Liberty, a very important concept in Western civilizations, is about pursuing life choices. For people with IDD, their choices may be limited, or they may not have a choice in important decisions, such as living arrangements, dating, marriage, childbearing, and employment. The position statement on inclusion from the American Association on Intellectual and Developmental Disabilities (AAIDD) says, "All our constituents have the right to participate fully in their diverse communities" (AAIDD, 2002, p. 1). This participation is limited, however, unless supports are made available and affordable for all people with IDD who need them.

Promotion of autonomy and self-determination are the goals that guide service to people with IDD. As Wehmeyer and Bolding (2001) concluded, the environment plays an essential role in enhancing self-determination. When the environment is "community-based and individually focused" (p. 371), there is a greater likelihood for inclusion and integration. Assistive technology devices that can help with organization of daily activities and home management skills could facilitate community living. The physical environment both at home and in the workplace can be structured to promote inclusion, decision making, and choice. Wehmeyer and Bolding (2001) found a significant difference in self-determination and autonomy measures between individuals living in noncongregate settings and those living in group homes and large congregate settings. However, Neely-Barnes, Marcenko, and Weber (2008a) found higher quality-of-life scores with those living in smaller living arrangements; they advocated for smaller living arrangements and offering choice to people regardless of degree of IDD to promote community inclusion (2008b).

In a content analysis of research literature since the 1970s, the authors saw a trend toward focusing on strengths versus challenges, acquisition of adaptive behaviors critical for community integration, and identification of factors influencing quality of life (Shogren, Wehmeyer, Buchanan, & Lopez, 2006). The ability to make a choice and communicate the choice is essential for community integration. Nurses need to be versed in ways to assess decision-making capacity and communication skills in order to teach/facilitate decision making and augment communication if necessary (Batorowicz, McDougall, & Shepherd, 2006).

In balancing the right to habilitation with the right to choose, Bannerman, Sheldon, Sherman, and Harchik (1990) proposed these strategies:

1. Teach independent living skills

2. Seek individuals' input into the skills they want to learn and their preferred teaching modalities

3. Teach individuals how to make a choice

4. Provide opportunities for individuals to make choices in their home setting and employment setting, both during work and at breaks

As the researchers aptly concluded, "All people have the right to eat too many doughnuts and take a nap" (Bannerman et al., 1990, p. 86).

Dignity of Risk

With choice comes risk, however, some questions the caregiver may have to ask include:

1. When is paternalism appropriate?

2. When should family and friends stand back and let a person with IDD make "bad" decisions?

3. Even when supports are available, what if individuals with IDD prefer not to use them and to make decisions on their own?

4. At what point should an advocate intercede or interfere?

The concept *dignity of risk* captures the positive tension between autonomy and paternalism. People with IDD should be able to make mistakes, "bad" decisions, or forgo making a decision—as those without IDD can do—and suffer the consequences. However, because they often live their lives under much scrutiny, individuals with IDD may not have the opportunity to make or exercise their choices. Tøssebro (2005) saw dilemmas in self-determination for people with IDD. He also supported the dignity of risk, but believed one can be powerless if one does not have the capacity to make choices and forecast consequences. Deinstitutionalization has occurred and community inclusion and integration continues, but as with other civil rights movements, there is a way to go before full participation and equality are achieved.

Opportunities for decision making, especially for increasingly important decisions, should be presented for individuals with IDD. Nurses can provide numerous opportunities for learning and practicing decisions, and can assess decision-making capabilities at those moments. Families or other caregivers closest to the person making the decision should refrain from abrogating the decision, except in dire circumstances in which great harm could be done.

Often, the family member accompanying the person with IDD to a medical appointment may be asked for consent when it is needed. In practice, there are three types of consents: *direct consent* from the person who is presumed to have the capacity to consent; *substitute consent* from a family member or guardian; and *concurrent consent,* which combines the direct and substitute (Turnbull, Turnbull, Bronicki, Summers, & Roeder-Gordon, 1989). When a person lacks capacity, substitute consent is sought. When capacity is questioned or the risk is higher, concurrent consent is sought. Many families have not gone through the guardianship process, often because the cost is prohibitive. However, some have not sought guardianship because they believe most of the time the person with IDD can make their own health care decisions. As with many people without IDD, family and friends advise and help make important decisions, so guardianship has not been necessary. Nurses need to be aware of the relevant laws in their state regarding obtaining informed consent and surrogate consent.

The Right to Bodily Integrity: Growth Attenuation

In 2006, a pediatrician/ethicist and pediatric endocrinologist published an article in which they described using high-dose estrogen to stunt the growth of a 6-year-old girl with significant developmental disabilities. Her uterus and breast buds were removed to avoid problems from the high-dose estrogen therapy. The combination of hormonal therapy, hysterectomy, and breast bud removal were coined the *Ashley treatment* by her parents. The parents sought this treatment as a way to keep Ashley smaller; they refer to her as their "pillow angel" because she remains on her pillow where they place her. The parents desired to care for Ashley at home without outsiders assisting and feared if Ashley grew to their height, she would be too big for them to care for her into her adulthood. Removal of the uterus was intended to prevent dysmenorrhea and removal of the breast buds was for ease in using a harness in her wheelchairs and to discourage sexual abuse that large breasts could "invite," according to her parents' blog (http://ashleytreatment.spaces.live.com).

Ashley's physicians went to the hospital's ethics committee for its review and approval. The parents maintain they received thousands of emails in support of the Ashley treatment. There was enormous media coverage and many professional groups issued statements. An investigation by Disability Rights Washington (2007) found the hospital and parents had broken the law regarding sterilization of a minor and violated Ashley's rights. The parents had been advised by an attorney that a court order for the hysterectomy was not required, and the hospital accepted this. As part of the settlement, the hospital agreed to include a disability rights advocate in any future meetings regarding the Ashley treatment or growth attenuation for children with disabilities.

Shannon (Shannon & Savage, 2007), a nurse and member of the ethics committee where Ashley was treated, wrote in support of the parents' decision. She acknowledged the "harsh social and economic realities" of caring for a child with significant disabilities and believed the parents were best suited to make decisions for Ashley. Terry and Campbell (2008) called for nurses to engage in "robust" discussions about the Ashley treatment and act as advocates for disabled children. Savage (Shannon & Savage, 2007) criticized the decision-making process and called for an independent advocate to represent the child in a due process hearing prior to this type of extensive life-altering treatment and surgeries. In further discussion, Kirschner, Brashler, and Savage (2007, p. 1028) questioned the use of surgery and hormonal therapy to treat a "lack of environmental support, negative social attitudes, and the way others see her [Ashley] or frame her possibilities."

The AAIDD board of directors drafted a position statement titled "Unjustifiable Non-Therapy: Response to the Issue of Growth Attenuation for Young People on the Basis of Disability" (Bersani et al., 2007). The authors argued that while the goal was to provide a better quality of life for Ashley, if her parents continued to care for her at home, comparisons could be made between growth attenuation treatment and involuntary sterilization and/or institutionalization. They viewed growth attenuation as "totally unacceptable" (p. 351), "bad medicine" (p. 353), and possibly opening doors to bariatric surgery, amputation therapy, or using psychoactive medication to ease caregiving. They concluded that they are "stunned and outraged by the very fact that the relative merits of growth attenuation could, in 2006, be a topic for serious debate in this forum... it distorts the concept of treatment and devalues the patient's personhood"(p. 353). Numerous disability organizations issued equally damning statements of the Ashley treatment (ADAPT Youth, 2007; Disability Rights Education and Defense Fund, 2007; Feminists Response in Disability Activism, 2007; Not Dead Yet, 2007; TASH, 2007).

The ethical issues in the Ashley treatment centered on the right of a person with significant cognitive and physical disabilities to bodily integrity. The interventions were directed not to treating a disease or illness, but to altering a child's body to permit ease in caregiving over her lifetime. There are times when interventions are used for the ease of caregiving, such as when children with feeding tubes who can also eat orally are fed by a tube to hasten the feeding process. Before some interventions are considered, though, less invasive interventions should be weighed. Dysmenorrhea, if it had occurred, could have been managed with less invasive treatment than a hysterectomy. Also, breast bud removal does not ensure that a harness will not be uncomfortable, or that Ashley would not be sexually abused. Viewing Ashley as a person with rights requires an analysis of her interests apart from her parents' interests. At times, family members make sacrifices for each other, but Ashley's sacrifice seemed excessive.

The Right of Sexual Expression and Reproduction

One of the criticisms of the Ashley treatment by Disability Rights Washington (2007) was the unlawful hysterectomy, thereby sterilizing Ashley. One might reason that Ashley's disabilities are so extensive that she is unlikely to ever be capable of deciding to bear children. Although dysmenorrhea was the other reason offered for the hysterectomy, there are other means to prevent pregnancy, such as abstinence, which in Ashley's case would be the method of choice because she is also likely to be incapable of consenting to sexual intercourse. Hysterectomies are usually not the first-line treatment for dysmenorrhea, as there are other more conservative treatments to be tried first. Sterilization of people with IDD has an ugly past and is only justified when the person with IDD makes an informed choice, or there has been an exhaustive review by appropriate bodies such as Protection and Advocacy agencies, elimination of less radical options, and all constitutional protections have been afforded the person with IDD (Reilly, 1991).

Myths persist that people with IDD are asexual or hypersexual. It is possible that they may have socially inappropriate expressions of sexual desires, so nurses can work with families and individuals with IDD to teach appropriate behaviors and recognize the person with IDD as a sexual being. With greater community inclusion and integration, people with IDD should have more opportunities to socialize and date. Sex education, consistent with the values of the family, is important; nurses can provide this sex education at an appropriate developmental level. Nurses also can be watchful for indications of sexual activity, which may indicate a need for particular education about birth control and prevention of sexually transmitted infection. Life skills can be taught to aid the person in finding appropriate sexual expression, protecting against abuse or harassment, and making decisions regarding marriage and bearing children. Ideally, life skills education will begin in childhood prior to the onset of puberty (Murphy, Elias, & the Council on Children with Disabilities, 2006).

One of the fundamental human rights is the right to reproduce. As we facilitate the full integration of people with IDD into society, we may pause to consider issues associated with people who require intensive support in caring for themselves having children. Their decision to have children affects not only themselves, but also the child. There is no "litmus test" for parenthood, though. Nurses can participate in the assessment of the needs of a person with IDD who wishes to become a parent and in securing resources for that person. Nurses also may connect families with organizations to provide information and resources regarding the rights of people with IDD to engage in sexual activity and to reproduce.

Freedom to Participate or Not Participate in Research

In addition to the history of sterilization of people with IDD, there is a history of exploitation of people with IDD in human subjects research. Smith and Mitchell (2001) described numerous instances in the 1950s during the polio vaccine trials in which children with IDD were used as research subjects and submitted to unknown risks. Institutionalized children were more appealing to researchers because chimpanzees and calves were costly to purchase for scientific use (Smith & Mitchell, 2001). One of the more notable experiments on institutionalized children is the Willowbrook hepatitis experiment (Levine, 1986). Children with IDD were admitted to a special unit at the Willowbrook State School in New York on the condition that their parents consented to the children's inclusion in a study of hepatitis. The children were given food with the stool of individuals with hepatitis and later received injections of the virus. The criticism of this study focused on the coercive recruitment and lack of informed consent. Institutions were able to raise revenue or barter for services in exchange for offering their patients as subjects in research (Hornblum, 1998).

People with IDD have also been excluded from participation in research (Yan & Munir, 2004). Another study of a vulnerable group occurred over a 40-year period in which African American sharecroppers who had syphilis were followed throughout the course of the disease and underwent nontherapeutic procedures under the pretense of treatment. They were prevented from getting treatment after penicillin was shown to be curative (Levine, 1986). The revelation about the Tuskegee syphilis study was the impetus for a Presidential commission to examine the ethics of biomedical and biobehavioral human subjects' research. The culmination of the commission's work, the Belmont Report, was a proposal for regulations pertaining to human subjects' research. The Belmont Report was adopted by 17 federal agencies as the Common Rule, but not in its entirety (Department of Health and Human Services, Office for Human Research Protections, 1979). There was no consensus on regulations pertaining to people with mental disorders, which included individuals with IDD. Children were covered in a separate category, as were prisoners, pregnant women, and their fetuses. The Belmont Report also calls for each institution conducting human subjects research to organize and convene an institutional review board (IRB) to review and approve research projects.

There are benefits to people with IDD for their participation in research. Programs, interventions, drugs, and medical devices should be tested in the population for whom they are intended. The Belmont Report emphasizes respect for individuals and justice as the fundamental principles in human subjects research. Respect for individuals is actualized in the informed consent process; justice in the recruitment and dissemination of research findings. There are a number of challenges in including people with IDD in research. The IRB requires that this "vulnerable" population is included only if the study is relevant to this population and the study could not be done without the inclusion of people from this population. The principal investigator must show how participants will be recruited and consented. As stated previously, capacity to consent is presumed if one has not been declared incompetent.

The researcher or designee must determine whether there is a guardian, get guardian consent to approach the person with IDD and for the person to participate, and then obtain assent, or affirmative agreement, from the person to participate. The principal investigator must demonstrate to the IRB through the research protocol how capacity will be assessed. There is no single method to assess capacity that is used or recommended. The process of obtaining informed consent should be structured to enhance the exchange of communication. Fisher (2003) called it the "goodness-of-fit" ethic when the emphasis is on the relationship between the researcher and potential participant rather than on the challenges of the potential participant. In a later study, Fisher, Cea, Davidson, and Fried (2006) demonstrated that people with mild to moderate intellectual disability can give consent, although they have some difficulties understanding the purpose of the research or reasoning whether or not to participate. She and colleagues stress using a format that addresses individual needs of the potential participants.

Once the person has agreed to participate, there is a familiarization process to the data collection. Exercise physiology researchers have estimated that it takes 9 hours to recruit and orient one person to a study (Savage, 2002). Given how time- and labor-intensive the process is, there is relatively little research involving people with IDD. Even if consent is obtained from the guardian or person with IDD, it is still necessary to elicit process consent (i.e., to ensure that the person is willing to participate once data collection has started). Should data collection occur over time, the researchers should determine the individual's understanding of the project and continued willingness to participate for each data collection. Other ethical issues in the research process are the use of a research partner to assess the responses of the person with IDD, especially if there are communication difficulties, and the use of incentives or honoraria for participation.

A research partner is a person selected by the participant to be present during data collection. It may be a family member, friend, or paid caregiver, but is usually someone who knows the research participant well, understands his or her mode of communication, and is trusted by the participant. If this person is expected to provide information about or on behalf of the participant, it is important to consider whether this partner is a secondary subject, and if consent should be obtained from the partner for participation in research.

There is also debate regarding the appropriate type of incentive or honoraria people with IDD should receive for participating in research. The IRB carefully scrutinizes incentives or honoraria so that they do not appear to entice people to participate when they otherwise would decline to participate. Often people with IDD who participate in research are recruited from facilities or agencies serving this population. They may be in a sheltered, supported work environment or day program where they receive no salary or earn below minimum wage. A number of questions then arise. What may be a typical honoraria (e.g., $30, a light lunch, and parking) would be in excess of a week's wages and therefore unduly influential. Some researchers argue, however, that based on equality, people with IDD who participate in research should receive the same amount and/or type of honoraria that other participants would receive (Savage, 2002).

Nurses who work with people with IDD can provide input into the design of a study in terms of recruitment, consent, familiarization process, process consent, and honoraria. They can also provide education to researchers about useful approaches to improve communication, recruitment, consent, and data collection. Serving on an IRB would aid in educating IRB members who may have myths about the abilities of people with IDD.

CONCLUSION

Ethical issues abound in caring for people with IDD. This chapter focused on four ethical issues in terms of the rights of people with IDD—the right to community inclusion, the right to bodily integrity (growth attenuation), the right to sexual expression and reproduction, and the freedom to participate or not in research.

This chapter provided an overview of key federal legislation aimed at enhancing the lives of individuals with IDD, as well as potential ethical and legal issues. State and local legislation provide additional protections and deserves study by nurses within their geographic area of practice. In addition, emerging ethical and legal issues present opportunities to explore best practices and to exercise advocacy on behalf of this vulnerable population.

REFERENCES

ADAPT Youth. (2007). *Adapt Youth appalled at parents surgically keeping disabled daughter childlike.* Retrieved November 30, 2008, from http://www.adapt.org/adapt pr/index.php?mode=A&id=253;&sort=D.

American Academy of Pediatrics, Committee on Children with Disabilities. (1996). The role of the pediatrician in implementing the Americans with Disabilities Act: Subject review. *Pediatrics, 98,* 146–148.

Americans with Disabilities Act Amendments Act of 2008, PL 110-325, 42 U.S.C. §§ 3406 *et seq.*

Americans with Disabilities Act of 1990, PL 101-336, 42 U.S.C. §§ 12101 *et seq.*

American Association on Intellectual and Developmental Disabilities. (2002). *Inclusion policy statement.* Retrieved November 29, 2008, from http://www.aaidd .org/content_161.cfm?navID=31.

Association of University Centers on Disabilities. (2007). *CCD Developmental Disabilities Assistance and Bill of Rights Act fact sheet.* Retrieved January 23, 2009, from http://search.aucd.org/cgi-bin/explhcgi? qry0988097101;aucd-03977.

Bannerman, D.J., Sheldon, J.B., Sherman, J.A., & Harchik, A.E. (1990). Balancing the right to habilitation with the right to personal liberties: The rights of people with developmental disabilities to eat too many doughnuts and take a nap. *Journal of Applied Behavior Analysis, 23,* 79–89.

Batorowicz, B., McDougall, S., & Shepherd, T.A. (2006). AAC and community partnerships: The participation path to community inclusion. *Augmentative and Alternative Communication, 22,* 178–195.

Bersani, H., Rotholz, D.A., Eidelman, S.M., Pierson, J.L., Bradley, V.J., Gomez, S.C., et al. (2007). Unjustifiable non-therapy: Response to the issue of growth attenuation for young people on the basis of disability. *Intellectual and Developmental Disabilities, 45,* 351–353.

Department of Health and Human Services, Office for Human Research Protections. (1979). *Belmont report.* Retrieved July 12, 2009, from http://www.hhs.gov/ohrp/ humansubjects/guidance/belmont.htm.

Developmental Disabilities Assistance and Bill of Rights Act of 1975, PL 94-103, 100 Stat. 840, 42 U.S.C. §§ 6000 *et seq.*

Developmental Disabilities Assistance and Bill of Rights Act Amendments of 2000, PL 106-402, 42 U.S.C. §§ 6000 *et seq.*

Disability Rights Education and Defense Fund. (2007). *Modify the system, not the person.* Retrieved November 30, 2008, from www.dredf.org/news/ashley.shtml.

Disability Rights Washington. (2007). *DRW (Disability Rights Washington [formerly Washington Protection and Advocacy System]) Progress Report: Taking seriously the saying: Nothing about us without us.* Retrieved November 30, 2008, from http://www.disability rightswa.org/about/DRW%20Progress% 20Report%202008.pdf.

Education of All Handicapped Children Act of 1975, PL 94-142, 20 U.S.C. §§ 1400 *et seq.*

Feminists Response in Disability Activism. (2007). *A disability community's response to Ashley's treatment.* Retrieved November 30, 2008, at www.ashleyx.info.

Fisher, C.B. (2003). Goodness-of-fit ethic for informed consent to research involving adults with mental retardation and developmental disabilities. *Mental Retardation and Developmental Disabilities Research and Review, 9,* 27–31.

Fisher, C.B., Cea, C.D., Davidson, P.W., & Fried, A.L. (2006). Capacity of persons with mental retardation to consent to participate in randomized clinical trials. *American Journal of Psychiatry, 163,* 1813–1820.

Hornblum, A.M. (1998). *Acres of skin: Human experiments at Holmesburg Prison.* New York: Routledge.

Individuals with Disabilities Education Act of 1990, PL 101-476, 20 U.S.C. §§ 1400 *et seq.*

Individuals with Disabilities Education Improvement Act of 2004, PL 108-446, 20 U.S.C. §§ 1400 *et seq.*

Kirschner, K.L., Brashler, R., & Savage, T.A. (2007). Ashley X. *American Journal of Physical Medicine and Rehabilitation, 86,* 1023–1029.

Levine, R.J. (1986). *Ethics and regulation of*

clinical research (2nd ed.). New Haven, CT: Yale University Press.

Mental Retardation Facilities and Community Mental Health Centers Construction Act of 1963, PL 88-164, 42 U.S.C. §§ 12501 et seq.

Mitka, M. (2008). Federal government seeks to clarify the Americans with Disabilities Act. JAMA, 300, 889.

Murphy, N.A., & Elias, E.R. (2006). Sexuality of children and adolescents with developmental disabilities. Pediatrics, 18, 398–403.

National Dissemination Center for Children with Disabilities. (2009a). Overview of early intervention. Retrieved February 5, 2009, from http://www.nichcy.org/babies/overview/Pages/default.aspx.

National Dissemination Center for Children with Disabilities. (2009b). The short and sweet IEP overview. Retrieved February 5, 2009, from http://www.nichcy.org/educatechildren/IEP/pages/overview.aspx.

Neely-Barnes, S., Marcenko, M., & Weber, L. (2008a). Does choice influence quality of life for people with mild intellectual disabilities? Intellectual and Developmental Disabilities, 46, 12–26.

Neely-Barnes, S., Marcenko, M., & Weber, L. (2008b). Community-based, consumer-directed services: Differential experiences of people with mild and severe intellectual disabilities. Social Work Research, 32, 55–64.

Nonverbal Learning Disorders Association. (2008). Section 504, the Americans with Disabilities Act (ADA) vs. the Individuals with Disabilities Education Act (IDEA); What is the Difference. Retrieved December 3, 2008, from http://www.nldline.com/iep_vs_504.com.

Not Dead Yet. (2007). Hastings Center Report: Article claims Ashley X "sacrificed for the disability rights agenda". Retrieved November 30, 2008, at http://notdeadyetnewscommentary.blogspot.com/search?q=ashley.

Rehabilitation Act Amendments of 1993, PL 103-73, 29 U.S.C. §§ 701 et seq.

Rehabilitation Act Amendments of 1998, PL 105-220, 29 U.S.C. §§ 701 et seq.

Rehabilitation Act of 1973, PL 93-112, 29 U.S.C. §§ 701 et seq.

Reilly, P.R. (1991). The surgical solution: A history of involuntary sterilization in the United States. Baltimore: Johns Hopkins University Press.

Savage, T.A. (2002). Obtaining informed consent from people with intellectual disabilities for participation in research: Current practices. Poster presented at the meeting of the American Association on Mental Retardation, Orlando, Florida.

Shannon, S.E., & Savage, T.A. (2007). The Ashley treatment: Two viewpoints. Pediatric Nursing, 33, 175–178.

Shogren, K.A., Wehmeyer, M.L., Buchanan, C.L., & Lopez, S.J. (2006). The application of positive psychology and self-determination to research in intellectual disability: A content analysis of 30 years of literature. Research & Practice for Persons with Severe Disabilities, 31, 338–345.

Smith, J.D., & Mitchell, A.L. (2001). Sacrifices for the miracle: The polio vaccine research and children with mental retardation. Mental Retardation, 39, 405–409.

TASH. (2007). Attenuating growth. Retrieved November 30, 2008, from www.tash.org/InTheNews/Attenuating-Growth.html.

Terry, L., & Campbell, A. (2008). Forever a child: Analysis of the Ashley case. Paediatric Nursing, 20, 21–25.

Tøssebro, J. (2005). Reflections on living outside: Continuity and change in the life of "outsiders." In K. Johnson, R. Traustadóttir (Eds.), Deinstitutionalization and people with intellectual disabilities: In and out of institutions (pp. 186–202). Philadelphia: Jessica Kingsley.

Turnbull, H.R., Turnbull, A.P., Bronicki, G.J., Summers, J.A., & Roeder-Gordon, C. (1989). Disability and the family: A guide to decisions for adulthood. Baltimore: Paul H. Brookes Publishing Co.

U.S. Department of Education. (2008a). Building the legacy: Idea 2004. Retrieved January 5, 2009, from http://idea.ed.gov.

U.S. Department of Education. (2008b). Protecting students with disabilities. Retrieved December 10, 2008, from http://www.ed.gov/print/about/offices/list/ocr/504faq.html.

U.S. Department of Health and Human Services. (2008). *Your rights under Section 504 of the Rehabilitation Act.* Retrieved November 26, 2008, from http://www.dhhs .gov/ocr/504.html.

U.S. Department of Justice. (2008). *Americans with Disabilities Act of 1990.* Retrieved August 5, 2008, from http://www.ada .gov.pubs.ada.htm.

U.S. Equal Opportunity Commission. (2009). *Americans with Disabilities Act: Disability discrimination.* Retrieved January 2, 2009, from http://www.eeoc.gov/types/ada.html.

WebAIM. (2008). *Overview of the Rehabilitation Act of 1973.* Retrieved November 26, 2008, from http://www.webaim.org/ articles/laws/usa/rehab.php.

Wehmeyer, M.H., & Bolding, N. (2001). Enhanced self-determination of adults with intellectual disability as an outcome of moving to community-based work or living environments. *Journal of Intellectual Disability Research, 45,* 371–383.

Yan, E.G., & Munir, K.M. (2004). Regulatory and ethical principles in research involving children and individuals with developmental disabilities. *Ethics & Behavior, 14,* 31–49.

Yell, M.L., Rogers, D., & Rogers, E.L. (1998). The legal history of special education. What a long, strange trip it's been. *Remedial and Special Education, 19,* 219–229.

Index

Page numbers followed by *f* indicate figures; those followed by *t* indicate tables.

AAFP, *see* American Academy of Family Physicians
AAIDD, *see* American Association on Intellectual and Developmental Disabilities
AAP, *see* American Academy of Pediatrics
Abbey Pain Scale, 126
ABR, *see* Auditory brainstem response
Abuse
  adults with IDD, 82, 262
  child abuse, 56, 76, 118
  elder abuse, 84, 85
  sexual, 262
Academic performance
  children with hearing impairment, 342
  see also Individualized education programs
Accessibility of health care
  for culturally diverse populations, 159–160, 205–206
  dental and mental health care, 207
  early detection of psychosocial problems, 118
  factors affecting, 79–80, 161–162
  nursing role in, 204
  Surgeon General's call to action, 163*t*–165*t*
Accidents
  as IDD etiology, 196
  prevention, 140, 141
Accommodations
  employment settings, 105, 356
  postsecondary education, 38, 77
  preschoolers, 58–59, 59*t*
  under Rehabilitation Act of 1973, 62, 360
  school-age children, 34–35, 62–63
ACOG, *see* American College of Obstetricians and Gynecologists
Acute lymphatic leukemia (ALL), 220
Acute megakaryoblastic leukemia (AMKL), 220
Acute myeloid leukemia (AML), 220
ADA, *see* Americans with Disabilities Act of 1990
ADA Amendments Act of 2008 (PL 110-325), 356

Adaptation strategies/functioning
  assessment and intervention, 201*t*, 324*t*
  normalization as, 23
Adaptive Behavior Assessment System, 324*t*
Adaptive equipment, 251
ADHD, *see* Attention-deficit/hyperactivity disorder
Administration on Developmental Disabilities, Kids as Self Advocates, 25
Adolescents
  autism spectrum disorders, 300
  Down syndrome, 224, 226–227
  employment resources, 36–37, 39*t*
  health care services, 35–36, 72–74, 103–104
  health promotion, 71–72
  income assistance, 37–38
  independence, development of, 71, 75
  intervention for IDD, 203
  lifestage-specific models of care, 27
  postsecondary education, 38
  prevalence of special health care needs, 70
  psychosocial development, 112
  puberty, 70–71, 153
  social relationships, 74–75
  transition to adult health care, 73–74, 103–104, 203, 227
  youth-centered care, 25
  see also Young adults
Adults with IDD
  aging and dying, 84–86, 125–127
  behavioral issues, 80
  emergency preparedness, 83–84
  employment, 39*t*, 40, 82
  family planning, 81–82
  futures planning, 81, 86
  health challenges, 79–80, 84–85
  housing, 40–41, 82–83, 361–362
  independent living centers (ILCs), 40–41
  intervention, 203–204
  leisure and recreation, 83, 85
  loss, coping with, 84, 85, 127
  person-centered planning, 81, 86
  psychosocial development, 112–113
  social relationships, 81–82, 84, 85

Adults with IDD—*continued*
    systems of care, 39–42, 104–105
    transportation, 83, 143, 203
    see also Young adults; *specific disorders*
Advanced practice nurses (APNs)
    education and certification, 92
    as public health nurses, 99
    research, involvement in, 162, 166*t*
    roles and responsibilities, 93
Advisory Committee on Immunization
        Practices, 225, 226, 229
After-school programs, 35
Agency for Healthcare Research and
        Quality, 95
*Ages & Stages Questionnaires® (ASQ-3): A
        Parent-Completed, Child Monitoring
        System (3rd ed.)* (Squires and
        Bricker), 120*t*, 201*t*
Aggressive behavior, 258, 300, 302, 342
Aging
    adults with IDD, 84–86, 125–127
    cerebral palsy, individuals with, 251
    Down syndrome, individuals with, 224,
        229
    hearing impairment and, 342–343
Alcohol abuse, 262
Alcohol toxicity, 207
Alliance for Self-Determination, 22
Alternative medicine, *see* Complementary
        and alternative medicine
Alzheimer's disease, *see* Dementia
Ambulation, individuals with cerebral
        palsy, 241, 251
American Academy of Family Physicians
        (AAFP)
    patient-centered medical home, 104, 280
    screening and immunization, 225, 226
    transition to adult health care, 73
American Academy of Pediatrics (AAP)
    cardiovascular assessment, 151
    family-centered care, 25
    fragile X syndrome, 325
    growth measurements, 148, 150
    head circumference measurements, 150
    medical home model of care, 24, 104,
        202, 280
    parent-physician partnerships, 49
    screening and immunization, 225, 226
    thyroid disease, screening for, 152
    transition to adult health care, 73
American Association on Intellectual and
        Developmental Disabilities (AAIDD)
    on growth attenuation, 364
    historical perspective, 2
    inclusion, position statement on, 361
    membership trends, 11–12
    nurse education and training, 95
    standards of care, 10, 157

terminology and classification systems,
        2–3, 193–194
American Association on Mental Defi-
        ciency, 2, 10
    see also American Association on Intellec-
        tual and Developmental Disabilities
American Cancer Society, 80
American College of Medical Genetics, 314
American College of Obstetricians and
        Gynecologists (ACOG), 227
American College of Physicians (ACP)
    patient-centered medical home, 104
    screening and immunization, 227
    transition to adult health care, 73
American Heart Association, 80
American Nurses Association
    delegation to UAPs, 160–161
    family-centered care, 25
    recognition of developmental disabilities
        specialty, 10
    standards of care, 95, 157
American Nurses Credentialing Center, 92
American Osteopathic Association, 104
American Psychiatric Association, 193
American Psychological Association, 193
American Sign Language (ASL), 341, 344
Americans with Disabilities Act of 1990
        (ADA; PL 101-336), 3, 56, 77,
        355–356
Americorps, 37, 78
Aneuploidies, 177–178
Angelman syndrome (AS), 188
Ankle clonus, 238
Anophthalmia, 337
Anticonvulsant medications, 316–317
Antidepressant medications, 267, 268
Antipsychotic medications, 267, 268
Anxiety
    antianxiety medications, 157, 268, 303
    assessment and intervention, 324*t*
    autism spectrum disorders, individuals
        with, 261*t*, 302
    fragile X syndrome, individuals with,
        314, 319, 324*t*
    IDD, individuals with, 261*t*, 262
    school-age children, 61, 117
    stranger anxiety, 54
    therapies for, 269
    toddlers, 56
    transfer anxiety, 204
Aortic root dilation, 316
APNs, *see* Advanced practice nurses
Arc of the United States, 11
ASDs, *see* Autism spectrum disorders
Ashley treatment, 363–364
ASL, *see* American Sign Language
Asperger syndrome
    assessment, 290*t*, 291*t*, 296*t*, 297*t*

overview, 228
sensitivity to touch, 336
Asperger Syndrome Diagnostic Scale, 290*t*
Aspiration
   causes of, 151, 152
   cerebral palsy and, 246
   preventing, 132
Aspirational Standards of Developmental Disabilities Nursing Practice (Willis), 10
ASQ, *see* Ages & Stages Questionnaires
   see also Autism Screening Questionnaire
ASSERT model of self-advocacy, 21
Assessment
   anxiety, 324*t*
   adaptive/emotional functioning, 201*t*
   attention-deficit/hyperactivity disorder, 324*t*
   autism spectrum disorders, 286–287, 288*f*–289*f*, 290*t*–298*t*
   bone density, 136*t*, 228*t*
   cardiovascular, 135*t*, 151
   cerebral palsy, 239, 241, 244–251, 244*t*
   chromosome analysis, 177, 199
   consciousness, 136*t*
   dental, 133*t*, 151
   depression, 119
   developmental screening, 200, 201*t*
   dyskinesia, 136*t*
   dysphagia, 133*t*–134*t*, 151–152
   endocrine system, 152–153
   feeding problems, 133*t*–134*t*, 151–152
   fragile X syndrome, 313–314, 324*t*–325*t*
   gastrointestinal, 151–152
   gastrointestinal system, 135*t*–136*t*
   general health, 148–150, 199, 245
   genitourinary tract, 153
   hearing impairments, 150–151, 200, 228*t*, 341, 343–344, 345–346
   IDD diagnosis, 198–200
   mental health, 258–260, 262–266, 264*t*
   metabolic studies, 199–200
   musculoskeletal, 154–155
   neurological, 154
   oral motor function, 133*t*–134*t*, 247
   pain, 126–127, 154
   physical, 132, 133*t*–136*t*
   psychosocial development, 117–119, 120*t*–122*t*, 123, 201*t*
   purpose and nature of, 148, 149*t*
   reproductive system, 153–154
   respiratory system, 134*t*, 151
   seizures, 154
   skin, 133*t*, 154
   speech and language disorders, 136*t*, 324*t*
   tardive dyskinesia, 136*t*
   vision impairments, 150–151, 200, 225, 228*t*, 337, 338–339
   vital signs, 133*t*

   see also Review of systems assessment process; *specific disorders*
Assessment, Evaluation, and Programming System, 122*t*
Assessment and diagnosis
   autism spectrum disorders, 286–287, 288*f*–289*f*, 290*t*–298*t*, 324*t*
Assistive technology
   ambulation, 251
   definition, 143–144
   hearing impairment, 344–345
   vision disorders, 338
   see also Accommodations
Assistive Technology Act of 1998 (PL 105-394), 143–144
Association of Rehabilitation Nurses, 92
Association of University Centers on Developmental Disability, *see* University Centers for Excellence in Developmental Disabilities
ASSQ, *see* Autism Spectrum Screening Questionnaire
Ataxic cerebral palsy, 241, 242*f*, 243*t*
Athetoid cerebral palsy, 240, 242*f*
Atlanta Down Syndrome Project, 217
Atlantoaxial instability, 218, 222–223
Atomoxetine, 317
Atrioventricular septal defect, 217
Attachment, mother-child, 48
Attention-deficit/hyperactivity disorder (ADHD)
   assessment and intervention, 324*t*
   Down syndrome and, 196
   fragile X syndrome and, 314, 315*t*, 317
   parents' expectations, 116
   school-age children, 61–62
   toddlers, 55
Auditory brainstem response (ABR), 343–344, 345
Auditory impairments, *see* Hearing impairments
Auditory neuropathy, 342, 344
Australian Scale for Asperger's Syndrome, 291*t*
Autism and Developmental Disabilities Monitoring Network, 279
Autism Diagnostic Interview, 292*t*, 318, 324*t*
Autism Diagnostic Observation Schedule, 293*t*, 318, 324*t*
Autism Screening Questionnaire (ASQ), 294*t*
Autism spectrum disorders (ASDs)
   approaches to care, 283–286
   assessment and diagnosis, 286–287, 288*f*–289*f*, 290*t*–298*t*, 324*t*
   brain growth, 150, 281
   clinical manifestations, 282–283
   complementary and alternative medicine, 304–305

Autism spectrum disorders (ASDs)—*continued*
  definitions and types of, 278–279
  Early Indicators/Red Flags Checklist, 287, 288f–289f
  epidemiology, 279
  etiology, 261t, 281–282
  food behaviors, 152
  health care surveillance, 303–304, 305f
  hypersensitivity to sound, 336
  immunizations and, 282
  impact of, 279–280
  life-span intervention and care
    adolescents, 300
    adults, 287, 300–301
    early intervention, 299
    school-age children, 287, 299–300
    toddlers, 54
  medications, 302, 303
  nonpharmacological intervention, 303–305, 324t
  nursing interventions, 261t, 306
  pathophysiology, 280–282
  preparation for medical procedures, 304
  range of severity in, 277
  secondary conditions and comorbidities
    Down syndrome, 196
    fragile X syndrome, 314, 315t, 316, 318–319
    gastrointestinal problems, 152, 301
    mental health disorders, 261t, 302
    overview, 261t, 282, 301–303, 305f
    seizures, 154, 282, 300, 302–303
    sleep disturbance, 301–302
Autism Spectrum Screening Questionnaire (ASSQ), 290t
Autonomy, *see* Independence
Autosomal dominant inheritance, 182–184
Autosomal recessive inheritance, 181–182

Bacterial meningitis, 196
Batelle Developmental Inventory, 120t
Bayley Infant Neurodevelopmental Screener, 201t
Bayley Scales of Infant Development, 122t, 201t
Beck Depression Inventory, 119
Behavior Rating Inventory of Executive Function, 201t, 324t
Behavioral problems
  adults with IDD, 80
  autism spectrum disorders, individuals with, 302
  Down syndrome, individuals with, 196, 218
  fragile X syndrome, individuals with, 314
  functional analysis, 266

hearing impairments, children with, 342
  medications for, 267–269
  parents' expectations and, 116
  prevalence, 142
  screening tests, 201t
  symptoms, 198
  toddlers, 55–56
Belmont Report, 366
Best Buddies program, 75
Biopsychosocial model of disability, 321–323, 321f, 322f, 323f, 325
Birth and delivery, *see* Perinatal period
Birth defects, 46–47
Bladder function, *see* Urinary incontinence
Blepharitis, 218
Blindness, *see* Deafblindness; Vision impairments
Bodily integrity, right to, 363–364
Bonding, *see* Attachment, mother–child
Bone density assessment, 136t, 228t
BPD, *see* Bronchopulmonary dysplasia
Braden Scale for Predicting Pressure Sore Risk, 140
Braille, 338
Brain development
  adolescence, 71
  autism spectrum disorders, 281
  cerebral palsy, 236
  head circumference and, 150
  pathophysiology, 197
  sensory systems and, 334
Brief Infant Toddler Social Emotional Assessment, 122t
Bright Futures program, 72
Bronchopulmonary dysplasia (BPD), 47, 49, 50
Bruxism, 151
Bullying, 62

Calgary Family Assessment Model, 285–286
CAM, *see* Complementary and alternative medicine
Carbamazepine, 268
Cardiovascular disorders
  assessment and intervention, 135t, 151
  cerebral palsy, 246
  Down syndrome, 217, 222
  fragile X syndrome, 315t
Care coordination, *see* Service coordination
Caregivers
  lifting and carrying safety, 141
  violent behavior experienced by, 258
  wellbeing of, 116, 124
CARS, *see* Childhood Autism Rating Scale
Case management, *see* Service coordination
Cataracts, 151, 218, 222
CCM, *see* Chronic care model

CDD, *see* Childhood disintegrative disorder
Celiac disease, 219
Centers for Disease Control and Prevention
   Centers for Autism and Developmental
      Disabilities Surveillance and Epide-
      miology, 282
   immunizations, 80
   National Survey of Children with Special
      Health Care Needs, 69
Cerebral palsy
   assessment, 239, 241, 244–251, 244*t*
   caregiver wellbeing, 116, 124
   causes and risk factors, 46–47, 236–237,
      237*t*
   classification, 239–240
   complementary and alternative medi-
      cine, 251–252
   definition, 235–236
   diagnosis, 238–239, 239*t*, 241
   epidemiology, 238
   growth, monitoring, 150, 245
   interdisciplinary services and supports,
      241
   mortality, 236, 238
   nursing roles, 244–251, 251*t*
   pathophysiology, 235–236
   quality of life, 251
   secondary conditions and comorbidities
      cryptorchidism, 153
      dental problems, 151, 245
      Down syndrome, 196
      overview, 237–238, 243*t*
      spasticity and posture, 154, 155,
         249–251, 250*t*
   types of, 240–241
Certified nurse midwives, 92
Certified nursing assistants (CNAs), 93
Certified registered nurse anesthetists, 92
Child abuse, 56, 76, 118
Child Behavior Checklist, 122*t*, 324*t*
Child care
   challenges, 56–57
   health consultants, 98
Child Find system, 53, 98
Child Sleep Habits Questionnaire, 325*t*
Childhood Autism Rating Scale (CARS),
   295*t*
Childhood disintegrative disorder (CDD),
   279
Children with special health care needs
   (CSHCN)
   definitions, 19, 33
   mental health problems, detection of,
      118–119
   prevalence, 69, 70
   Title V, 33, 35
Children's Bureau
   nurse consultants, employment of, 11
   training for nurses, 10

Children's Depression Inventory, 119
Choice, *see* Decision making
Choreoathetotic cerebral palsy, 240,
   242*f*
Chromosomal abnormalities, 175,
   176–179, 197*t*, 211–212, 213*f*
Chronic care model (CCM), 104
Chronic sorrow, 49
Clinical nurse specialists (CNSs), 92, 100
Clonidine, 318
CNAs, *see* Certified nursing assistants
CNSs, *see* Clinical nurse specialists
COBRA, *see* Consolidated Omnibus Recon-
   ciliation Bill Act
Cochlear implants, 344–345
Cognitive behavioral therapies, 269
Cognitive disabilities
   cerebral palsy, 238, 243*t*
   classification of mental retardation,
      193–194
   Down syndrome, 218
   fragile X syndrome, 315*t*, 319–320
   intervention, 324*t*
   screening tests, 201*t*
   see also Intellectual and developmental
      disabilities (IDD), individuals with
Collaboration, *see* Interdisciplinary
   practice
College attendance, *see* Postsecondary
   education
Combating Autism Act of 2006
   (PL 109-416), 306
Communication disorders, *see* Speech and
   language disorders
Community care, nursing roles and
   responsibilities, 98–100
Community inclusion, right to, 361–362
Community living
   independent living centers, 40–41
   see also Housing and living arrangements
Comorbid conditions, *see* Dual diagnosis;
   specific disorders
Compassion, need for, 205
Complementary and alternative medicine
   (CAM)
   autism spectrum disorders, 304–305
   cerebral palsy, 251–252
   IDD, 204
   mental health disorders, 269
Conductive hearing loss, 342
Connors' Rating Scales–Revised, 324*t*
Consciousness, assessment, 136*t*
Consent
   for research participation, 365–367
   types of, 363
Consolidated Omnibus Reconciliation Bill
   Act (COBRA), 36
Constipation, 152, 247, 249
Consultants, *see* Nurse consultants

Continuing education, historical perspective, 9–10
Continuing Education Needs for Nurses Caring for Children with Special Health Care Needs (Austin and Donohoe), 10
Contractures, positioning for, 137, 138*f*
Coordination of care, *see* Service coordination
Cornelia de Lange syndrome, 150
Cortical blindness/cortical deafness, 334
Cortisol, 319
Court cases
    Mills v. Board of Education, 3
    Pennhurst State School v. Halderman, 4
    Pennsylvania Association for Retarded Children v. Commonwealth of Pennsylvania, 3
    Wyatt v. Aderholt, 3
    Wyatt v. Stickney, 3
Crossing the Quality Chasm initiative, 26
Cryptorchidism, 153
CSHCN, *see* Children with special health care needs
Cultural sensitivity, 159–160, 205–206, 284–285, 347
Curriculum, nursing programs
    core knowledge base, 93–95, 94*t*
    historical perspective, 8–9
Cystic fibrosis, 71
Cytomegalovirus, 334

Daytrana, 317
DC-LD, *see Diagnostic Criteria for Psychiatric Disorders for Use with Adults with Learning Disabilities/Mental Retardation*
DDNA, *see* Developmental Disabilities Nurses Association
DDS, *see* Disability determination services
Deaf community, 341, 344, 347
Deafblindness, 347–348
Deafness, *see* Hearing impairments
Death and dying, 85–86, 125–127
Decision making
    adolescents, development of skills, 75, 103
    dignity of risk, 362–363
    end-of-life care, 126
    ethical considerations, 126, 362–363
    person-centered planning and, 81, 86
    see also Independence; Self-advocacy/self-determination
Decubitus ulcers, 140, 154, 248, 249
Deinstitutionalization, 3–4
Delegation by nurses
    in child care settings, 98
    in group homes and institutions, 100
    rights of, 161

in schools, 102
to unlicensed assistive personnel (UAPs), 160–161
Deletions, chromosomal, 179
Dementia, 80, 85, 142, 211, 218, 224, 229
Dental health
    access to care, 207
    assessment and intervention, 133*t*, 151
    care and monitoring, 141, 225, 229
    cerebral palsy, 151, 245, 249
    Down syndrome, 219–220, 225, 229
    periodontal disease, 220
    types of problems, 151
Denver II Developmental Screening Test, 120*t*, 201*t*
Denver Prescreening Developmental Questionnaire II, 201*t*
Depression
    assessment, 119
    autism spectrum disorders, 302
    cerebral palsy and, 251
    fragile X syndrome, 314
    IDD, individuals with, 203, 260, 263
    risk factors, 260
Development
    developmental screening, 200, 201*t*
    infants, 50–51
    preschool period, 57–58
    psychosocial, 109–113
    school-age children, 61–62
    speech and language, 51, 54, 61, 341–342, 346
    toddlers, 54
    see also Brain development; Motor development
Developmental Disabilities Assistance and Bill of Rights Act Amendments of 2000 (PL 106-402), 357–358
Developmental Disabilities Assistance and Bill of Rights Act of 1975 (PL 94-103), 357
Developmental Disabilities Nurses Association (DDNA)
    certification, 92
    membership trends, 11–12
    nurse education and training, 95
    standards of care, 10
Developmental disabilities nursing, definition, 8
Developmental model of care, 7–8
Developmental Observation Checklist System, 120*t*
Developmental screening, 200, 201*t*
Devereux Early Childhood Assessment Program, 122*t*
Diabetes
    adolescents with, 71
    Down syndrome, 219, 223
Diagnostic and Statistical Manual of Mental

Disorders (DSM-IV-TR; American Psychiatric Association), 2, 263–264, 266, 283, 287
Diagnostic Criteria for Psychiatric Disorders for Use with Adults with Learning Disabilities/Mental Retardation (DC-LD; Royal College of Psychiatrists), 265
Diagnostic Manual–Intellectual Disability (DSM-ID; Fletcher et al.), 264
Diagnostic overshadowing, 80, 117–118, 162, 258
Diarrhea, 152
Diazepam, 157, 303
Dignity of risk, 362–363
Dilantin (phenytoin), 317
Diplegia, 240, 242*f*, 243*t*
Disabilities, individuals with
  barriers to employment, 82
  biopsychosocial model, 321–323, 321*f*, 322*f*, 323*f*, 325
  census data, 79, 84
  definition, 356
  prevalence of disorders, 142
  Surgeon General's call to action, 163*t*–165*t*
Disability care coordination organizations (DCCOs), 24
Disability determination services (DDS), 41
Disability Distress Assessment Tool, 126
Disability Rights Washington, 363, 364
Disability support services (DSS), 38, 77
Discharge planning, 51–52, 101–102
Disruptions of metabolism, 282
Divalproex sodium, 268
Doctor of Nursing Practice (DNP) degree, 92
Down syndrome
  chromosomal abnormalities, 176, 179, 196, 211–212, 213*f*
  clinical features, 178, 214, 215*t*
  diagnosis, 217
  epidemiology, 195, 196, 214, 216–217
  etiology, 213–214, 261*t*
  growth charts, use of, 149–150
  historical perspective, 211
  interdisciplinary services and supports, 223–224
  life-span intervention and care
    adolescents, 224, 226–227
    adults, 227, 228*t*, 229
    aging, 224, 229
    infants, 223, 224–225
    preschool and school-age children, 223–224, 226
  mortality, 216
  nursing roles, 224–227, 229, 261*t*
  risk factors, 212
  screening guidelines, 228*t*
  secondary conditions and comorbidities

    cardiovascular problems, 151, 217, 222
    communication difficulties, 125–126
    dementia, 80, 85, 142, 211, 218, 224, 229
    dental problems, 151, 219–220, 225, 229
    dermatologic problems, 221
    gastrointestinal problems, 152, 219, 222
    growth and obesity, 221
    hearing disorders, 151, 196, 219, 222
    immune system deficiencies, 219
    leukemias, 220
    mental health disorders, 261*t*
    musculoskeletal problems, 218
    neurodevelopmental issues, 218
    overview, 80, 196, 217–223, 225, 261*t*
    respiratory problems, 218
    seizures, 221
    sleep problems, 221–222
    solid tumors, 220–221
    thyroid disease, 152
    vision problems, 218
  societal expectations about, 116
Drugs, *see* Medications
DSM-ID, *see Diagnostic Manual–Intellectual Disability*
DSM-IV-TR, *see Diagnostic and Statistical Manual of Mental Disorders*
DSS, *see* Disability support services
Dual diagnosis
  diagnostic overshadowing, 80, 117–118, 162, 258
  mental illness and IDD, 56, 80, 258
Duchenne muscular dystrophy, 185
Duplications, chromosomal, 179
Dyskinesia, 136*t*, 268, 303
Dyskinetic cerebral palsy, 240, 242*f*, 243*t*
Dyslexia, 334
Dysphagia
  aspiration prevention, 132
  assessment and intervention, 133*t*–134*t*, 151–152
  preterm infants, 50
Dystonic cerebral palsy, 240–241, 242*f*

Early and periodic screening, diagnosis and treatment (EPSDT) services, 33–34
Early Head Start, 59
Early Indicators/Red Flags of ASD Checklist, 287, 288*f*–289*f*
Early intervention programs
  autism spectrum disorders, individuals with, 280, 299
  Down syndrome, children with, 225
  eligibility for services, 32
  hearing impairment, children with, 341

Early intervention programs—*continued*
    individualized family service plans, 32,
        53, 202
    legislative mandate, 32, 53, 202,
        358–359
    nursing roles and responsibilities, 97–98
    transition from, 57, 299
Early Language Milestone Scale 2, 201*t*
Early Learning Accomplishment Profile,
    122*t*
Ears
    Down syndrome abnormalities, 215*t*
    see also Hearing impairments
Ecological intervention model, 27, 258
Education and training for nurses
    in autism spectrum disorders, 280
    core knowledge base, 93–95, 94*t*
    historical perspective, 8–10
    IDD nurses, 8–10, 11, 12
    interdisciplinary training, 26
    need for, 161–162
Education for All Handicapped Children
        Act of 1975 (PL 94-142), 3, 23, 358
Education of the Handicapped Act Amend-
        ments of 1986 (PL 99-457), 3, 53
Educational considerations, *see* Individual-
        ized education programs; School-age
        children
Edwards syndrome, 178
Elder abuse, 84, 85
Electronic records, benefits of, 74
Emergency preparedness, 83–84, 348, 349
Emotional development
    screening tests, 201*t*
    see also Behavioral problems; Psycho-
        social development
Employment
    adolescents and young adults, 36–37,
        78
    autism spectrum disorders, adults with,
        280, 300, 301
    cerebral palsy, adults with, 251
    Down syndrome, adults with, 229
    health-related accommodations, 105
    reasonable accommodations, 356
    under Rehabilitation Act, 360
    settings for IDD nurses, 11, 91
    Social Security Administration programs,
        39*t*
    vocational rehabilitation, 36, 40, 300
Enamel hypoplasia, 151
End-of-life care, 86, 125–127
Endocardial cushion defects, 151
Endocrine system disorders
    cerebral palsy, 248
    Down syndrome, 219
    fragile X syndrome, 316
    overview, 152–153
Enteral feeding, 137–138

Environmental concerns
    lead toxicity, 46, 196, 207
    mercury toxicity, 46, 196, 207, 282
    teratogens, 46
Epilepsy, *see* Seizures
EPSDT, *see* Early and periodic screening,
        diagnosis and treatment (EPSDT)
        services
Ethical issues
    community inclusion, right to, 361–362
    dignity of risk, 362–363
    growth attenuation, 363–364
    research participation, 162, 167,
        365–367
Ethnic differences, *see* Racial/ethnic differ-
        ences
Eugenics, 5
Every Child Deserves a Medical Home (AAP),
    74
Evidence-based care
    physical nursing care, 132
    research, need for, 95–96
    training in, need for, 12
    wheelchair positioning, 137
Exercise,adolescents, 72
Eyberg Child Behavior Inventory, 120*t*
Eyes
    Down syndrome abnormalities, 215*t*
    physical abnormalities, 198
    see also Vision impairments

Fagan Test of Infant Intelligence, 201*t*
Families
    child care challenges, 56–57
    child–parent relationships, 74
    educating, 156, 200, 202
    futures planning, 81, 86
    grieving process, 49
    impact of autism spectrum disorders on,
        280
    parent support groups, 53, 97, 200, 202
    perinatal period, 49
    preschool period, challenges of, 59–60
    school-age children, challenges, 63
    single-parent families, 49, 52, 202
    stress, effects of on young children,
        55–56
    stress and coping, 115–116
    see also Parents
Family management styles, 22–23
Family Needs Scale, 120*t*
Family planning, 81–82
Family Resource Scale, 120*t*
Family Support Program, 358
Family Support Scale, 120*t*
Family Voices, 53
Family-centered care
    in NICU environment, 49

nursing roles and responsibilities, 97, 103–104, 206

theoretical model, 21*t*, 24–25, 72, 284

Fathers

characteristics linked with birth anomalies, 46

paternal age and chromosome abnormalities, 180

Federal agencies, nursing representation in, 11

Federal legislation, *see* Legislation; *specific statutes*

Feeding problems

arched palate and, 151

assessment and intervention, 133*t*–134*t*, 151–152

cerebral palsy, 247

dysphagia, 50, 132, 151–152

enteral feeding, 137–138

positioning for, 137, 139*f*

Feet

Down syndrome abnormalities, 215*t*

physical abnormalities, 198

Fenobam, 326

Fetal alcohol syndrome, 195, 261*t*

Fetal development, *see* Prenatal period

Fine motor function, 51, 55*t*, 154–155

FMR1 gene, 311–312

Fragile X-associated primary ovarian insufficiency (FXPOI), 311, 312, 322*f*

Fragile X-associated tremor/ataxia syndrome (FXTAS), 311, 313, 314, 322*f*

Fragile X syndrome (FXS)

biopsychosocial model, 321–323, 321*f*, 322*f*, 323*f*, 325

clinical manifestations, 314, 315*t*

diagnostic testing, 313–314

epidemiology, 195, 196, 312

etiology, 261*t*

food behaviors, 152

genetic mutation, 189, 311–313, 312*f*, 313*f*

head circumference measurements, 150

medications, 325–326

nursing interventions, 261*t*

secondary conditions and comorbidities

assessment of, 324*t*–325*t*

autism spectrum disorders, 282, 314, 315*t*, 316, 318–319

cognitive disabilities, 319–320

dental problems, 151

macroorchidism, 153, 315*t*

mental health disorders, 261*t*

overview, 261*t*, 316–319

seizures, 154, 316–317

speech and language delay, 315*t*, 320–321

FRAXA Research Foundation, 325

Free appropriate education mandate, 3, 202, 299

Functional behavioral analysis, 266

Functional Emotional Assessment Scale, 122*t*

Futures planning, 81, 86

FXPOI, *see* Fragile X-associated primary ovarian insufficiency

FXS, *see* Fragile X syndrome

FXS Clinic Consortium, 325

FXTAS, *see* Fragile X-associated tremor/ataxia syndrome

Gabapentin, 317

Ganaxolone, 326

GARS, *see* Gilliam Autism Rating Scale

Gastroesophageal reflux disease (GERD), 152, 246, 249, 316

Gastrointestinal system disorders

assessment and intervention, 135*t*–136*t*

autism spectrum disorders, 301

cerebral palsy, 246–247

Down syndrome, 152, 219, 222

types of, 140, 151–152

Gastrostomy tube feeding, 98, 247

Gender differences

autism spectrum disorders, 277

Down syndrome, 216

fragile X syndrome, 312

IDD and, 194, 195

General health assessment, 148–150, 199, 245

see also Assessment

Genetic disorders

autism spectrum disorders, 281

categories of, 173–174, 196

as causes of IDD, 46, 195, 196, 197*t*

chromosomal disorders, 176–179, 197*t*

delayed manifestation, 174

genetic counseling, 47, 153, 189, 202, 314, 323

mitochondrial inheritance, 186–187

multifactorial/polygenic inheritance, 186, 197*t*

nontraditional inheritance, 187–189

single-gene/inherited biochemical disorders, 179–186, 197*t*

Genetics, overview, 174–176

Genetics/Genomics Nursing: Scope & Standards of Practice (International Society of Nurses in Genetics), 10

Genitalia, physical abnormalities, 153, 198

Genitourinary tract

assessment, 153

cerebral palsy, 248

Genomes, 174, 179

Genotypes, 179

GERD, *see* Gastroesophageal reflux disease

Gilliam Asperger's Disorder Scale, 296*t*

Gilliam Autism Rating Scale (GARS), 296*t*

Glasgow Depression Scale for People with a Learning Disability, 264t, 265
Glucose-6-phosphate dehydrogenase deficiency, 185
GMFCS, see Gross Motor Function Classification System
Gold Standards Framework, 127
Gonadal (germline) mosaicism, 189
Grieving process
    adults with IDD, 84, 85, 127
    families, 49
    as risk factor for depression, 260
Gross motor function, 51, 55t, 154
Gross Motor Function Classification System (GMFCS), 244t
Group homes, 78, 100
    see also Independent living centers
Growth attenuation, 363–364
Growth measurements
    cerebral palsy, 150, 245, 248
    as components of general health assessment, 148–150
    Down syndrome, 221
A Guide to Family-Centered Care (Lewandowski and Tesler), 25
Guidelines for Continuing Education in Developmental Disabilities (Haynes et al.), 10
Gynecologic care, see Reproductive care

Hair
    assessment and intervention, 133t
    physical abnormalities, 198
Haldol, 303
Hands
    Down syndrome abnormalities, 215t
    physical abnormalities, 198
Head circumference measurements, 150, 198, 245
Head Start, 59
Health disparities, eliminating, 159–160
Health history, obtaining, 148, 149t, 199, 259
Health insurance
    adolescents and young adults, options for, 35–36
    adults with IDD, 79, 80
    disenrollment in SSI and, 38, 41
    in family-centered care model, 25
    Medicare, 42
    preexisting conditions, 74, 80
    reluctance to pay for interdisciplinary services, 96
    State Health Insurance Program (SCHIP), 33, 35
    transition to adulthood and, 74, 78–79
    see also Medicaid
HealthSoft, 93

Healthy People 2010, 73, 159
Hearing aids, 344
Hearing impairments
    assessment, 343–344, 345–346
    causes and risk factors, 334, 335, 342–343, 345t, 347
    cerebral palsy, 237, 243t, 245
    classification of, 342, 343t
    Down syndrome, 151, 196, 219, 222
    incidence, 333
    infants, 123–124, 340, 342
    interventions, 123–124
    language development, 341–342, 346
    prevention, 347
    school-age children, 346
    screening for, 150–151, 200, 228t, 341, 343–344
    sign language, use of, 340–341, 344
    signs and symptoms, 343, 346
    telephone relay systems, 256
    toddlers, 54, 55
    treatment and intervention, 344–345, 346–347
Helicobacter pylori, 140
Hemiplegia, 240, 242f, 243t
Hemophilia, 185
Hip disorders, 249
Hirschsprung disease, 152
Holistic models of care
    family-centered care, 21t, 24–25
    patient-centered care, 26–27
    youth-centered care, 25
Home care nursing, 99
Home Observation for Measurement of the Environment, 120t
Home schooling, 61
Home visiting programs, 99–100
Hospice care, 125
Hospitalization
    children's experiences, 115
    individuals with communication disorders, 101
    person-centered planning, 143
Hospitals, nursing roles and responsibilities, 101–102
Housing and living arrangements
    adults with IDD, 82–83
    autism spectrum disorders, adults with, 300, 301
    cerebral palsy, adults with, 251
    Down syndrome, adults with, 229
    group homes, 78, 100
    independent living centers (ILCs), 40–41
    promoting autonomy and self-determination, 361–362
    Section 8 assistance (HUD), 41
    young adults, 78
HUD, see U.S. Department of Housing and Urban Development

Human papillomavirus (HPV) vaccine, 227
Humane care, right to, 3
Huntington disease, 189
Hydrocephalus, 150, 245
Hyperarousal, fragile X syndrome, 315t, 318, 320
Hyperphagia, 152–153
Hypersensitivity, 336
Hyperthyroidism, 219, 259
Hypothyroidism, 152, 219, 223, 259
Hypotonia
    Down syndrome, 178, 214, 218, 222
    fragile X syndrome, 316
    IDD, individuals with, 154, 198, 199
Hypotonic cerebral palsy, 241
Hypoxic-ischemic injuries, 50, 236

ICD-10, see International Classification of
        Diseases 10
ICF, see International Classification of
        Functioning
IDD, see Intellectual and developmental
        disabilities (IDD), individuals with
IDDNS, see Intellectual and Developmental
        Disabilities Nursing Standards
IDEA, see Individuals with Disabilities Edu-
        cation Act of 1990; Individuals with
        Disabilities Education Improvement
        Act of 2004
Identity-focused ecological intervention
        model, 27
IEPs, see Individualized education programs
IFSPs, see Individualized family service
        plans
ILCs, see Independent living centers
Immune system deficiencies, 219
    see also Endocrine system disorders
Immunizations
    autism spectrum disorders and, 282
    Down syndrome, individuals with, 225,
        226, 227
Imprinting, genomic, 188
Inborn errors of metabolism, 153
Inclusion, 21t, 23, 116–117, 361–362
Incontinentia pigmenti, 186
Independence
    autonomy, promoting, 361–362
    development of in adolescents, 71
    see also Self-advocacy/self-determination
Independent living centers (ILCs), 40–41
    see also Housing and living arrangements
Individualized education programs (IEPs)
    adolescents, 36, 71, 73
    autism spectrum disorders, students
        with, 299–300
    compared to Section 504 plan, 361t
    Down syndrome, students with, 226
    nurse participation, 102

overview, 34, 202, 359
    transition IEPs, 227, 359
Individualized family service plans (IFSPs),
        32, 53, 225, 299, 358–359
Individualized plans for employment
        (IPEs), 40
Individuals with Disabilities Education
        Act (IDEA) of 1990 (PL 101-476),
        358
Individuals with Disabilities Education
        Improvement Act (IDEA) of 2004
        (PL 108-446)
    early intervention services, 32, 53, 202,
        225, 358–359
    inclusion, 23
    individualized education programs, 359
    school-based services under, 59t, 359
    transition from Part C to Part B, 57, 299
Infant-Toddler Developmental Assessment,
        122t
Infant Toddler Social Emotional Assess-
        ment, 122t
Infant/Toddler Symptom Checklist, 201t
Infants
    development, 50–51
    Down syndrome, 223, 224–225
    early intervention programs, 32–34, 53
    family challenges and coping, 52–53
    hearing disorders, 342
    home care nursing, 99
    number with disability or developmental
        delay, 31
    preterm, common conditions, 49–50
    psychosocial development, 110
    vision disorders, 335, 336
    see also Perinatal period; Toddlers
Infection control, 142–143
Informed consent, 363, 365–367
Inherited biochemical disorders
    autosomal dominant inheritance,
        182–184
    autosomal recessive inheritance,
        181–182
    as causes of IDD, 197t
    overview, 179–181
    X-linked inheritance, 184–186
    Y-linked (holandric) inheritance, 186
Injuries
    accident prevention, 140, 141
    children in special education programs,
        56
    as IDD etiology, 196
    lifting and carrying, 141
    personal safety strategies, 72
    sensory impairments, causes of, 335
Institute of Medicine
    interdisciplinary services, 26
Institutional care
    historical perspective, 6–8

Institutional care—*continued*
  nursing roles and responsibilities,
    100–101
  percentage of individuals in, 100
  research, participation of residents in,
    365
Institutional review boards (IRBs), 162,
  167, 366
Insurance, *see* Health insurance
Intellectual ability, *see* Cognitive disabilities
Intellectual and Developmental Disabilities
  (journal), 95
Intellectual and developmental disabilities
    (IDD), individuals with
  abuse, risk of, 262
  alternative and complementary treat-
    ments, 204
  attitudes about, 93, 161, 260
  core knowledge base for nurses, 93–95,
    94*t*
  diagnosis of, 198–200, 207
  end-of-life care, 125–127
  ethical issues, 361–367
  etiologies, 45–47, 165–196
  historical perspective, 1–4, 81
  mental illness distinguished from mental
    retardation, 5–6
  overview of issues, 1–4
  participation in research, 162, 167,
    365–367
  posttraumatic stress disorder, 262
  prevalence and epidemiology, 194–195
  psychosocial development, 113–117
  research, nursing, 95–96, 162, 166*t*, 167
  risk factors, 195
  secondary conditions, 142, 206–207
  social isolation, 260
  standards of care, 10, 157, 158*t*
  substance abuse, 262
  symptoms, 197–198
  terminology and classification, 1–3, 4,
    193–194
  see also specific disorders
Intellectual and Developmental Disabilities
    Nursing: Scope & Standards of Practice
    (Nehring et al.), 10, 95, 158*t*
Intellectual and Developmental Disabilities
    Nursing Standards (IDDNS), 157,
    158*t*, 159
Intelligence tests
  classification of mental retardation,
    193–194
  screening tests, 201*t*
  see also Cognitive disabilities
Interdisciplinary practice, 97*t*, 99, 159
  theoretical model of care, 21*t*, 26, 285
International Classification of Diseases 10
    (ICD-10; World Health Organiza-
    tion), 264–265

International Classification of Functioning
    (ICF), 321–323, 321*f*, 322*f*, 323*f*, 325
International Journal of Nursing In Intellectual
    and Developmental Disabilities, 95
Interpersonal relationships, *see* Social rela-
    tionships
Intestinal flow
  assessment and intervention, 135*t*
  see also Gastrointestinal system disorders
Intraventricular hemorrhages, 50, 116,
    236–237
IPEs, *see* Individualized plans for employ-
    ment
IQ tests, *see* Cognitive disabilities; Intelli-
    gence tests
IRBs, *see* Institutional review boards

Job Corps, 37
Jobs, *see* Employment
Joint Commission on Accreditation of
    Healthcare Organizations, 95
Joint Committee on Infant Hearing, 347

KADI, *see* Krug Asperger's Disorder Index
Kansas Infant Development Scales, 201*t*
Karyotypes, 177, 211
Kaufman Brief Intelligence Test-2, 201*t*
Keratoconus, 218, 222
Kids as Self Advocates, 25
Kindergarten
  private schools, 61
  transition to, 60–61, 299
Klinefelter syndrome, 178
Krug Asperger's Disorder Index (KADI),
    297*t*

Lactic acidosis, 187
Language
  derogatory, 4
  interpretation and translation, need for,
    284
  people first, 71, 163*t*
  see also Speech and language disorders
Lead toxicity, 46, 196, 207
Leadership roles
  IDD nurses, 11–12
  special health care needs, individuals
    with, 22
Learning disabilities, *see* Intellectual and
    developmental disabilities (IDD),
    individuals with
Leber optic neuropathy, 187
Legislation
  overview, 3–4, 355–361
  see also specific statutes
Leigh syndrome, 187

Leisure and recreation, *see* Recreation and leisure
Leukemias, Down syndrome and, 220
Licensed practical nurses (LPNs), 93
Licensed vocational nurses (LVNs), 93
Licensure, registered nurses, 91–92
Lifestage-specific models of care, 27, 72, 259
Linguistic competence, 284
Lisdexamfetamine (Vyvanse), 317
Lithium, 268, 303, 325
Liverpool Care Pathway, 127
Living arrangements, *see* Housing and living arrangements
Lorazepam, 157
Loss, coping with
  adults with IDD, 84, 85, 127
  of typically developing child, 49, 63
Low birth weight infants, 48, 195, 236
LPNs, *see* Licensed practical nurses (LPNs)
LVNs, *see* Licensed vocational nurses

Macrocephaly, 150
Macroorchidism, 153, 315*t*
Macular degeneration, 337
Making Action Plans, 81
Maltreatment, *see* Abuse
Managed care, impact on patient services, 11
Manual Ability Classification System, 244*t*
March of Dimes Foundation, 11
Maternal and Child Health Bureau (MCHB)
  care coordination, 99
  interdisciplinary training programs, funding for, 26
  Kids as Self Advocates, 25
  Leadership in Neurodevelopmental and Related Disabilities program, 9
  medical home concept, 202
  National Survey of Children with Special Health Care Needs, 69
  pediatric nurse practitioner training, funding for, 9
Maternal characteristics, *see* Mothers
MCHB, *see* Maternal and Child Health Bureau
McLean Asylum (Somerville, Massachusetts), 8–9
Measles, mumps, rubella (MMR) vaccine, 282
Medicaid
  adult services, 41
  beneficiary categories, 33, 34*t*
  billing for related services, 63
  disability care coordination organizations, 24
  early and periodic screening, diagnosis

and treatment (EPSDT) services, 33–34
  functional analysis, coverage of, 266
  nursing assistants, use of, 161
  redetermination for, 35, 41
  reluctance to pay for interdisciplinary services, 96
  waivers for home care, 51–52, 99
Medical home model, 21*t*, 24, 73–74, 104–105, 202, 280
Medical jargon, 119, 125
Medical model of care, 7, 22
Medicare, 42, 266
Medications
  adverse effects, monitoring, 157, 246
  attention-deficit/hyperactivity disorder, 317
  autism spectrum disorders, 302, 303
  child care staff administration of, 98
  fragile X syndrome, 325–326
  for mental health and behavior disorders, 267–269
  polydrug use, 157, 267
  prescriptive authority, 156
  rights of administration, 157
  seizures, 316–317
  unlicensed assistive personnel, administration by, 156
Melatonin, 318, 339
Mendelian patterns of inheritance, *see* Inherited biochemical disorders
Ménière's disease, 343
Meningitis, 196, 237, 335
Mental health disorders
  access to care, 207
  adolescents, 74
  autism spectrum disorders and, 302
  case management, 269–270
  cognitive behavioral therapies, 269
  complementary and alternative medicine, 269
  diagnosis, 263–266, 264*t*
  diagnostic overshadowing, 80, 117–118, 162, 258
  distinguished from mental retardation, 5
  Down syndrome and, 196
  dual diagnosis with IDD, 56, 80, 257, 258
  evaluation of care, 270
  fragile X syndrome and, 314
  grieving and, 84, 260
  interdisciplinary services and supports, 258, 269–270
  lack of care, 258
  medications, 267–269
  nursing roles, 258–259, 266–270
  prevalence, 117, 142, 257
  risk and contributing factors, 260, 262–263

Mental health disorders—*continued*
  screening and early detection, 118, 263, 264*t*
  toddlers, 56
  see also Psychosocial development
Mental retardation, *see* Intellectual and developmental disabilities (IDD), individuals with
Mental Retardation Facilities and Community Mental Health Centers Construction Act of 1963 (PL 88-164), 357
Mercury toxicity, 46, 196, 207, 282
Metabolic assessment, 199–200
Microcephaly, 150
Microdontia, 151
Middle ear infections, *see* Otitis media
Middle school, transition to, 63–64
Mills v. Board of Education, 3
Minocycline, 325
Mitochondrial inheritance, 186–187
Mitral valve prolapse, 151, 217, 222, 316
MMR vaccine, 282
Models of care, *see* Theoretical models of care
Modifications
  school-age children, 63
  see also Accommodations
Monoamine oxidase inhibitors, 268
Monoplegia, 240
Monosomies, 178
Mood stabilizing medications, 268
Mosaicism, 176, 177, 189, 212, 213*f*
Mothers
  age and chromosomal disorders, 176, 180
  attachment, 48
  characteristics linked with birth anomalies, 46–47
  risk factors for children with IDD, 195
  see also Families; Parents
Motor development and disorders
  assessment, 154–155
  early warning signs, 55*t*
  infants, 51
  school-age children, 61
  toddlers, 54
  see also Cerebral palsy
Mouth
  Down syndrome abnormalities, 215*t*
  physical abnormalities, 198
Mouth breathing, 151
Mullen Scales of Early Learning, 324*t*
Multidimensional Anxiety Scale for Children, 324*t*
Multifactorial/polygenic inheritance, 186, 197*t*
Musculoskeletal assessment, 154–155
  see also Motor development

Musculoskeletal problems
  Down syndrome, 218
  fragile X syndrome, 316
  see also Cerebral palsy
Mutations, genetic, 176
Myoclonic epilepsy, 187
Myotonic dystrophy, 189

National Center of Medical Home Initiatives for Children with Special Needs, 73–74
National Center on Child Abuse and Neglect, 76
National Center on Health Statistics, use of growth charts, 149
National Center on Physical Activity and Disability, 72, 79
National Committee for Mental Hygiene, 2
National Council Licensure Examination for Registered Nurses, 91
National Council of State Boards of Nursing (NCSBN), delegation to UAPs, 160–161
National Disability Rights Network, 357
National Down Syndrome Congress, 11
National Fragile X Foundation, 325
National Institute for Occupational Safety and Health, lifts and carrying, 141
National Institute on Deafness and Other Communication Disorders, 346
National Institutes of Health, 80, 312
National Institutes of Health State of the Science Conference, 125
National League for Nursing Practice, 9
National Survey of Children with Special Health Care Needs, 69, 118
National Survey of Children's Health, 117
National United Cerebral Palsy Association, 238
NCSBN, *see* National Council of State Boards of Nursing
Neck
  assessment and intervention, 134*t*
  Down syndrome abnormalities, 215*t*
  physical abnormalities, 198
Neonatal intensive care units (NICUs)
  care in, 48, 49
  transition from, 49–50, 51–52
Neonatal period, *see* Infants; Perinatal period
Neonatal sepsis, 47
Neural tube defects, 116
Neurodevelopmental issues
  cerebral palsy, 236, 242*f*, 249
  Down syndrome, 218
  see also Brain development
Neuroleptic medications, 303
Neurological assessment, 154

NICUs, *see* Neonatal intensive care units
Nondisjunction, chromosomal, 176–177,
  212, 213*f*, 214, 216
Normalization theoretical model, 21*t*,
  22–23
Nose
  Down syndrome abnormalities, 215*t*
  physical abnormalities, 198
Nurse consultants, 11, 92, 131, 156
Nurse practitioners, 92
Nurse specialists, 92, 101
Nursing care and practice
  accessibility of care, factors affecting,
    161–162, 204
  assessment process/review of systems,
    148–155, 149*t*
  collaboration, 159
  community care, 98–100
  core knowledge base, 93–95, 94*t*
  cultural sensitivity, 159–160, 205–206,
    284–285, 347
  delegation, 98, 100, 102, 160–161
  early intervention programs, 97–98
  education and training, 8–10, 11, 12, 26,
    91–93, 161–162
  employment settings, changes in, 11
  genetic disorders, 189
  historical perspective, 4–8
  hospitals and specialty clinics, 101–102
  institutional care, 100–101
  interdisciplinary practice, 97*t*, 99
  leadership issues, 10–12
  medication administration, 156–157
  organizations, 11–12
  outcome identification, 155
  planning and coordination of care,
    155–156, 204–205
  primary health care, 102
  research, 95–96, 162, 166*t*, 167
  self-awareness of nurses, 285
  shortage of professionals, 95, 160
  standards of care, 10, 95, 157, 158*t*
  *see also specific disorders; specific specialties
    and training*
Nutrition
  autism spectrum disorders, 302
  cerebral palsy, 246–247
  dysphagia and, 50, 132
  infants, 50
  maternal, 46, 47, 195
  mental and behavioral disorders, 269
Nystagmus, 151, 218, 237, 243*t*, 338

OAEs, *see* Otoacoustic emissions
Obesity
  adolescents, 72
  cerebral palsy, 247
  Down syndrome, 221, 223

fragile X syndrome, 316
  maternal, 47
  Prader-Willi syndrome, 152–153
Obsessive-compulsive disorder (OCD), 61,
  115, 261*t*, 287, 302
Obstructive sleep apnea, 221–222, 223,
  246
OCD, *see* Obsessive-compulsive disorder
Office of Women's Health, 227
Older Americans Act of 1965 (PL 89-73),
  85
Oral intake, *see* Feeding problems
Oral motor function assessment, 133*t*–134*t*,
  247
Orthopedic problems, *see* Musculoskeletal
    problems
Osteoporosis, 250
Otitis media, 151, 219, 249, 316
Otoacoustic emissions (OAEs), 343, 345
Outcome identification, 155
Outpatient specialty clinics, 102
Overweight, *see* Obesity

Pain
  assessment, 126–127, 154
  cerebral palsy, 251
  cerebral palsy and, 249
  sources of, 154
Palliative care, 125
Parent Interview for Autism (PIA), 298*t*
Parent support groups, 53, 97, 200, 202
Parenting Stress Index, 121*t*
Parents
  communication with, 119, 123–125
  concerns about psychosocial develop-
    ment, 117
  in diagnostic process, 198–199
  of Down syndrome children, 224–225
  parenting style, 114
  single parents, 49, 52, 202
  stress and coping, 52–53, 115–116
  see also Families
Parents and Friends of Mentally Retarded
    Children, *see* Arc of the United
    States
Parents' Evaluation of Developmental
    Status, 121*t*, 201*t*
Parkinson's disease, 187
Partners in Policymaking, 75
PAS-ADD 10, *see* Psychiatric Assessment
    Schedule for Adults with Develop-
    mental Disabilities 10
Paternal age, genetic disorders and, 180
Patient-centered care model, 26–27, 81, 86
Patient-centered medical home (PCMH),
  104–105
PDD-NOS, *see* Pervasive developmental
    disorder-not otherwise specified

Peabody Developmental Motor Scale 2, 244*t*
Peabody Picture Vocabulary Test-4, 201*t*
Pediatric Evaluation of Disability Inventory, 244*t*
Pediatric Outcome Data Collection Instrument, 244*t*
Pediatric Sleep Questionnaire, 325*t*
Pediatric Symptom Checklist, 121*t*, 201*t*
Penetrance, genetic, 180
Pennhurst State School v. Halderman, 4
Pennsylvania Association for Retarded Children v. Commonwealth of Pennsylvania, 3
People First, 20
People first language, 71, 163*t*
Perinatal chorioamnionitis, 46–47
Perinatal period
    birth and delivery problems, 47–48, 196
    causes of sensory impairments during, 335
    family challenges, 49
Periodontal disease, 133*t*, 141, 220
Periventricular leukomalacia, 50, 236, 237
Person-centered care, *see* Patient-centered care model
Personal safety, *see* Safety
Pervasive developmental disorder-not otherwise specified (PDD-NOS), 278
Pharmacological interventions, *see* Medications
Phenobarbital, 157, 317
Phenotypes, 179
Phenytoin (Dilantin), 157, 317
Phthalates, 46
Physical nursing care
    accidents, preventing, 140, 141
    assessment and intervention, 132, 133*t*–136*t*
    dysphagia and prevention of aspiration, 132, 151–152
    enteral feeding, 137–138
    evidence base for, 132, 137
    gastrointestinal disorders, 141
    monitoring and supporting tasks, 141–144
    positioning and contractures, 137, 138*f*, 139*f*
    seizures, 139–140
    skin and wound care, 140, 154
    tracheostomies, 138
PIA, *see* Parent Interview for Autism
PL 74-271, *see* Social Security Act of 1935
PL 88-164, *see* Mental Retardation Facilities and Community Mental Health Centers Construction Act of 1963
PL 89-73, *see* Older Americans Act of 1965
PL 93-112, *see* Rehabilitation Act of 1973
PL 94-103, *see* Developmental Disabilities Assistance and Bill of Rights Act of 1975
PL 94-142, *see* Education for All Handicapped Children Act of 1975

PL 99-457, *see* Education of the Handicapped Act Amendments of 1986
PL 101-336, *see* Americans with Disabilities Act of 1990
PL 101-476, *see* Individuals with Disabilities Education Act (IDEA) of 1990
PL 103-73, *see* Rehabilitation Act Amendments of 1993
PL 105-220, *see* Rehabilitation Act Amendments of 1998; Rehabilitation Act of 1973
PL 105-394, *see* Assistive Technology Act of 1998
PL 106-402, *see* Developmental Disabilities Assistance and Bill of Rights Act Amendments of 2000
PL 108-446, *see* Individuals with Disabilities Education Improvement Act (IDEA) of 2004
PL 109-416, *see* Combating Autism Act of 2006
PL 110-325, *see* ADA Amendments Act of 2008
Planning Alternative Tomorrows with Hope, 81
Plans of care, developing, 155–156
Polychlorinated biphenyls, 46
Polydrug use, 157, 267
Polymorphisms, genetic, 176, 188–189
Position Statement on Family-Centered Care Content in the Nursing Curriculum (Curry), 25
Positioning, 137, 138*f*, 139*f*, 248
Postsecondary education, 38
Posttraumatic stress disorder, 262
Posture control problems, 155
Prader-Willi syndrome (PWS)
    endocrine system disorders, 152–153
    epidemiology, 195
    etiology, 261*t*
    food behaviors, 152
    informing children about prognoses, 123
    mental health disorders, 261*t*
    nursing interventions, 261*t*
    obesity, 152–153
    psychosocial development, 114–115
    secondary conditions, 261*t*
Preferred Priorities of Care, 127
Pregnancy, *see* Family planning
Premature ovarian failure (POF), *see* Fragile X-associated primary ovarian insufficiency (FXPOI)
Prenatal period
    brain development, 197
    causes of sensory impairments during, 335
    screening and diagnosis, 47, 314
    teratogens and causes of IDD during, 45–47, 195
Presbyterian Hospital (Chicago), 9

Preschool and Kindergarten Behavioral
     Scales–Second Edition, 121*t*
Preschool Language Scale 4, 201*t*
Preschool period
   accommodations, 58–59, 59*t*
   behavioral disorders, 58
   common conditions, 58
   development, 57–58
   family challenges, 59–60
   intervention for IDD, 202
   private schools, 59
   psychosocial development, 111
   transition to kindergarten, 60–61
President's Committee for Persons with
     Intellectual Disabilities, 11
Pressure sores, 140, 154, 248, 249
Preterm infants
   ages of presentation for developmental
      abnormalities, 51*t*
   IDD and, 195
   perinatal period, 48
   transition from NICU, 49–50, 51–52
Primary health care, nursing roles and
     responsibilities, 102
Private schools
   kindergarten, 61
   preschool, 59
Projects of National Significance, 358
Psychiatric Assessment Schedule for Adults
     with Developmental Disabilities 10
     (PAS-ADD 10), 265
Psychiatric disorders, *see* Mental health
     disorders
Psychopathology Instrument for Mentally
     Retarded Adults, 264*t*
Psychosocial development
   cerebral palsy, individuals with, 251
   end-of-life care, 125–127
   IDD, individuals with, 113–117
   interventions, 123–125
   screening and assessment, 117–119,
      120*t*–122*t*, 123, 201*t*
   stages of, 109–113
   underidentification of problems, 118
Puberty, 70–71, 153, 226–227, 248
Public health nursing, 99
Pulmonary assessment, *see* Respiratory
     system
PWS, *see* Prader-Willi syndrome

Quadriplegia, 240, 242*f*, 243*t*, 245
Quality of life
   cerebral palsy, 251
   Down syndrome, 229
   living arrangements and, 362
   sensory impairments, 333

Racial/ethnic differences
   cultural sensitivity, 159–160, 205–206

Down syndrome, 216
   IDD and, 194–195
Recreation and leisure
   adolescents, 75
   adults with IDD, 83, 85
   school-age children, 35, 202–203
Registered nurses (RNs)
   education and licensure, 91–92
   roles and responsibilities, 93
   as UAP supervisors, 161
Rehabilitation Act Amendments of 1993
     (PL 103-73), 360
Rehabilitation Act Amendments of 1998
     (PL 105-220), 360
Rehabilitation Act of 1973 (PL 93-112)
   overview, 23, 360
   postsecondary institutions, 77
   Section 504, 3, 62, 62*t*, 360–361, 361*t*
Reiss Scale for Children's Dual Diagnosis,
     264*t*
Reiss Screen for Maladaptive Behaviors, 264*t*
Related services, 63
Relocation stress, 204
Reproduction, right to, 364–365
Reproductive care
   assessment, 153–154
   cerebral palsy, 248
   Down syndrome, individuals with, 229
   see also Sexuality
Research
   institutional review boards (IRBs), 162,
      167, 366
   by nurses, 95–96, 162, 166*t*, 167
   participation in by individuals with IDD,
      162, 167, 365–367
   research partners, 367
Respiratory system disorders
   assessment and intervention, 134*t*, 151
   cerebral palsy, 246
   Down syndrome, 218
Respite care, 52, 57
Retinoblastoma, 335
Retinopathy of prematurity, 50, 335
Rett syndrome, 278
Review of systems assessment process
   autism spectrum disorders, 301–303,
      305*t*
   cerebral palsy, 244–251
   Down syndrome, 217–223
   overview, 148–155
Reynolds Depression Scale, 119
Ring chromosome, 14, 179
RNs, *see* Registered nurses
Royal College of Psychiatrists, 265
Rubella, congenital, 282

Safety
   accident prevention, 140, 141
   for caregivers, 141

Safety—*continued*
  emergency preparedness, 83–84, 348,
    349
  strategies for adolescents, 72
SCHIP, *see* State Health Insurance Program
School-age children
  accommodations, 62–63
  autism spectrum disorders, 287, 299–300
  common conditions, 61–62
  development, 61–62
  Down syndrome, 223–224, 226
  family challenges, 63
  hearing impairment, 346
  intervention for IDD, 202
  psychosocial development, 111–112
  services for, 34–35, 102–103
  transition to middle school, 63–64
  see also specific disorders
School nurses, 34–35, 102–103, 299–300,
    302–303
School Nursing: Scope & Standards of Practice
    (National Association of School
    Nurses), 10
Scoliosis, 249
Screen for Childhood Anxiety Related
    Emotional Disorders, 324*t*
Screening
  autism spectrum disorders, individuals
    with, 286–287, 288*f*–289*f*
  Down syndrome, individuals with, 225,
    227, 228*t*
  hearing impairments, 150–151, 200, 341
  mental health disorders, 263, 264*t*
  psychosocial development, 117–119,
    120*t*–122*t*, 123
  vision disorders, 150–151, 200, 225, 337
  see also Assessment
Screening Tool for Autism in Two-Year-
    Olds (STAT), 298*t*
Secondary conditions
  prevention of, 141–142
  types of, 206–207
  see also Dual diagnosis; *specific disorders*
Secondhand smoke, 207
Section 504, *see* Rehabilitation Act of 1973
Seizures
  assessment, 154
  autism spectrum disorders, 154, 282,
    300, 302–303
  cerebral palsy, 238, 243*t*, 249
  Down syndrome, 196, 221
  fragile X syndrome, 314, 315*t*, 316–317
  myoclonic epilepsy, 187
  prevalence, 142
  prevention and control, 139–140
Selective serotonin reuptake inhibitors,
    267, 268
Self-advocacy/self-determination, 20–22,
    21*t*, 75, 77, 81, 361–362

Self-awareness, of nurses, 285
Self-injurious behavior, 258, 300, 302
Self-Report Depression Questionnaire, 264*t*
Sensorineural hearing loss, 342
Sensory impairments
  deafblindness, 347–348
  Down syndrome and, 196
  emergency preparedness, 348, 349
  incidence, 333
  nursing roles, 348–349
  prevalence, 142
  suggestions for nurses, 340, 346–347,
    349–350
  see also Hearing impairments; Vision
    impairments
Sepsis, 237
Septal defects, 151, 217
Service agencies, *see* Systems of care
Service coordination
  autism spectrum disorders, 303–304,
    305*f*
  disability care coordination organiza-
    tions, 24
  early intervention, 98
  mental health disorders, 269–270
  as nursing approach to care, 155–156,
    204–205
  by public health nurses, 99
  sensory impairments, 348–349
Sex chromosome variations, 178
Sexual abuse, 262
Sexuality
  adolescents, 70–71, 153
  autism spectrum disorders, individuals
    with, 300
  cerebral palsy, individuals with, 248
  Down syndrome, individuals with,
    226–227
  family planning, 81–82, 153, 154
  right to sexual expression and reproduc-
    tion, 364–365
  young adults, 76, 153–154
Shaken baby syndrome, 196
Sialorrhea, 246
Siblings, 60
Sickle-cell disease, 181, 182
Single nucleotide polymorphisms, 176
Single-gene disorders, *see* Inherited bio-
    chemical disorders
Single-parent families
  challenges of, 52, 202
  premature infants in, 49
Skin
  assessment and intervention, 133*t*, 154
  care of and wound treatment, 140, 154
  cerebral palsy, 248
  Down syndrome, 221
  physical abnormalities, 198
Sleep problems

adolescents, 72
autism spectrum disorders, 301–302
cerebral palsy, 237, 246
Down syndrome, 196, 223
Down syndrome and, 221–222
fragile X syndrome, 317–318
intervention, 325t
symptoms, 259
vision disorders, 339
Smell, sense of, 336
Smoking, 262
Social anxiety, fragile X syndrome, 315t,
    318, 319, 320
Social isolation, 260
Social norms theoretical models
    normalization, 21t, 22–23
    self-advocacy, 20–22, 21t
Social relationships
    adolescents, 74–75
    adults with IDD, 81–82, 84, 85
    autism spectrum disorders, 282–283,
        300–301
    school-age children, 61, 62
    young adults, 76
    see also Psychosocial development
Social role valorization, 22
Social Security Act of 1935 (PL 74-271), 3,
    99
Social Security Administration (SSA)
    disability determination services (DDS),
        41
    employment support programs, 39t
    Social Security Disability Insurance
        (SSDI), 37
    Supplemental Security Income (SSI),
        37–38, 41
Social Security Disability Insurance (SSDI),
    37
Social Skills Rating System, 122t
Society of Pediatric Nurses (SPN), 25, 92
Socioeconomic status, IDD and, 194
SORF, see Systematic Observation of Red
        Flags for Autism Spectrum Disorders
        in Young Children
Spastic cerebral palsy, 240, 242f, 243t
Spasticity, 51, 154, 155, 249, 250t
Special education, see Individualized educa-
        tion programs
Specialty clinics, 102
Speech and language development
    hearing impairment and, 51, 54,
        341–342, 346
    infants, 51
    school-age children, 61
Speech and language disorders
    assessment and intervention, 136t, 324t
    autism spectrum disorders, 282–283
    cerebral palsy, 238, 245
    fragile X syndrome, 315t, 320–321

hospitalization of individuals with, 101
school-age children, 62
screening tests, 201t
symptoms, 198
toddlers, 54
SPN, see Society of Pediatric Nurses
SSA, see Social Security Administration
SSDI, see Social Security Disability Insur-
        ance
SSI, see Supplemental Security Income
SSPs, see Support service providers
Standards for State Residential Institutions for
        the Mentally Retarded (Leboiteux), 10
Standards of care
    current standards, 10, 95, 157, 158t
    historical perspective, 3–4, 10
Stanford-Binet Intelligence Scales, 5th edi-
        tion, 201t, 324t
STAT, see Screening Tool for Autism in
        Two-Year-Olds
State councils on developmental disabili-
        ties, 357
State Health Insurance Program (SCHIP),
        33, 35
State-run institutions, see Institutional care
Stereotypical motor patterns, 283
Stigmatization, 4, 161, 205, 260
Stimulant medications, 303, 317
Strabismus, 151, 218, 237, 243t, 316
Strengths and Difficulties Questionnaire,
        121t
Streptococcus infections, 47
Stress
    families of individuals with IDD, 115–116
    families with infants transitioning from
        NICU, 52–53
    in young children, 55–56
Strohmer-Prout Behavior Rating Scale,
        264t
Substance abuse, 262
Supplemental Security Income (SSI),
        37–38, 41
Support groups
    nurse involvement in, 11
    parental, 53, 97, 200, 202
Support service providers (SSPs), 348
Supported living programs, 100
Supravalvular aortic stenosis, 151
Surgeon General's Call to Action to Improve the
        Health and Wellness of Persons with
        Disabilities (U.S. Department of
        Health and Human Services), 72,
        163t–165t
Sutter-Eyberg Behavior Inventory-Revised,
        120t
Swallowing problems, see Dysphagia
Systematic Observation of Red Flags for
        Autism Spectrum Disorders in
        Young Children (SORF), 298t

Systems of care
  adolescents and young adults, 35–38
  adults, 39–42
  inclusion, 21*t*, 23
  infants and toddlers, 31–34
  medical home model, 21*t*, 24
  school-age children, 34–35

Tanner scale, 153
Tardive dyskinesia, 136*t*, 268, 303
Tay-Sachs disease, 174, 181, 182
Team nursing, 7
Telephone relay systems
Teratogens, 45, 46, 195
Tetrasomy disorders, 177
Theoretical models of care
  biopsychosocial model of disability,
    321–323, 321*f*, 322*f*, 323*f*, 325
  family-centered care, 24–25, 284
  inclusion, 23
  interdisciplinary services, 26, 285
  International Classification of Function-
    ing, 321–323, 321*f*, 322*f*, 323*f*, 325
  lifestage-specific models, 27
  medical home model, 24
  normalization, 22–23
  nursing framework of care, 285–286
  overview, 19–20, 21*t*, 284
  patient-centered care, 26–27
  self-advocacy/self-determination, 20–22
  youth-centered care, 25
Thimerosal, 282
Thorazine, 303
Thrombophlebitis, 151, 246
Thyroid disease, 152, 219, 314
Title V for Children with Special Health
  Care Needs, 33, 35, 99
Toddlers
  behavioral concerns, 55–56
  common conditions, 54
  development, 54
  family challenges, 56–57
  motor development, 54, 55*t*
  number with disability or developmental
    delay, 31
  psychosocial development, 110–111
  transition to preschool, 57
  see also Early intervention programs
Toileting, 116, 285
Topiramate, 268
TORCH infections, 47
Touch, sense of, 336
Toxic chemicals, 46
Tracheostomies, 138
Transfer anxiety, 204
Transient leukemia (TL), 220
Transition plans
  for adolescents, 73, 103–104, 227, 300

  to middle school, 59
  to preschool, 32, 57
Transition to adult health care, 73–74,
  78–79, 103–104, 203, 227
Translocation, chromosomal, 178, 179,
  212, 214, 216
Transportation, 83, 143, 203
Traumatic brain damage, 196
Tricyclic antidepressants, 268
Triple X syndrome, 178
Triplegia, 240
Triplet/trinucleotide repeats, 188–189
Trisomy disorders, 175, 176, 178, 179, 212,
  213*f*
  see also Down syndrome
Tuberous sclerosis, 282
Tumors, Down syndrome and, 220
Turner syndrome, 175, 176, 178
Tuskegee syphilis study, 366
Tympanometry, 345

UAPs, *see* Unlicensed assistive personnel
Uniparental disomies, 188
United Cerebral Palsy Association, 11
Universal design, 143
Universal newborn hearing screening, 150,
  341
University Affiliated Programs, 9, 26
University Centers for Excellence in Devel-
  opmental Disabilities (UCEDDs), 9,
  26, 93, 95, 97*t*, 357
University of Colorado Health Sciences
  Center, 9, 93
University of Minnesota School of Nursing,
  93
University of Washington, 9
Unlicensed assistive personnel (UAPs)
  administration of medications, 156
  delegation of tasks to, 160–161
Urinary catheterization, 98
Urinary incontinence, 153, 248
U.S. Census (2000), distribution of disabili-
  ties, 79, 84
U.S. Department of Education
  Office of Special Education Programs, 358
  Office of Vocational Rehabilitation, 300
U.S. Department of Housing and Urban De-
  velopment, Section 8 assistance, 41
U.S. Food and Drug Administration, 345
U.S. Public Health Service, nurse consult-
  ants, employment of, 11
Usher syndrome, 337, 345*t*

Vaccines, *see* Immunizations
Valium (diazepam), 157, 303
Vanderbilt Rating Forms, 324*t*
Very low birth weight infants, 48, 50

Vineland II: Social-Emotional Early Child-hood Scales, 201*t*
Vineland II: Vineland Adapative Behavior Scales, Second Edition, 122*t*, 324*t*
Vision impairments
    assessment and screening, 150–151, 200, 225, 228*t*, 337, 338–339
    causes and risk factors, 334–335, 334*t*, 335*t*, 337
    cerebral palsy, 237, 243*t*, 245
    Down syndrome, 196, 218, 222, 225
    facial expressions of individuals with blindness, 336–337
    incidence, 333
    infants, 336
    interpersonal strategies, 340
    parent-child interactions, 336
    prevention of, 340
    treatment and intervention, 337–338, 339–340
Vital signs, assessment, 133*t*
Vocational rehabilitation (VR), 36, 40, 300
Volunteerism
VR, *see* Vocational rehabilitation
Vyvanse (lisdexamfetamine), 317

Waardenburg syndrome, 183, 335, 345*t*
Web-based instruction, 12
Weschler Intelligence Scale for Children IV Integrated, 201*t*
Wheelchairs
    positioning in, 137, 138*f*, 248
    self-propelling, friction from, 248

WIA, *see* Workforce Investment Agencies (WIA) programs
Williams syndrome, 150, 151, 152, 261*t*
Willowbrook State School, New York, 365
Work, *see* Employment
Workforce Investment Agencies (WIA) programs, 36–37, 40
Wyatt v. Aderholt, 3
Wyatt v. Stickney, 3

X-linked inheritance, 184–186, 311
    see also Fragile X syndrome
Xanax, 303

Y-linked (holandric) inheritance, 186
Young adults
    behavioral issues, 76
    developmental tasks, 75–76
    employment, 36–37, 39*t*, 78
    health care services, 35–36, 78–79, 103–104
    housing, 78
    income assistance, 37–38
    intervention for IDD, 203
    postsecondary education, 38, 77
    psychosocial development, 112
    self-advocacy, 77
    social relationships, 76
    transition to adult health care, 73–74, 78–79, 103–104, 227
    see also Adolescents; Adults
Youth-centered care, 25